PATHOLOGY OF WILDLIFE AND ZOO ANIMALS TEXTBOOK 2026

A Clinical Reference Covering Necropsy Methodology, Cross-Taxa Lesion Recognition, & Comparative Diagnostic Reasoning for ACVP Candidates

Ramon C. Henson, MD

the use, misuse, or application of any information, recommendation, protocol, or clinical guidance contained in this publication.

TABLE OF CONTENT

PREFACE

The pathologist opening a carcass of a species they have never before autopsied faces a cognitive challenge unique to this discipline. The gross specimen offers its findings without regard for the pathologist's prior exposure. The lesion is what it is; the responsibility to interpret it correctly is what it is; and the antemortem history is often sparse, delayed, or absent. Repetition-built pattern recognition, the foundation on which diagnostic pathology of domestic species rests, is not available. Wildlife and zoo animal pathology is instead a discipline of reasoning across taxa — of holding in mind that hepatic hemosiderosis in a captive lemur is not the same clinical event as iron storage disease in a rhinoceros, that multifocal hepatic necrosis in a psittacine looks very like the same lesion in a viverrid but points to different agents and different reportability obligations, and that the meaningful diagnostic anchor is often the one detail the taxonomically inexperienced observer misses.

This book is written to make that reasoning tractable. It sits alongside the taxonomically organized references that dominate the field but approaches the material along a different axis. Content is organized by lesion pattern first, taxon second. Every major topic in every chapter carries a named callout — the Comparative Necropsy Pattern — that isolates the lesion pattern, states its cross-taxa signature (the species where the pattern appears and the features that identify it), gives the single diagnostic anchor that locks the interpretation, names the look-alike lesion that most often produces the wrong answer, and flags reportable or zoonotic implications. These callouts recur through the book at the same structural position and in the same five-part format, so the pathologist begins to recognize the pattern of the pattern-callout itself — a scaffold on which cross-taxa recognition can be built even in the absence of repetition-based exposure.

The book closes with The Comparative Necropsy Pattern Master Atlas, a dedicated back-of-book section that consolidates every Pattern introduced in the chapters into two parallel indexes — by lesion type (hepatic, renal, pulmonary, cardiac, neurologic, integumentary, musculoskeletal, hematolymphatic, gastrointestinal, endocrine, reproductive, ocular, generalized) and by taxonomic group (carnivores, ungulates, primates, marine mammals, small mammals, birds, reptiles, amphibians, fish). The Atlas is the reference the pathologist reaches for at the cutting board or before signout: not a chapter-length narrative but a structured navigator, cross-referenced back to the parent chapter where the mechanism and evidence live.

The primary audience is the anatomic pathology resident whose training program carries a wildlife or zoo caseload, and the diplomate whose diagnostic laboratory receives occasional non-domestic species submissions. Candidates preparing for the American College of Veterinary Pathologists Phase II examination will find the pattern-recognition scaffolding aligned with the cognitive demands of unfamiliar-species interpretation under exam conditions. Zoo veterinarians preparing submissions and interpreting reports, wildlife disease investigators at USDA APHIS, the USGS National Wildlife Health Center, and state wildlife health programs, veterinary students on pathology electives, and field biologists doing necropsy work will find the book usable both as a chapter-by-chapter reference and as an atlas navigator.

A statement on what this book is not. It is not a question bank, a mock examination, or a drill workbook. It contains no multiple-choice items, no answer keys, and no self-assessment sections. It is a clinical reference, written to teach reasoning through narrative case presentations and structured pattern callouts. Where diagnostic decisions are given, they are given in the vocabulary of medicine — probabilities and associations, first-line and preferred, characteristic and pathognomonic — because the discipline itself does not operate on the certainty a lettered answer choice implies.

The reader is invited to work through the chapters in order on first reading and to return to the Atlas thereafter. The Pattern callouts will begin to feel familiar somewhere in the second or third chapter. That familiarity is the scaffold this book was written to build.

CHAPTER 1: PRINCIPLES OF WILDLIFE AND ZOO ANIMAL PATHOLOGY

Learning Objectives

1. Define the scope, cognitive demands, and disciplinary boundaries of non-domestic species pathology relative to domestic species diagnostic practice.
2. Apply lesion-first diagnostic reasoning when antemortem clinical history is absent, unreliable, or delayed.
3. Recognize the comparative pathology framework as the primary cognitive tool for cross-taxa lesion interpretation.
4. Identify the regulatory, zoonotic, and one-health obligations attached to wildlife and zoo necropsy findings.
5. Use the Comparative Necropsy Pattern callout structure as a scaffold for pattern recognition when repetition-based recognition is unavailable.
6. Distinguish body condition interpretation, postmortem interval assessment, and lesion morphology as the three primary interpretive channels available when clinical history is absent.

The pathologist who elects to work with non-domestic species inherits a discipline that behaves differently from every other branch of veterinary diagnostic pathology. In domestic species practice, the accumulated case volume of any one pathologist — thousands of canine biopsies, hundreds of feline necropsies, and repeated exposure to the same limited set of species — permits pattern recognition built by repetition. Wildlife and zoo animal pathology grants no such privilege. A given zoo pathologist may autopsy an individual member of a rare species only once in a career; a wildlife disease investigator may encounter a novel host-pathogen combination each field season; a diagnostic laboratory pathologist called to interpret a chelonian necropsy from a private practice submission may have no prior slide exposure to that taxonomic group. What must substitute for repetition is reasoning: reasoning across taxa, reasoning from lesion morphology backward toward disease process, and reasoning about what is normal for a species whose normal has not been recorded.

The discipline is unified by the necropsy as the point where clinical, epidemiologic, and pathologic reasoning converge. Antemortem workup, when it exists, is often abbreviated by the animal's cryptic clinical presentation, its position on the population continuum from managed captive to free-ranging, and the logistical constraints of remote fieldwork or exhibit conditions. The pathologist is frequently the first observer to generate a diagnostic hypothesis, and that hypothesis carries downstream implications far beyond the individual case: population-level intervention, regulatory reporting, zoonotic surveillance, conservation policy, and the well-being of the animals that share the affected animal's environment. This chapter introduces the disciplinary framework on which the remainder of the book is built, defines the interpretive tools available when history is absent, positions comparative pathology as a cognitive method rather than a taxonomic reference, and describes the regulatory interfaces the pathologist is obligated to recognize at the cutting board.

Scope and Discipline of Non-Domestic Species Pathology

Historical Emergence of the Discipline

Wildlife and zoo animal pathology emerged from two initially separate threads. The zoo pathology tradition developed within urban zoological gardens of the late nineteenth and early twentieth centuries, where the deaths of exhibited animals prompted institutional pathologists to describe lesions in species that had no precedent in the veterinary literature. Descriptions were often anatomically framed because the underlying etiology could not be identified: hepatic necrosis in a psittacine, encephalitis of undetermined cause in a nonhuman primate, or generalized amyloidosis in a captive cheetah were reported as morphologic findings first, mechanistic interpretations second. Free-ranging wildlife pathology developed later, driven by the recognition that disease processes in wild populations were both important to species conservation and relevant to human public health. The consolidation of these two threads into a single discipline occurred as diagnostic techniques improved and as institutions such as the C.L. Davis Foundation, the American Association of Zoo Veterinarians, and the Wildlife Disease Association created a shared professional literature.

Institutional and Programmatic Landscape

The contemporary discipline is distributed across a network of institutions whose case flow determines the pathologist's day-to-day work. Zoological pathology programs at Species Survival Plan institutions provide sustained access to managed captive populations across taxonomic breadth. Wildlife diagnostic laboratories at state departments of natural resources, at universities affiliated with the Southeastern Cooperative Wildlife Disease Study, and at the United States Geological Survey National Wildlife Health Center concentrate free-ranging case volume. The United States Department of Agriculture Animal and Plant Health Inspection Service Wildlife Services coordinates surveillance for diseases of regulatory concern. Private zoological consulting services, aquarium pathology programs, and marine mammal stranding networks fill the remaining institutional space. A resident training program that intends to prepare a pathologist for wildlife and zoo caseload will typically rotate through several of these institutions during the anatomic pathology residency, because no single institution provides adequate taxonomic breadth.

Case Diversity and Cognitive Load

The taxonomic diversity carried by a wildlife or zoo pathologist is difficult to overstate. A single week of case flow may include a marine mammal stranding, a psittacine sudden death, a chelonian systemic illness, an ungulate herd mortality event, and a nonhuman primate necropsy from a research institution. Each of those cases requires the pathologist to recognize the boundaries of their species-specific knowledge, to reason from comparative anatomic and physiologic principles when species-specific data are absent, and to know when to defer to specialty consultation. The cognitive load is not principally a matter of memorization; it is a matter of recognizing which interpretive framework the case belongs to. A hepatic mass in a canine is interpreted through a well-mapped set of neoplastic and non-neoplastic differentials; the same gross lesion in a Sumatran orangutan requires an entirely different interpretive path because the differential list is not identical, the ancillary testing options are constrained, and the population-level implications differ.

Distinction From Domestic Species Practice

Several structural distinctions separate non-domestic species pathology from domestic species diagnostic work. The reference range problem is the most immediate: reliable species-specific ranges for hematologic, biochemical, and histologic parameters exist for only a minority of the species a wildlife pathologist will encounter, so the interpretive baseline is often extrapolated from the closest available taxonomic relative. The autopsy technique itself varies substantially by species — chelonian necropsy requires plastron removal, avian necropsy requires attention to air sac and syrinx anatomy, cetacean necropsy is performed by flensing pattern rather than dorsal-to-ventral incision, and elasmobranch necropsy requires familiarity with cartilaginous skeletal anatomy that no domestic species approaches. The ancillary testing landscape is similarly non-standard: many diagnostic assays validated in domestic species have not been validated in the species under examination, and the pathologist must reason about the interpretive weight to grant a test whose sensitivity and specificity in that species are unknown.

KEY POINT: Wildlife and zoo animal pathology substitutes cross-taxa reasoning for repetition-based pattern recognition. The pathologist who accepts this substitution — and who builds explicit interpretive scaffolds for cases in taxonomically unfamiliar species — will develop diagnostic competence faster than the pathologist who attempts to memorize species-specific patterns one taxon at a time.

Procedural Necropsy Sequence: Non-Domestic Terrestrial Mammal

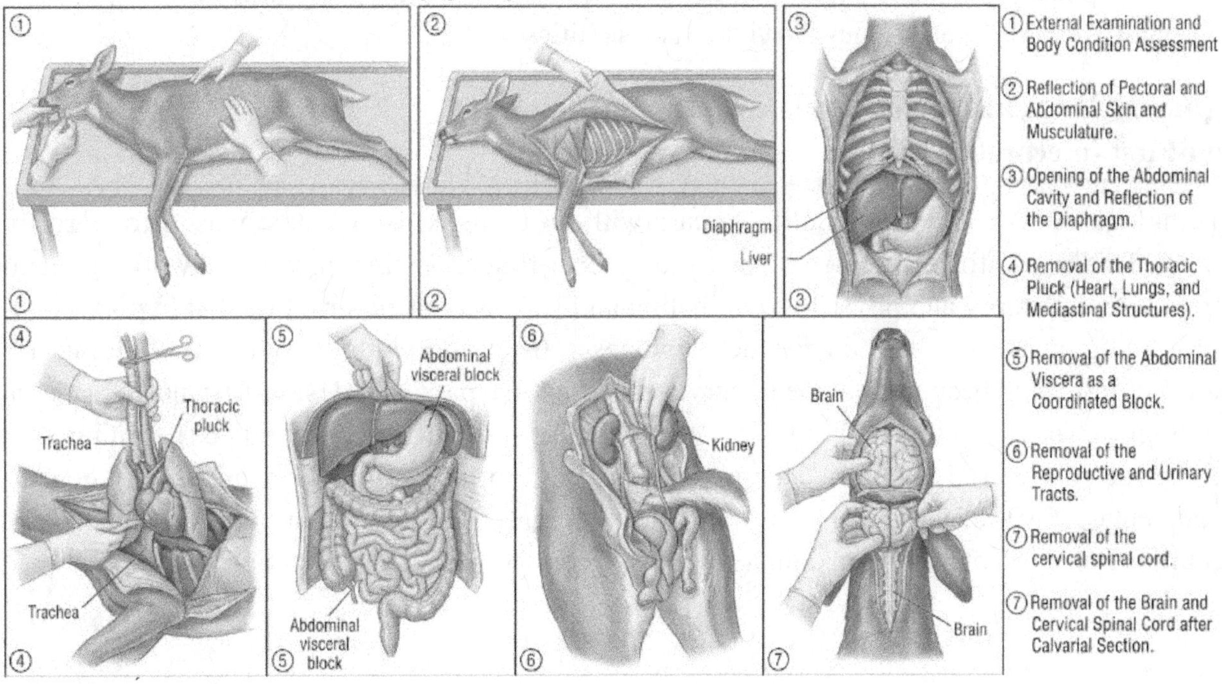

THE COMPARATIVE NECROPSY PATTERN SYSTEM — Cross-Taxa Hepatic Necrosis of Herpesviral Origin

The Pattern: Multifocal to coalescing hepatic necrosis with intranuclear viral inclusion bodies at the periphery of necrotic foci, occurring as sudden mortality with minimal antemortem clinical warning.

Cross-Taxa Signature: Recognized across at least four taxonomic groups: nonhuman primates (herpes B-related lesions in macaques, callitrichid herpesvirus in marmosets), elephant calves (elephant endotheliotropic herpesvirus with cardiac and hepatic hemorrhage), captive psittacines (psittacid herpesvirus 1 producing Pacheco disease with hepatic necrosis), and free-ranging cervids and mustelids (malignant catarrhal fever variants). The gross lesion is remarkably similar across taxa: pale to red-tinged, well-demarcated, randomly distributed foci of necrosis on all hepatic surfaces, typically 2 to 8 mm in diameter, sometimes coalescing to larger regions.

Diagnostic Anchor: Cowdry type A intranuclear inclusion bodies (eosinophilic, glassy, with peripheral chromatin margination) in hepatocytes at the periphery of necrotic foci, confirmed by immunohistochemistry or polymerase chain reaction targeting the taxon-appropriate herpesvirus.

Trap Logic: The look-alike is bacterial hepatic necrosis (particularly Yersinia pseudotuberculosis in psittacines and elephants, and Clostridium piliforme in nonhuman primates and marsupials). Discrimination: bacterial necrotic foci contain neutrophil-rich exudate and gram-stainable bacteria within necrotic tissue, and Cowdry type A inclusions are absent.

Zoonotic/Reportable Flag: Herpes B (Macacine alphaherpesvirus 1) in macaques is a hard-stop biosafety concern with human fatal encephalitis potential; contact institutional biosafety officer before further tissue handling. Elephant endotheliotropic herpesvirus and psittacine herpesviruses are non-zoonotic but institutionally reportable at Species Survival Plan facilities.

Diagnostic Reasoning Without Antemortem History

Lesion-First Interpretive Logic

The pathologist who receives a wildlife carcass with no clinical history must reason forward from the specimen. This is a distinct cognitive mode from clinical-first reasoning, in which a working diagnosis is constructed from history and physical examination and lesions confirm or refute that hypothesis. Lesion-first reasoning constructs the diagnostic hypothesis from morphology outward, holding no prior probability until the specimen has been surveyed. The first pass of a lesion-first necropsy is a broad morphologic characterization: distribution (focal, multifocal, diffuse, generalized), timing (peracute, acute, subacute, chronic), and pattern (necrotizing, proliferative, inflammatory, degenerative, developmental). Each of these axes constrains the differential in specific and predictable ways, and the reasoning is transportable across taxa in a way that species-specific memorization is not.

Body Condition Scoring as Baseline Interpretive Data

Body condition is a channel of interpretive data available on every carcass regardless of history availability. In free-ranging wildlife, body condition often carries the disease process in itself: chronic wasting disease in cervids, mycobacterial disease in cervids and bovids, and any chronic infectious or neoplastic process characteristically produce a cachectic carcass with serous atrophy of the pericardial and epicardial adipose stores. In managed captive populations, body condition disproportionate to the terminal event points toward a chronic underlying process the clinical team may not have recognized. Scoring is species-specific — a 5-point scale developed for a domestic species does not apply to a giraffe or a rhinoceros — and reference is made to species-appropriate scoring systems where they exist, or to comparative ungulate or carnivore scales where the species-specific system has not been published. Serous atrophy of adipose stores, when present, is worth noting on the gross report because it dates the disease process to weeks rather than days.

Postmortem Interval and Autolysis Interpretation

Postmortem interval interpretation is a routine cognitive task in wildlife pathology because the interval between death and necropsy is frequently longer than in a hospital setting and is often unknown at the time of tissue receipt. Autolytic change follows a predictable progression that is modified by ambient temperature, carcass position, presence of scavenger predation, and integumentary characteristics of the species. Distinguishing autolysis from antemortem lesions is essential because autolytic softening, mucosal sloughing, and hemoglobin imbibition of endothelial surfaces can mimic disease processes: postmortem sloughing of gastrointestinal mucosa is easily misread as antemortem enteritis, and hemoglobin imbibition of vascular walls can be misread as vasculitis. Two principles guide interpretation: an antemortem lesion is bordered by an inflammatory response of some kind, however subtle, whereas an autolytic change is not; and antemortem hemorrhage contains fibrin and platelet-rich material, whereas postmortem hemoglobin release does not.

Reconstructing Presumptive Clinical Course From Lesions

The pathologist practiced in lesion-first reasoning can reconstruct a presumptive clinical course from the specimen that closely approximates the actual clinical narrative when it eventually becomes available. Body condition dates the disease process. Organ-specific lesions constrain the anatomic system involved. The presence or absence of inflammatory response constrains the timing. The distribution of lesions constrains the mechanism of insult: hematogenous distribution suggests a bloodborne agent, mucosal-surface distribution suggests an inhaled or ingested agent, and dependent lung distribution suggests aspiration. This reconstruction is not a substitute for antemortem history when history is available; it is the interpretive framework applied when history is not.

Figure 1.2. Cachexia With Serous Fat Atrophy: Comparative Gross Appearance Across Free-Ranging Ungulate Taxa

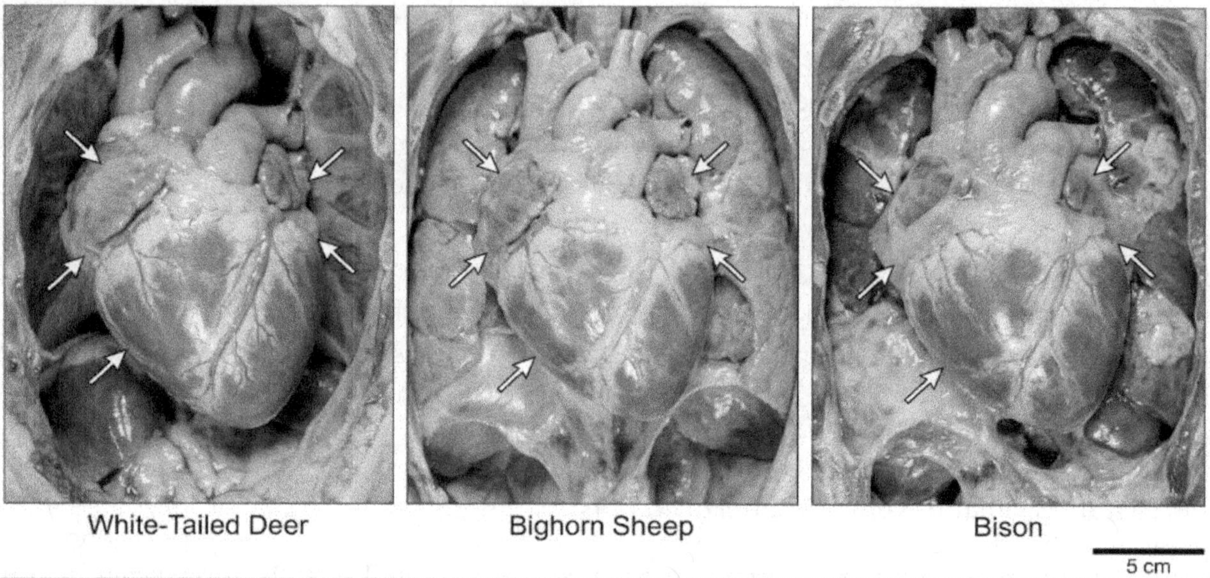

THE COMPARATIVE NECROPSY PATTERN SYSTEM — Cachexia With Serous Fat Atrophy Across Free-Ranging Ungulates

The Pattern: Marked underweight body condition with gelatinous, translucent serous atrophy of the pericardial, epicardial, coronary groove, and perirenal adipose stores in a carcass without acute terminal event lesions.

Cross-Taxa Signature: Recognized in cervids (chronic wasting disease, chronic hepatic capillariasis), bovids (mycobacterial disease, mycoplasmal pneumonia, chronic parasitism), suids (chronic Streptococcus suis disease, atrophic rhinitis progression), and camelids (chronic paratuberculosis, chronic gastric parasitism). The lesion is a signal of a chronic disease process that has depleted the animal's energy reserves over weeks; the terminal event that brought the carcass to the pathologist is typically the endpoint of that chronic depletion rather than an acute independent event.

Diagnostic Anchor: The transition of pericardial adipose from opaque white to translucent, gelatinous, and easily deformed under gentle pressure is the anchor. When present, the disease process is dated to at least two to four weeks in duration regardless of terminal event lesions.

Trap Logic: The look-alike is postmortem autolytic softening of adipose stores in a carcass with prolonged postmortem interval, or dehydration-associated adipose loss in a recently deceased carcass exposed to warm ambient temperature. Discrimination: autolytic softening involves the entire carcass symmetrically and is accompanied by other autolytic changes (mucosal sloughing, epithelial detachment); serous atrophy involves the adipose stores specifically and is accompanied by other chronic disease markers (reduced skeletal muscle mass, dull haircoat, ectoparasite burden).

Zoonotic/Reportable Flag: In cervid submissions, chronic wasting disease is a reportable condition in most jurisdictions and requires obex and retropharyngeal lymph node submission for prion testing before further tissue handling. In bovid and cervid submissions, mycobacterial disease requires biosafety containment and state animal health authority notification before continued dissection.

CLINICAL PEARL: The presence of serous atrophy of adipose stores dates the disease process to weeks in duration regardless of the terminal event that brought the carcass to necropsy. A carcass with acute terminal lesions and unremarkable adipose stores is a different disease event from a carcass with acute terminal lesions and serous fat atrophy; the second is a chronic disease process with an acute terminal event, and both must be worked up.

Comparative Pathology as a Cognitive Framework

Cross-Taxa Lesion Pattern Recognition

Comparative pathology as practiced in this discipline is not a reference activity of looking up how a given disease presents in a given species; it is a cognitive framework of holding in mind that a lesion pattern observed in one species predicts, with meaningful reliability, the interpretation of a similar lesion pattern observed in a taxonomically distant species. The predictive reliability is not absolute — species-specific modifications occur — but the framework carries the pathologist across the gap between familiar taxa and unfamiliar ones. Multifocal random hepatic necrosis in a canine narrows the differential to a bloodborne infectious agent, a hematogenous embolic process, or an ingested hepatotoxin. That same interpretive frame applies without substantive modification to a psittacine, a chelonian, an ungulate, or a marine mammal. What varies is the identity of the likely agents; what remains constant is the interpretive path.

Anatomic Variation and Its Interpretive Weight

Anatomic variation across taxa modifies interpretation in specific and predictable ways, and knowledge of the variation is prerequisite to correct interpretation. Avian species have air sacs that traverse the coelomic cavity and terminate in the pneumatized skeleton; a respiratory infection in a bird is not confined to the parenchyma of the lung and must be interpreted with air sac involvement in mind. Reptiles have variable degrees of ventricular septation and a functionally three-chambered heart in most non-crocodilian species; a cardiac lesion in a squamate cannot be interpreted through the mammalian four-chamber frame. Ruminant compartmentalized stomachs, marine mammal countercurrent thermoregulatory retia, marsupial reproductive anatomy with paired uteri and paired lateral vaginas, and the extensive lymphoreticular tissue in the fish head kidney each modify lesion interpretation in the systems where they occur. The pathologist working in a taxonomically unfamiliar species must first ask what the normal anatomic frame is before asking what the lesion means.

Species-Specific Reference Ranges and Their Absence

Reference range data for non-domestic species are, for most species, either absent or based on samples too small to support confident inference. The interpretive workaround is comparative reference: reference ranges for a species that has not been characterized are extrapolated from the closest available taxonomic relative, with the extrapolation flagged in the report as such. A serum biochemistry value in a giraffe interpreted against published bovid ranges is defensible with explicit acknowledgment of the extrapolation; the same value interpreted as if giraffe-specific ranges were available is not. The same reasoning applies to histopathologic interpretation: characteristics of the hepatic sinusoid in a species whose normal has not been described are interpreted against the closest available comparator, with explicit acknowledgment.

Comparative Case Reasoning at Signout

The signout discussion is where the comparative framework is transmitted between pathologists in practice. A senior pathologist reviewing an unfamiliar-species case with a resident routinely thinks aloud through the comparative reasoning: what would this lesion mean in a canine, what modifications does the species-specific anatomy demand, what is the closest previously characterized species, and what ancillary tests are informative in that species. Residents who develop the habit of asking these four questions on every case in a taxonomically unfamiliar species will build the comparative framework more efficiently than residents who wait to encounter a case that duplicates one they have seen before.

Applied Framework: A Worked Case in Cross-Taxa Reasoning

A 14-year-old female Aldabra tortoise (Aldabrachelys gigantea), a long-established member of an institutional collection, was found deceased in her outdoor enclosure on a temperate spring morning. Keepers reported no antemortem clinical signs; the animal had eaten normally the previous day. Ambient overnight temperature had reached 4°C, within the animal's documented seasonal tolerance range. The carcass reached the pathologist five hours after discovery, refrigerated during transport. External examination showed body condition assessed against the closest published comparative reference (Galápagos tortoise scoring, applied with explicit acknowledgment of extrapolation) as one to two grades below appropriate. Mucous membranes were pink; oral cavity, cloacal opening, and shell surface were unremarkable; there was no evidence of external trauma.

Chelonian necropsy was performed by standard plastron removal after skin reflection. Serous atrophy of the coelomic adipose stores was noted immediately upon plastron removal, a finding that dated the disease process to weeks in duration regardless of the absence of antemortem clinical signs recognized by keepers. The liver appeared enlarged and pale-tan throughout with rounded margins. The lungs contained multiple firm, tan, discrete nodules ranging from 3 to 12 mm scattered throughout both faveolar surfaces. The remaining coelomic viscera were grossly unremarkable. Body condition, chronic hepatic pallor, and multifocal pulmonary nodules together constrained the lesion-first differential to a chronic systemic infectious or infiltrative process.

The pathologist reasoned lesion-first because antemortem history was uninformative. The differential for a chronically ill chelonian with hepatic pallor and multifocal pulmonary nodules in a temperate managed captive population included chronic mycobacterial disease, ranavirus infection, chronic parasitism with granulomatous inflammatory response, chelonian herpesvirus disease, hepatic lipidosis secondary to unrecognized anorexia, and, in an elderly individual, chronic hepatocellular or biliary neoplasia. The pulmonary distribution — multifocal, discrete, and firm — argued against acute viral or bacterial pneumonia and toward a chronic granulomatous or neoplastic process.

Comparative reasoning was the interpretive bridge. The pulmonary pattern in the chelonian resembled the pattern observed in chronic mycobacterial disease in other reptile species and, at a greater taxonomic distance, in nonhuman primate and ungulate mycobacterial disease: multifocal, well-demarcated, firm granulomas distributed across the pulmonary parenchyma. The hepatic pattern in isolation was nonspecific for chronic hepatic disease of many etiologies. What distinguished the case for further comparative interpretation was the concurrent involvement of two organ systems (liver and lung) with morphologically compatible lesions, a distribution pattern that pointed toward a systemic infectious agent rather than a two-hit process of independent disease. In domestic species reasoning, concurrent hepatic and pulmonary granulomatous disease in a mammal narrows the differential quickly toward mycobacteriosis; the framework transported to the chelonian without substantive modification.

Histopathology confirmed multifocal granulomatous hepatitis and pneumonia with central caseation, epithelioid macrophage cuffs, and multinucleate giant cells. Ziehl-Neelsen acid-fast staining demonstrated numerous rod-shaped acid-fast bacilli within macrophages at granuloma centers. Polymerase chain reaction targeting the hsp65 gene identified Mycobacterium chelonae. The final diagnosis was chronic disseminated Mycobacterium chelonae infection with hepatic and pulmonary granulomatous disease.

Regulatory pathway activation followed the diagnostic finding through institutional and biosafety channels appropriate to this specific pathogen. Chelonian mycobacterial disease is not federally reportable in the United States, but Mycobacterium chelonae is a documented human opportunistic pathogen with cutaneous and pulmonary disease potential in immunocompromised humans. Institutional biosafety protocols required immediate notification of the collection veterinarian and the institutional biosafety officer. Keepers who had handled the animal during the preceding months received occupational health follow-up including baseline interferon-gamma release testing. Remaining animals in the collection were placed on enhanced surveillance for compatible clinical signs, environmental sampling of the shared enclosure surfaces and water features was initiated, and the necropsy report was distributed to the institution's veterinary team and pathology archive with explicit notation of the biosafety-relevant diagnosis.

This case demonstrates the four elements of the cognitive framework in application. Absent antemortem history was addressed by lesion-first characterization by distribution (multifocal), timing (chronic, dated by serous fat atrophy), and pattern (granulomatous). Comparative reasoning across reptile, primate, and ungulate mycobacterial disease provided the interpretive frame for a chelonian pattern the pathologist had not previously encountered in this species. Body condition and postmortem interval interpretation dated the disease process to weeks in duration and separated antemortem from postmortem changes. Regulatory pathway activation followed the diagnostic finding through institutional and biosafety channels appropriate to a non-federally-reportable but occupationally significant condition. The reasoning would apply, with agent-specific modification, to a captive nonhuman primate presenting with the same distribution pattern, to a captive artiodactyl, or to a free-ranging carnivore.

Figure 1.3. Histopathological photomicrograph paired panel: Hepatic hemosiderosis in captive lemur (*Eulemur* species).

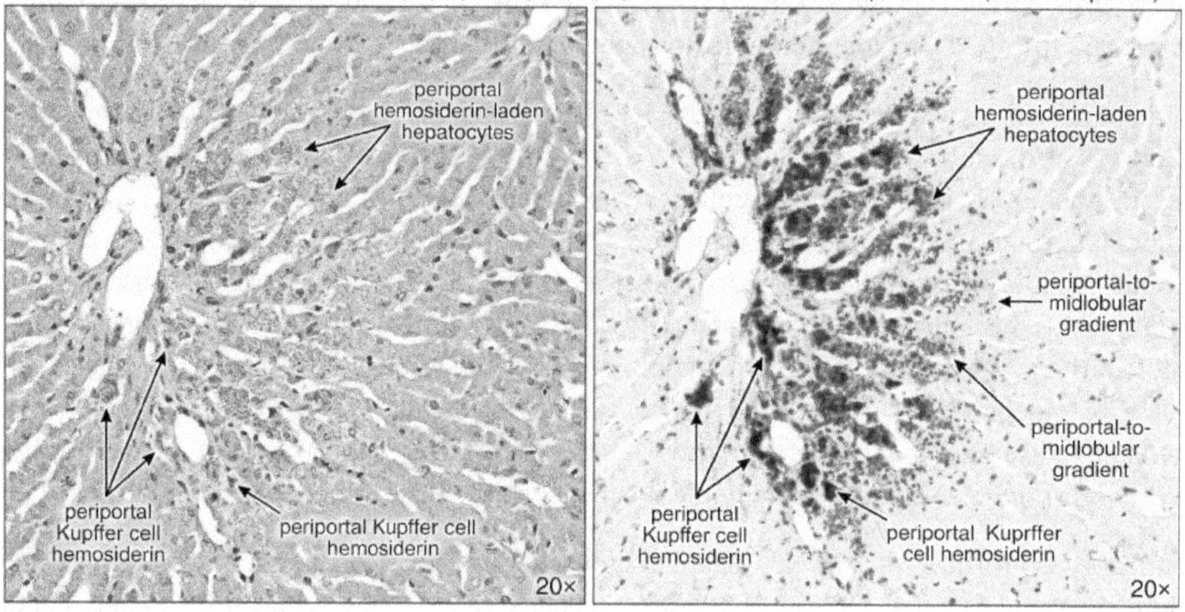

Figure 1.3. Histopathological photomicrograph paired panel, hepatic hemosiderosis in a captive lemur (*Eulemur* species).

THE COMPARATIVE NECROPSY PATTERN SYSTEM — Hepatic Hemosiderosis Across Frugivorous Primates and Perissodactyls

The Pattern: Marked accumulation of iron-positive, refractile, golden-brown pigment within hepatocyte cytoplasm and periportal Kupffer cells, with a periportal-to-midlobular distribution and, in advanced cases, associated hepatocellular necrosis and periportal fibrosis.

Cross-Taxa Signature: Recognized in captive frugivorous primates (lemurs, marmosets, tamarins), Southeast Asian and Indian frugivorous bats, black rhinoceros, tapirs, and, less prominently, several passerine species. The unifying etiologic feature is chronic dietary iron overload in species with intestinal absorptive machinery adapted to iron-poor natural diets; captive diets containing pelleted, iron-supplemented feed or iron-rich fruit substitutes exceed the animal's regulatory capacity to downregulate absorption.

Diagnostic Anchor: Prussian blue (Perls) staining confirms the pigment as ferric iron. Quantitative hepatic iron measurement, where available, distinguishes physiologic accumulation from pathologic overload; species-specific thresholds are published for black rhinoceros and a limited number of lemur species and are approximated by extrapolation elsewhere.

Trap Logic: The look-alike is hemosiderosis secondary to chronic hemolytic disease or transfusion, which produces a similar pigment distribution but is confined to macrophages of the reticuloendothelial system rather than accumulating within hepatocytes. Discrimination: dietary iron storage disease demonstrates prominent hepatocyte cytoplasmic hemosiderin; hemolytic hemosiderosis demonstrates hemosiderin in Kupffer cells and splenic macrophages with relative sparing of hepatocytes.

Zoonotic/Reportable Flag: Not zoonotic and not regulatorily reportable. Institutionally reportable at Species Survival Plan facilities managing black rhinoceros or lemurs because dietary reformulation is the population-level intervention required to prevent recurrence.

Iron-Associated Hepatic Lesion	Primary Distribution	Cell Population Affected	Species Predisposed	Distinguishing Feature
Dietary iron storage disease	Periportal to midlobular	Hepatocyte cytoplasm predominant	Frugivorous primates, black rhinoceros, tapirs, frugivorous bats	Hepatocyte-dominant distribution; dietary iron history
Hemolytic hemosiderosis	Diffuse, macrophage-associated	Kupffer cells and splenic macrophages	Any species with recent hemolytic event or transfusion	Kupffer cell dominance; hepatocyte relative sparing
Iatrogenic parenteral iron accumulation	Periportal Kupffer cell prominent	Kupffer cells; hepatocytes late	Species receiving parenteral iron supplementation	Injection or infusion history; Kupffer cell early involvement
Hereditary hemochromatosis analog	Diffuse hepatocyte cytoplasm	Hepatocyte cytoplasm	Not well characterized in non-domestic species; suspected in a small number of captive lineages	Family history clustering; absence of dietary or hemolytic explanation
Postmortem hemoglobin imbibition artifact	Endothelial surface staining	Vascular endothelium	Any species with prolonged postmortem interval	Endothelial pattern; absent cytoplasmic granular pigment

CAUTION: Interpretation of hepatic iron content in a species without published reference thresholds requires the pathologist to state the extrapolation explicitly in the report. Reporting an iron-associated lesion as diagnostic of iron storage disease in a species whose thresholds have not been characterized is a common source of overinterpretation, and downstream population-level dietary reformulation may be initiated based on the report.

One-Health and Regulatory Interfaces

Zoonotic Disease Recognition and Reporting

Wildlife and zoo carcasses carry a nontrivial baseline probability of zoonotic pathogen presence, and the necropsy is frequently the point of first detection. The pathologist working in the discipline maintains a running list of zoonotic disease patterns that must be recognized before continued dissection, because continued dissection may pose direct risk to the pathologist and to laboratory personnel. Highly pathogenic avian influenza in mammalian spillover is the most prominent contemporary example; hemorrhagic multifocal necrosis of the brain, lungs, and liver in a mustelid or marine mammal received during an active avian outbreak requires biosafety escalation before further tissue handling. Rabies in a wildlife carnivore, tuberculosis in an ungulate, brucellosis in a marine mammal or ungulate, herpes B in a macaque, monkey pox in a nonhuman primate, and Nipah virus in a fruit bat represent the recurring baseline of zoonotic patterns the wildlife pathologist is obliged to recognize before continuing.

Reportable Wildlife Disease Pathways

The regulatory reporting landscape differs from domestic species veterinary practice in specific and important ways. Federally reportable wildlife diseases in the United States include highly pathogenic avian influenza, foot-and-mouth disease in cloven-hoofed wildlife, chronic wasting disease in cervids, and several others, with the specific list updated by the Animal and Plant Health Inspection Service. State-reportable diseases vary by jurisdiction and include diseases with significant wildlife-livestock interface implications: bovine tuberculosis, brucellosis, pseudorabies. Institutionally reportable conditions at accredited zoos are governed by the Association of Zoos and Aquariums and by Species Survival Plan protocols and include a broad range of diseases relevant to captive population management. The pathologist working in this discipline maintains contact information for the state wildlife health veterinarian, the state animal health official, the institutional biosafety officer, and the appropriate federal authority, and knows which regulatory pathway is activated by which diagnostic finding.

USDA APHIS, USGS NWHC, and State Wildlife Health Programs

The institutional actors in the wildlife regulatory landscape have distinct but overlapping roles. The United States Department of Agriculture Animal and Plant Health Inspection Service holds regulatory authority for diseases of livestock importance, including diseases whose wildlife reservoirs pose a risk to domestic livestock. The United States Geological Survey National Wildlife Health Center in Madison, Wisconsin, is the principal federal diagnostic laboratory for free-ranging wildlife disease investigation and receives submissions for mortality events, emerging disease investigation, and surveillance in wild populations. State wildlife health programs, typically embedded within state departments of natural resources or state game and fish agencies, are the first responders to free-ranging mortality events and coordinate submissions with federal partners. Institutional zoo pathology programs coordinate with the Association of Zoos and Aquariums and with Species Survival Plan coordinators for population-level events. Tribal wildlife programs hold sovereign authority over wildlife on tribal lands and are the appropriate contact for events involving those populations.

Sample Chain of Custody and Legal Considerations

Wildlife necropsy findings frequently carry legal weight beyond the diagnostic report. Federal wildlife protection statutes, including the Migratory Bird Treaty Act, the Bald and Golden Eagle Protection Act, the Marine Mammal Protection Act, and the Endangered Species Act, criminalize specific interactions with wildlife, and necropsy findings may become evidence in enforcement action. The pathologist working with a case that may enter legal proceedings maintains chain of custody documentation from receipt through report issuance, secures tissue archives against tampering, and coordinates with federal law enforcement partners at United States Fish and Wildlife Service or National Oceanic and Atmospheric Administration Fisheries Office of Law Enforcement when a case is designated as an investigative submission. Photodocumentation of external lesions before internal examination is a standard step for these cases, because external lesions relevant to cause of death may be altered by the necropsy itself.

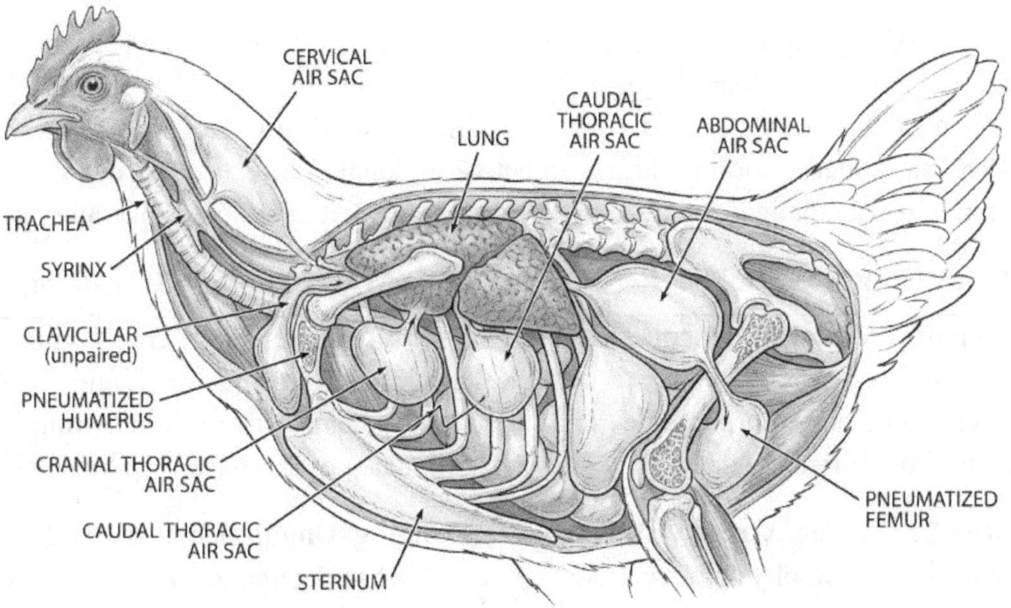

Figure 1.4: Comparative Coelomic Anatomy of the Domestic Chicken: Air Sac Distribution

THE COMPARATIVE NECROPSY PATTERN SYSTEM — Multifocal Hepatic and Splenic Necrosis Signaling HPAI in Mammalian Spillover

The Pattern: Multifocal to coalescing hepatic and splenic necrosis with meningoencephalitis in a carnivorous mammal received during an active regional highly pathogenic avian influenza outbreak in birds.

Cross-Taxa Signature: Recognized since 2022 across multiple mammalian taxa exposed to infected avian carrion or prey: mustelids (mink, otters, fishers), procyonids (raccoons), ursids (black bears, brown bears), pinnipeds (harbor seals, gray seals, elephant seals), and domestic and wild carnivores (foxes, coyotes). The unifying epidemiologic context is exposure to infected avian carcasses or aerosols, and the unifying pathologic feature is a systemic hemorrhagic and necrotizing lesion pattern with prominent central nervous system involvement.

Diagnostic Anchor: Detection of influenza A virus antigen in affected tissues by immunohistochemistry, or detection of H5-clade viral RNA by polymerase chain reaction on brain, lung, or spleen. Histopathologic anchor: necrotizing encephalitis with viral antigen positivity in neurons and glial cells.

Trap Logic: The look-alike in a carnivorous mammal is bacterial septicemia with disseminated intravascular coagulation (Yersinia pestis in mustelids, Streptococcus phocae in pinnipeds), which produces a similar hemorrhagic multifocal pattern but lacks the encephalitic component and lacks viral antigen positivity.

Zoonotic/Reportable Flag: Highly pathogenic avian influenza in mammalian spillover is a federally reportable condition with human zoonotic potential; biosafety escalation to BSL-3 practices and immediate notification of state animal health official and USDA APHIS are required before further dissection. Do not proceed with unfixed tissue handling until confirmation of biosafety containment.

EVIDENCE: The 2022 through 2025 highly pathogenic avian influenza panzootic produced documented mammalian spillover in more than a dozen carnivore and marine mammal species across multiple continents, with mustelid outbreaks in farmed mink demonstrating documented mammal-to-mammal transmission. The pathologist working during an active regional outbreak treats hemorrhagic multifocal disease in an exposed mammalian carcass as HPAI until refuted, and escalates biosafety accordingly.

THE COMPARATIVE NECROPSY PATTERN SYSTEM — Chapter 1 Reasoning Foundations

Cross-Taxa Hepatic Necrosis of Herpesviral Origin: Multifocal hepatic necrosis with Cowdry type A intranuclear inclusions across nonhuman primates, elephants, psittacines, and cervids. Anchor: intranuclear inclusion body morphology. Trap: bacterial hepatic necrosis discriminated by absent inclusions and neutrophil-rich exudate. Flag: herpes B in macaques is a hard-stop biosafety concern.

Cachexia With Serous Fat Atrophy Across Free-Ranging Ungulates: Gelatinous pericardial and epicardial adipose serous atrophy across cervids, bovids, suids, and camelids. Anchor: pericardial adipose transition to translucent gelatinous consistency. Trap: postmortem autolytic adipose softening discriminated by symmetric distribution and accompanying autolytic changes. Flag: chronic wasting disease and mycobacterial disease require regulatory notification.

Hepatic Hemosiderosis Across Frugivorous Primates and Perissodactyls: Periportal-to-midlobular hepatocyte and Kupffer cell hemosiderin across lemurs, marmosets, black rhinoceros, tapirs, and frugivorous bats. Anchor: Prussian blue confirmation of ferric iron in hepatocyte cytoplasm. Trap: hemolytic hemosiderosis discriminated by Kupffer cell dominance and hepatocyte relative sparing. Flag: institutionally reportable at Species Survival Plan facilities for dietary intervention.

Multifocal Hepatic and Splenic Necrosis Signaling HPAI in Mammalian Spillover: Systemic hemorrhagic and necrotizing lesion pattern with meningoencephalitis across mustelids, procyonids, ursids, pinnipeds, and wild carnivores exposed to infected avian carrion. Anchor: influenza A antigen positivity in neurons and glial cells. Trap: bacterial septicemia with disseminated intravascular coagulation discriminated by absent encephalitis and absent viral antigen. Flag: federally reportable with human zoonotic potential; biosafety escalation before continued dissection.

Summary and Key Concepts

Wildlife and zoo animal pathology substitutes cross-taxa reasoning for repetition-based pattern recognition because taxonomic diversity in caseload precludes repetition as a learning mechanism.

Lesion-first diagnostic reasoning is the routine cognitive mode when antemortem clinical history is absent or unreliable; morphologic characterization by distribution, timing, and pattern constrains the differential without species-specific memorization.

Body condition scoring, postmortem interval interpretation, and lesion morphology are the three interpretive channels available on every carcass regardless of history availability, and serous atrophy of adipose stores dates the disease process to weeks in duration.

Comparative pathology as a cognitive framework holds that lesion pattern interpretation is transportable across taxa with species-specific modifications, and that anatomic variation, reference range absence, and signout discussion are the routine tools for applying the framework.

The one-health and regulatory landscape in wildlife and zoo pathology includes zoonotic biosafety obligations, federal and state reportable disease pathways coordinated through USDA APHIS, USGS NWHC, and state wildlife health programs, and chain of custody requirements for cases with potential legal weight.

The Comparative Necropsy Pattern callout structure — Pattern, Cross-Taxa Signature, Diagnostic Anchor, Trap Logic, and Zoonotic/Reportable Flag — is the recurring scaffold on which cross-taxa pattern recognition is built throughout the remainder of this book.

CHAPTER 2: NECROPSY METHODOLOGY IN NON-DOMESTIC SPECIES

Learning Objectives

1. Apply the systematic necropsy sequence to a non-domestic species carcass with attention to the interpretive channels each step provides.
2. Modify necropsy technique appropriately for mammals across body size ranges from small mustelids to megavertebrates.
3. Perform avian necropsy with attention to air sac anatomy, syrinx, and the pneumatized skeleton.
4. Perform reptile and amphibian necropsy with correct plastron removal in chelonians and appropriate approach in squamates and anurans.
5. Perform fish and aquatic invertebrate necropsy with attention to gill, kidney, and swim bladder anatomy in teleosts and to species-specific approaches in cephalopods and cnidarians.
6. Interpret findings from decomposed or field-necropsy carcasses distinguishing autolytic change from antemortem lesions.

The necropsy is the single most consequential procedure in wildlife and zoo animal pathology because it generates almost all of the primary interpretive data on which diagnosis rests. A necropsy performed poorly cannot be repeated; the specimen has been altered irreversibly, and the diagnostic questions the necropsy failed to answer will remain unanswered. This chapter presents the systematic necropsy sequence as it applies across the taxonomic breadth encountered in wildlife and zoo practice. The general principles of systematic necropsy — external examination, systematic organ removal, and standardized tissue collection — apply across every taxonomic group with species-specific technical modifications. Those modifications are consequential: an avian necropsy approached as a mammalian necropsy will destroy air sac architecture before it can be examined; a chelonian necropsy approached without plastron removal cannot access most coelomic viscera; a cetacean necropsy approached by the dorsal-to-ventral incision appropriate for terrestrial mammals will miss the blubber-associated lesions that carry the marine mammal pathologist's most important interpretive data.

The chapter organizes technique by taxonomic group and closes with a section on decomposed carcass and field-necropsy interpretation because the wildlife pathologist frequently receives carcasses in states that would be considered unusable in domestic species diagnostic practice. Autolytic softening, scavenger predation, freeze-thaw artifact, and prolonged postmortem interval do not exclude the case from diagnostic investigation; they modify the interpretive weight the pathologist grants to findings and require explicit acknowledgment of the modifications in the necropsy report.

General Principles of Systematic Necropsy

Pre-Necropsy Preparation and Documentation

Pre-necropsy preparation begins with case documentation before the carcass is opened. The submission form is reviewed for signalment, clinical history where available, gross observations by field or clinical staff, and any regulatory or law-enforcement designations. The pathologist confirms the species identification if it is not obvious from morphology; misidentification of species is a recurring source of downstream diagnostic error, particularly in juvenile animals and in taxa with cryptic species complexes (small mustelids, tropical frogs, some fish species). Photographic documentation of the intact carcass in dorsal and ventral views precedes any incision, because external lesions relevant to cause of death may be altered or obscured during subsequent steps.

External Examination as an Interpretive Channel

External examination is a substantive interpretive channel and is not a preliminary step to be rushed. Body condition is assessed by palpation of skeletal prominences and adipose stores over the sternum, the paralumbar region, and the tail base, with reference to species-appropriate scoring systems where available and to comparative reference where they are not. Integument is examined systematically for wounds, scars, ectoparasites, and areas of alopecia or dermatitis; ectoparasite identification is important because tick and flea species carry epidemiologic weight for vector-borne disease workup. The oral cavity is examined for mucosal lesions, foreign material, and dental condition; dental attrition or malocclusion in the young of species with monophyodont dentition may account for chronic anorexia. Ocular condition, ear canal cleanliness, and cloacal or perineal appearance complete the external survey.

Systematic Organ Removal and Tissue Collection

Systematic organ removal follows a standardized sequence that varies by taxonomic group but shares a common logic: cavities are opened before their contents are removed, organs are examined in situ before removal, and the removal sequence proceeds from most easily displaced structures to those most anchored to the body wall. In terrestrial mammals, the sequence typically proceeds from external examination through opening the abdominal and thoracic cavities, in-situ examination of the pluck, removal of the thoracic block, removal of the abdominal viscera, examination of the reproductive and urinary systems, and finally examination of the brain and cervical spinal cord after calvarial section. Standardized tissue collection follows: samples for histopathology are collected from every major organ regardless of gross appearance, because the histologic interpretation of a grossly unremarkable organ is a routine source of diagnostic finding. Tissues for ancillary testing are collected fresh (frozen, refrigerated, or preserved in appropriate medium) before any tissue is fixed, because fixation renders many ancillary assays uninterpretable.

Ancillary Sample Collection and Preservation Strategy

Ancillary sample collection is planned before the first incision because samples that were not collected during the necropsy cannot be added afterward, and samples that were collected incorrectly are frequently uninterpretable. A standardized panel of representative samples from every major organ system is the baseline collection strategy on every case regardless of gross findings; lesion-targeted samples are added when specific lesions are identified. The standard panel typically includes formalin-fixed samples of liver, spleen, kidney, heart, lung, brain, gastrointestinal tract at three anatomically standardized levels, adrenal gland, thyroid, pancreas, and lymph nodes representative of the anatomic drainage regions. Formalin fixation at a tissue-to-fixative ratio of at least one to ten is required for adequate penetration; tissue sections greater than 5 mm in thickness will fix inadequately at the center regardless of fixation duration.

Fresh-frozen tissue is collected in parallel with formalin-fixed tissue because many ancillary diagnostic tests require unfixed material. A minimum fresh-frozen panel of liver, spleen, kidney, and lung permits downstream polymerase chain reaction, viral isolation, toxicological analysis, and molecular diagnostics on the most commonly targeted organ systems. Fresh-frozen brain is added when neurologic disease is suspected. Fresh-frozen bone marrow is added when hematologic or systemic disease is suspected. Storage at negative 80 degrees Celsius is preferred; storage at negative 20 degrees Celsius is acceptable for shorter intervals and for tissues destined for polymerase chain reaction rather than for viral isolation. Microbiologic samples require sterile collection technique with instruments changed or heat-sterilized between organs to prevent cross-contamination; aerobic and anaerobic bacterial culture, mycologic culture, and mycobacterial culture require distinct transport media, and the sample plan is determined by the anticipated differential rather than by reflex.

Toxicological sample collection follows separate rules driven by the analytical requirements of the anticipated toxicants. Liver and kidney are the workhorse tissues for heavy metal analysis. Adipose tissue is required for organochlorine and persistent organic pollutant analysis. Whole blood or serum is required for anticoagulant rodenticide analysis and for cholinesterase-inhibitor pesticide analysis. Vitreous humor is a robust sample for postmortem electrolyte, glucose, urea, and creatinine analysis and retains interpretive value in decomposed carcasses when serum has been lost. Bone is required for chronic lead exposure analysis. Sample volumes must meet the receiving laboratory's requirements; a submission with inadequate sample volume cannot be analyzed and may not be flagged for the pathologist until weeks after the specimen has been discarded.

Necropsy Report Structure and Communication

The necropsy report structures the pathologist's observations for downstream users who did not attend the necropsy. A report structured as gross findings, histopathologic findings, ancillary test results, morphologic diagnoses, and interpretive comments permits the reader to reconstruct the reasoning from primary observation through interpretive conclusion. Morphologic diagnoses are the operative diagnostic statement of the report: they describe the lesion in standardized morphologic terminology (distribution, timing, severity, and cellular process), identify the affected organ, and, where possible, name the etiologic agent or process. An interpretive comment that ties the morphologic diagnoses together into a coherent clinical narrative is the point where the pathologist's reasoning is made explicit to the reader.

Communication of the report follows the case's regulatory and institutional context. Routine case reports are distributed to the submitting clinician and archived in the pathology database. Cases with regulatory implications require distribution to appropriate federal or state authorities on defined timelines. Cases with institutional implications at collection facilities are distributed to the collection veterinarian, curator, and biosafety officer as warranted. Cases with law-enforcement implications require secure archival of the report and of tissue samples pending investigative direction. The pathologist's obligation extends beyond report issuance to timely communication of findings that require immediate action; a suspect zoonotic or reportable disease finding is communicated by direct contact with the appropriate authority rather than by report distribution alone.

THE COMPARATIVE NECROPSY PATTERN SYSTEM — Multifocal Organ Involvement Recognized During Systematic Necropsy

The Pattern: Concurrent, morphologically compatible lesions involving three or more anatomically separate organs identified during systematic necropsy, without an anatomic connection that would explain contiguous spread.

Cross-Taxa Signature: Recognized across every taxonomic group examined. In carnivores, concurrent hepatic, splenic, and renal necrosis suggests hematogenous infectious spread. In birds, concurrent hepatic, splenic, and pulmonary necrosis suggests a systemic infectious agent transported through the air sac and vascular systems together. In reptiles, concurrent hepatic, splenic, and coelomic serosal involvement suggests systemic bacterial or ranaviral disease. The pattern is recognized during systematic necropsy specifically because organ-by-organ examination in isolation may miss the multifocal distribution that carries the diagnostic weight.

Diagnostic Anchor: Explicit noting of the multifocal distribution in the necropsy report is the anchor. Ancillary workup differs from single-organ disease workup: samples from every involved organ are submitted for histopathology, bacteriology, and molecular diagnostics; a differential based on multifocal distribution is constructed and worked from the top down.

Trap Logic: The look-alike is postmortem autolytic change producing pseudo-multifocal pallor, softening, or hemorrhage across multiple organs simultaneously in a carcass with prolonged postmortem interval. Discrimination: antemortem multifocal lesions demonstrate inflammatory response at lesion margins on histopathology; autolytic change does not.

Zoonotic/Reportable Flag: Multifocal disease patterns are disproportionately likely to reflect zoonotic agents. Systemic mycobacterial disease, systemic salmonellosis, disseminated tuberculosis, systemic tularemia, and systemic HPAI in mammals all present as multifocal disease; biosafety awareness during dissection of a multifocal case is warranted from the first identification of the pattern.

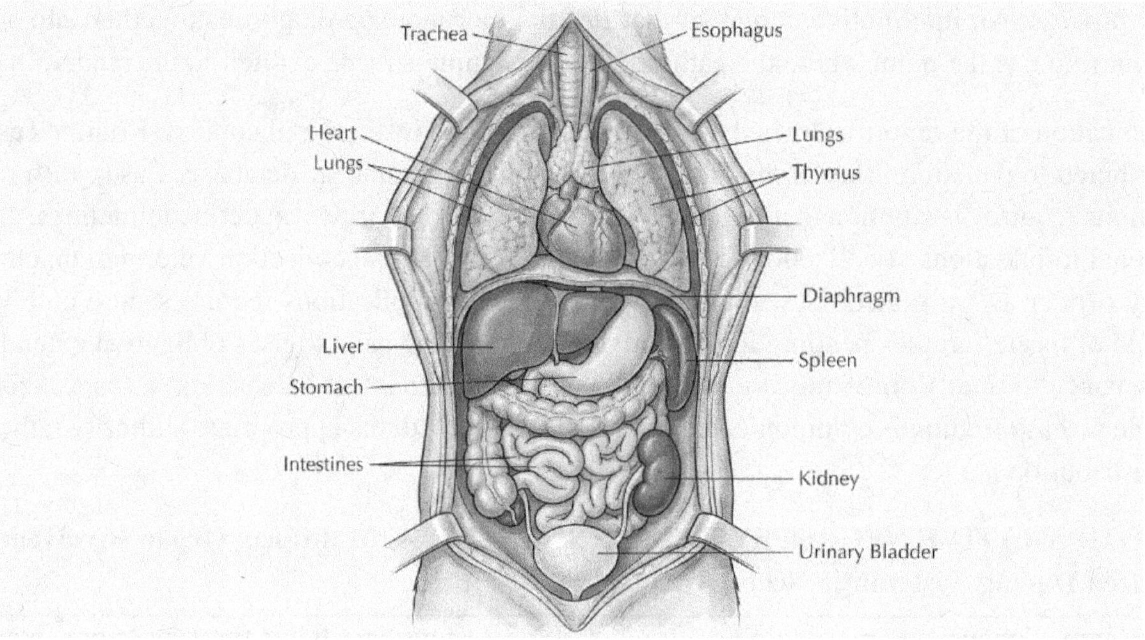

KEY POINT: The systematic necropsy is the primary tool for identifying multifocal organ involvement. Organ-by-organ examination in isolation, without a preceding in-situ survey of all cavities, will miss the multifocal distribution that separates single-organ disease from systemic disease and that carries most of the interpretive weight for infectious and neoplastic differentials.

Species-Specific Necropsy Approaches: Mammals

Small and Medium Terrestrial Mammals

Small and medium terrestrial mammals — carnivores from mustelid size through canid size, rodents from mouse size through capybara size, small ungulates, insectivores, and primates through cercopithecine size — follow the general mammalian necropsy sequence with only minor species-specific modifications. Positioning in dorsal recumbency with limbs abducted permits systematic access to both cavities. Skin reflection through a ventral midline incision extends from mandibular symphysis to pubis; the pectoral and abdominal musculature is reflected to expose the body wall. The rib cage is cut on both sides through the costochondral junctions to lift the sternum free; the diaphragm is inspected and released. In-situ organ examination precedes removal of the thoracic pluck as a coordinated unit including heart, lungs, mediastinal structures, and cervical viscera to the level of the tongue. The abdominal viscera are removed as a coordinated block with attention to preserved relationships between adjacent organs.

Large Terrestrial Mammals and Megavertebrates

Large ungulates, large carnivores, large primates, and megavertebrates (elephants, rhinoceros, giraffe, large ratites) require necropsy technique adapted to the physical constraints of the carcass. Positioning is typically lateral recumbency because the animal cannot be maintained in dorsal recumbency. The uppermost limb is removed to expose the flank; a paracostal incision through skin and musculature exposes the intact abdominal wall, which is opened along the linea alba. The thoracic wall is cut through the ribs to expose the pluck. Organ removal proceeds systematically but is often limited by carcass position and size: whole-organ removal may not be practicable for the liver, gastrointestinal tract, and heart of an elephant or a large rhinoceros, and systematic sampling from anatomically standardized sites within the intact organ replaces whole-organ removal in these cases. Documentation of sample sites is essential because the pathologist reviewing the histology will interpret the sample against the standardized site rather than the whole organ.

Marine Mammals and Cetacean-Specific Approach

Marine mammals require necropsy techniques that differ substantially from terrestrial mammalian technique because of the thermoregulatory blubber layer, the coelomic architecture, and the relative size of the animal. Cetaceans are approached by flensing pattern: parallel incisions through the skin and blubber are made in defined lines that permit removal of the blubber layer as intact sheets, which preserves the interpretive value of the blubber for evaluation of thermoregulatory function, prey energy status, and contaminant burden. Blubber thickness at standardized sites (typically at the level of the axilla, mid-body, and peduncle) is measured and recorded because blubber thickness is a body condition metric in cetaceans. Pinniped necropsy is closer to terrestrial mammalian technique but requires attention to the extensive subcutaneous adipose layer and to the aquatic-specific respiratory anatomy including reinforced tracheal cartilages. Sirenian necropsy shares elements of both cetacean and pinniped approaches.

THE COMPARATIVE NECROPSY PATTERN SYSTEM — Fatal Trauma Pattern Recognition in Free-Ranging Mammals

The Pattern: Concurrent skeletal fracture, soft tissue hemorrhage, and internal organ laceration in a distribution pattern consistent with a specific external mechanism of injury (vehicular collision, projectile injury, entanglement, intraspecific or interspecific trauma, predation).

Cross-Taxa Signature: Recognized across free-ranging mammals of all body sizes. Vehicular collision produces a characteristic pattern of long-bone fractures, thoracic and abdominal wall bruising with underlying organ contusion, and skin abrasion in the direction of impact. Projectile injury produces entrance and exit wounds with intervening organ pathology along the projectile path. Predation produces perimortem soft tissue damage with characteristic tooth or claw pattern; scavenger consumption after death produces postmortem tissue damage without vital reaction. Entanglement produces circumferential dermal lesions with associated skeletal deformation and secondary myoglobinuric renal injury.

Diagnostic Anchor: Documentation of vital reaction at wound sites (hemorrhage, inflammatory cell infiltrate, fibrin deposition) distinguishes antemortem from postmortem tissue disruption. Documentation of directional injury pattern (vehicular strike direction, projectile trajectory, entanglement wrap direction) supports the mechanism of injury conclusion.

Trap Logic: The look-alike is postmortem scavenger predation superimposed on antemortem disease death, which produces gross tissue disruption without a fatal traumatic mechanism. Discrimination:

postmortem scavenger damage lacks vital reaction and is confined to accessible surfaces; antemortem trauma demonstrates vital reaction and follows a mechanism-consistent pattern.

Zoonotic/Reportable Flag: Federally protected species (bald eagle, golden eagle, migratory birds, marine mammals, endangered species) with traumatic mortality require notification of federal law enforcement (US Fish and Wildlife Service or NOAA Fisheries Office of Law Enforcement) because the case may enter investigative proceedings. Chain of custody documentation is initiated at case receipt.

Species-Specific Necropsy Approaches: Birds

External Examination and Feather Interpretation

Avian external examination adds feather condition to the standard external survey because plumage condition carries substantial interpretive weight. Feather quality reflects nutritional and hormonal status over the interval since the last molt; broken or stress-barred feathers may reflect trauma, chronic illness during feather development, or captive husbandry inadequacies. The ceres, eyes, and beak are examined for lesions, discoloration, and overgrowth. The keel is palpated for body condition assessment; keel prominence is the primary body condition metric across most avian orders. Vent examination completes the external survey.

Coelomic Necropsy and Air Sac Preservation

Avian coelomic necropsy is approached with the animal in dorsal recumbency and the ventral body wall opened through a longitudinal incision from the caudal keel to the cloaca. The pectoral musculature is reflected and the keel bone is removed by cutting through the coracoid, clavicular, and sternal articulations on both sides; the intact keel is lifted free to expose the coelomic cavity. Air sac architecture is examined in situ before any organ is displaced, because air sac walls are thin, delicate, and easily disrupted; air sacculitis manifests as thickening, opacity, or exudate accumulation on the normally transparent air sac walls. The pericardial sac, liver, and spleen are examined in situ. The proventriculus and ventriculus are opened after removal to examine mucosal surfaces and contents; foreign material, ulceration, and impaction findings are recorded.

Syrinx, Trachea, and Pneumatized Skeleton

The syrinx is examined because it is the anatomic site of several important avian pathogens. The trachea is opened longitudinally from the larynx to the syrinx, and the syrinx is opened at the tracheal bifurcation to expose the tympanic membranes and internal syringeal surface. The pneumatized skeleton is inspected: the humerus, femur, and portions of the vertebral column contain air sac extensions and may harbor infectious material contiguous with air sacculitis or systemic infection. Bone marrow of non-pneumatized bones (typically the tibiotarsus in most species) is examined for color, consistency, and lesions; a red bone marrow in a mature bird suggests either chronic hematologic demand or infiltrative disease.

Figure 2.2: Avian Coelomic Anatomy in Situ: Air Sac Distribution Relevant to Systematic Necropsy

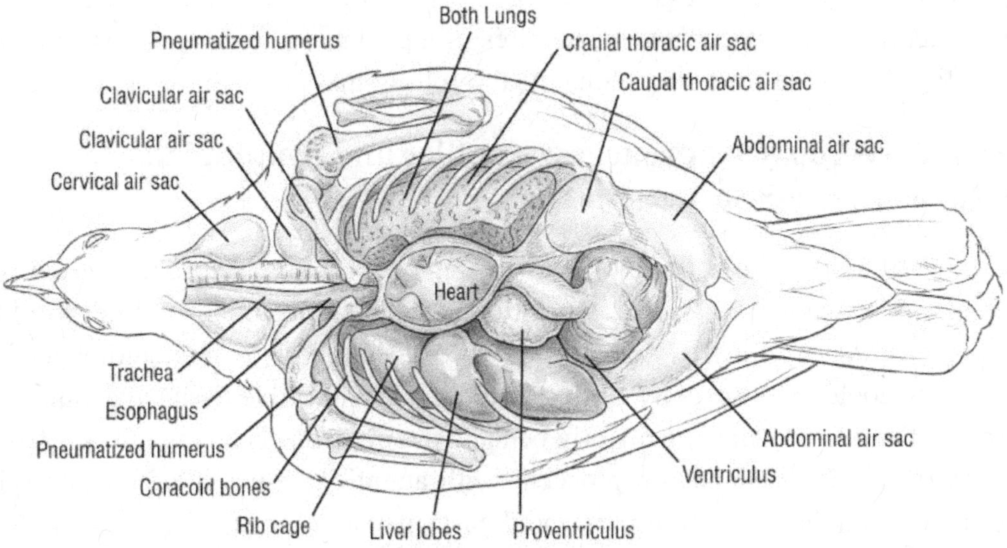

THE COMPARATIVE NECROPSY PATTERN SYSTEM — Air Sacculitis Pattern in Avian Necropsy Across Orders

The Pattern: Thickening, opacification, or fibrinous exudate accumulation on the normally transparent air sac walls, identified during in-situ coelomic examination before organ displacement.

Cross-Taxa Signature: Recognized across all avian orders. In psittacines and passerines, air sacculitis is prominently associated with aspergillosis, chlamydiosis, and mycobacterial disease. In poultry and gallinaceous birds, air sacculitis is prominently associated with Mycoplasma gallisepticum, Escherichia coli, and Ornithobacterium rhinotracheale. In waterfowl, air sacculitis is prominently associated with aspergillosis, avian cholera, and, during outbreaks, highly pathogenic avian influenza. In raptors, air sacculitis is prominently associated with aspergillosis and, historically, with trichomoniasis-related disease. The gross appearance across orders is remarkably similar; the etiologic differential varies by order and by epidemiologic context.

Diagnostic Anchor: Identification of air sacculitis during in-situ examination triggers systematic sampling of air sac wall for histopathology, bacteriology, mycology, and molecular diagnostics before any organ is disturbed. Delayed sampling after coelomic disruption compromises interpretive value because environmental contamination from opened viscera reaches the air sac surfaces.

Trap Logic: The look-alike is postmortem air sac desiccation and secondary opacification in a carcass with prolonged postmortem interval, which produces air sac appearance changes without antemortem disease. Discrimination: antemortem air sacculitis demonstrates inflammatory cell infiltrate on histopathology; postmortem change does not. Additionally, aspiration of yolk material in a hen at end of lay produces yolk peritonitis that can secondarily involve the abdominal air sac but is distinguished by the presence of yolk material and characteristic granulomatous inflammation.

Zoonotic/Reportable Flag: Air sacculitis in a psittacine, columbid, or free-ranging bird received during an active regional highly pathogenic avian influenza outbreak requires biosafety escalation before further dissection. Air sacculitis with mycobacterial features in a psittacine or ratite is institutionally reportable at collection facilities and requires occupational health follow-up.

Species-Specific Necropsy Approaches: Reptiles and Amphibians

Chelonian Necropsy and Plastron Removal

Chelonian necropsy requires plastron removal as the first substantive step because the plastron blocks access to all coelomic viscera. The animal is positioned in dorsal recumbency; the skin bridge between the plastron and the carapace is incised on both sides from the axillary to the inguinal notch. The plastron is separated from the coelomic viscera by cutting through the connective tissue attachments; care is taken to preserve the heart and liver which lie directly beneath the plastron. The plastron is lifted free to expose the coelomic cavity. In-situ examination proceeds with attention to the coelomic serosal surfaces, the heart, the liver lobes, and the multi-compartmented gastrointestinal tract. The lungs are located dorsally against the carapace and are accessed after the coelomic viscera are removed; chelonian lungs are faveolar rather than alveolar and are examined as a distinct organ system.

Squamate and Crocodilian Approaches

Squamates (lizards and snakes) are approached by ventral midline incision without any bony structure to remove. In snakes, the incision extends from the cloaca cranially to a level appropriate for the target organs; systematic examination proceeds from the caudal end forward because the reproductive tract and kidneys are located caudally, the intestines and stomach midbody, the liver and heart cranially. Species-specific attention to venom gland and hemipenal anatomy is required in venomous species. Crocodilians are approached by ventral midline incision with attention to the reinforced ventral scute pattern; the incision is made lateral to the midline scutes to avoid the reinforced keratinized structures.

Anuran and Caudate Amphibian Approaches

Anurans and caudates are approached by ventral midline incision. In small amphibians, the entire necropsy is performed under a dissecting microscope because organ size precludes gross examination of small organs without magnification. The abdominal wall is thin and easily disrupted; care is taken to avoid contamination of coelomic viscera by cutaneous flora. Skin is examined systematically for chytridiomycosis-compatible lesions before dissection because cutaneous involvement is the primary lesion of chytridiomycosis, and postmortem handling that disrupts the epidermis may compromise diagnostic interpretation.

Figure 2.3: Chelonian Necropsy: Plastron Removal and In-Situ Coelomic Examination

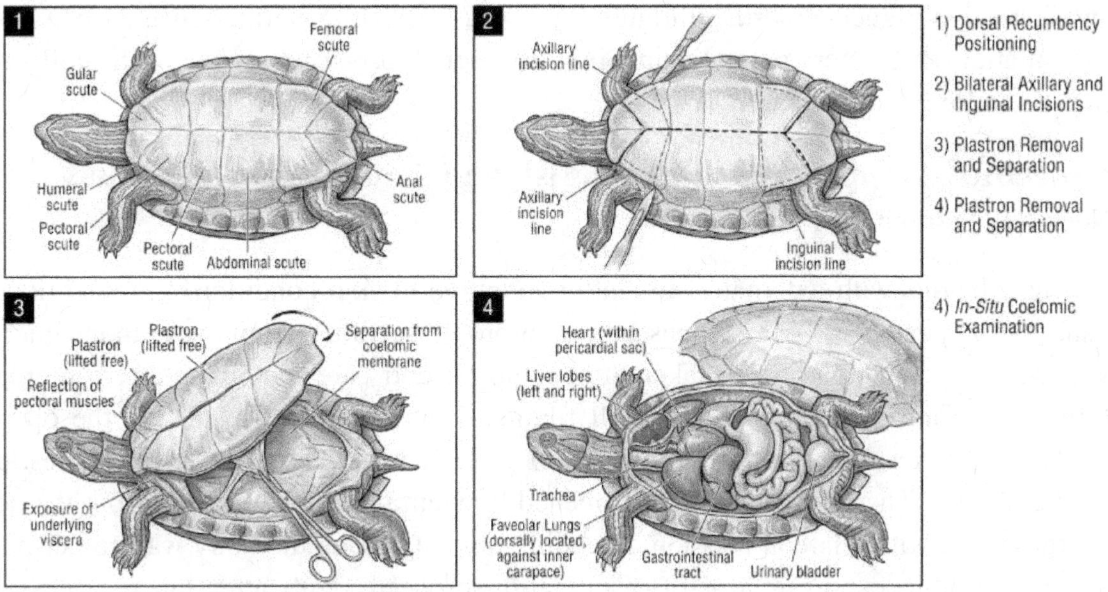

THE COMPARATIVE NECROPSY PATTERN SYSTEM — Multifocal Hepatic and Splenic Necrosis Signaling Ranavirus in Chelonians and Anurans

The Pattern: Multifocal hepatic and splenic necrosis with intracytoplasmic viral inclusion bodies and prominent basophilic to eosinophilic paracrystalline arrays visible on histopathology in chelonians and anurans, often accompanied by cutaneous ulceration in anurans and by oral or ocular lesions in chelonians.

Cross-Taxa Signature: Recognized across chelonians (Frog virus 3-like ranavirus in North American chelonians, Testudinid herpesvirus 3 as a look-alike differential requiring distinction), anurans (Frog virus 3 across North American anurans, Bohle iridovirus in Australian anurans), caudates (Frog virus 3 in North American caudates, Ambystoma tigrinum virus in tiger salamanders and related species), and elasmobranchs and teleosts (Santee-Cooper ranavirus in largemouth bass, epizootic hematopoietic necrosis virus in redfin perch). The pattern crosses across ectothermic vertebrate classes in a way few other agents do.

Diagnostic Anchor: Polymerase chain reaction targeting the ranavirus major capsid protein gene from affected tissue confirms the agent. Histopathologic anchor: intracytoplasmic basophilic viral inclusions with associated hepatic and splenic necrosis; electron microscopy demonstrates paracrystalline arrays of icosahedral virions in affected cells.

Trap Logic: The look-alike in chelonians is Testudinid herpesvirus 3 disease, which produces stomatitis-rhinitis-conjunctivitis with hepatic necrosis and can overlap grossly with ranavirus. Discrimination: herpesvirus produces intranuclear (not intracytoplasmic) Cowdry type A inclusion bodies. The look-alike in anurans is chytridiomycosis with secondary bacterial septicemia, which produces cutaneous lesions and hepatic necrosis. Discrimination: chytridiomycosis demonstrates fungal thalli in the epidermis on histopathology; ranavirus does not.

Zoonotic/Reportable Flag: Ranavirus is a World Organisation for Animal Health-notifiable disease of amphibians. Detection triggers reporting through state wildlife health veterinarian and USDA APHIS. Not zoonotic. Population-level intervention (source investigation, biosecurity review of the collection or field site) follows detection.

Species-Specific Necropsy Approaches: Fish and Aquatic Invertebrates

Teleost Necropsy Sequence

Teleost necropsy begins with external examination attentive to skin condition, fin condition, gill cover position, and eye appearance. Skin scrapes taken before dissection permit wet-mount microscopy for ectoparasite identification; skin scrapes taken after coelomic entry are contaminated by internal fluid and are uninterpretable for external parasitism. Gill filaments are examined by lifting the operculum and examining the gill arches; wet-mount microscopy of gill filaments identifies gill parasites, hyperplasia patterns, and clubbing. The coelomic cavity is opened by ventral midline incision from the pelvic girdle to the pectoral girdle, with a lateral incision extending dorsally along the body wall to permit body wall reflection and coelomic exposure. In-situ examination proceeds with attention to the swim bladder (species-specific: physostomous or physoclistous), the liver, the anterior kidney (containing hematopoietic and lymphoid tissue), the posterior kidney (renal excretory tissue), the spleen, the gastrointestinal tract, and the reproductive organs.

Elasmobranch Approaches

Elasmobranchs (sharks, rays, and skates) require necropsy technique adapted to cartilaginous skeletal anatomy. Ventral midline incision opens the coelomic cavity; in-situ examination is attentive to the spiral valve intestine, the paired liver lobes (which in sharks are large and constitute a substantial proportion of body weight), the pancreas, and the paired kidneys. The rectal gland is examined in situ because it has osmoregulatory function and may harbor lesions. Cartilaginous vertebrae are examined for skeletal disease including spondylosis-like lesions and neoplasia.

Cephalopod and Cnidarian Approaches

Cephalopod necropsy is performed with attention to the mantle cavity anatomy including the gills, the heart complex (systemic heart plus paired branchial hearts), the digestive gland, and the ink sac. Ventral mantle incision permits mantle cavity access without disruption of the gills. Cnidarian necropsy in captive scyphozoan and anthozoan collections is typically approached by whole-animal fixation followed by systematic sectioning because gross dissection of small or delicate cnidarians is uninformative; cross-sectional examination of fixed specimens permits identification of infectious agents, environmental contaminants, and tissue integrity changes.

THE COMPARATIVE NECROPSY PATTERN SYSTEM — Gill Pathology Pattern in Teleost Necropsy Interpretation

The Pattern: Gill lamellar hyperplasia, clubbing, fusion, or necrosis identified during systematic gill examination, with distribution across gill arches informing the underlying etiology.

Cross-Taxa Signature: Recognized across teleosts of all ecological types. Freshwater teleosts commonly present with lamellar hyperplasia secondary to environmental water quality (ammonia, nitrite, low dissolved oxygen). Marine teleosts commonly present with lamellar hyperplasia secondary to amoebic gill disease (Neoparamoeba perurans in salmonids), gill flukes, or environmental hypoxia. Ornamental and aquarium teleosts commonly present with hyperplasia secondary to chronic water quality inadequacies; symmetric bilateral involvement suggests environmental cause, while asymmetric or focal involvement suggests infectious cause.

Diagnostic Anchor: Wet-mount microscopy of gill filaments taken before formalin fixation confirms the presence and identification of parasitic agents. Histopathology confirms lamellar architecture and inflammatory cell infiltrate. Water quality history from the case submitter contextualizes environmental versus infectious etiology.

Trap Logic: The look-alike is postmortem gill autolysis and epithelial sloughing in a carcass with prolonged postmortem interval, which produces gill filament changes without antemortem disease. Discrimination: antemortem gill hyperplasia demonstrates lamellar architectural change on histopathology with inflammatory infiltrate; autolytic change demonstrates loss of epithelial adherence without underlying architectural change.

Zoonotic/Reportable Flag: Amoebic gill disease and several viral pathogens of teleosts (viral hemorrhagic septicemia virus, spring viremia of carp virus, infectious salmon anemia virus) are World Organisation for Animal Health-notifiable diseases requiring reporting through state animal health authorities. Not zoonotic.

Field Necropsy and Decomposed Carcass Interpretation

Field-Necropsy Constraints and Adapted Technique

Field necropsy is performed at the site of carcass discovery when the carcass cannot be transported to a laboratory. Field-necropsy constraints include ambient temperature affecting tissue quality, absence of laboratory instrumentation, limited sample preservation capacity, and safety considerations at the discovery site. Adapted technique prioritizes sample collection over comprehensive gross examination: representative tissue samples from every major organ system are collected in appropriate preservative for later histopathologic and ancillary examination, and gross observations are documented photographically and in written notes. A field-necropsy kit typically includes 10% neutral buffered formalin, cassettes for tissue placement, cryotubes with liquid nitrogen or dry ice for fresh-frozen samples, appropriate transport media for microbiologic samples, and personal protective equipment appropriate to the anticipated pathogen risk.

Decomposed Carcass Interpretation

Decomposed carcasses retain diagnostic value if interpretive limits are recognized. Autolysis progresses from mucosal surfaces inward; the deep parenchymal tissue of solid organs may retain histologic architecture long after mucosal surfaces have sloughed. Bone marrow is a robust tissue for both toxicological and microbiological analysis in decomposed carcasses because it is protected within the osseous cavity. Vitreous humor is similarly protected within the ocular globe and retains value for postmortem chemistry and toxicological analysis. The pathologist working a decomposed carcass explicitly documents which tissues were compromised and which were preserved, and grants interpretive weight accordingly.

Freeze-Thaw and Scavenger Modification

Freeze-thaw modification of tissue produces characteristic artifact: ice crystal formation disrupts cellular architecture and can produce apparent vacuolation, cellular disruption, and pseudo-hemorrhage that must be distinguished from antemortem lesions. Freeze-thawed tissue submitted for histopathology is flagged for the histopathologist because the interpretive threshold for morphologic change is different in frozen-thawed than in fresh-fixed tissue. Scavenger modification produces characteristic gross patterns: raptor consumption typically produces defleshing of soft tissue and eye orbits; canid consumption typically produces limb removal and thoracic entry; corvid and gull consumption typically produces eye and cloacal orifice consumption. The pattern of scavenger modification is often diagnostic of the scavenger species and helps constrain the postmortem interval.

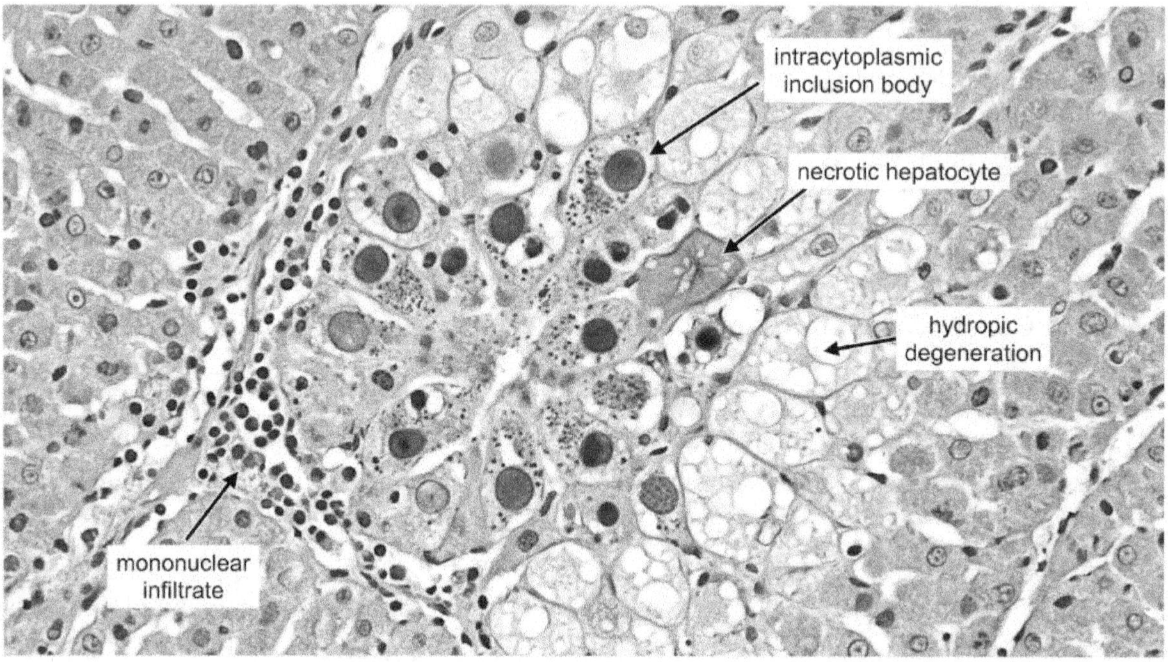

THE COMPARATIVE NECROPSY PATTERN SYSTEM — Postmortem Interval Interpretation Across Necropsy Findings

The Pattern: Systematic evaluation of tissue autolysis progression across multiple organ systems to estimate postmortem interval and to distinguish antemortem lesions from postmortem change.

Cross-Taxa Signature: Autolysis progression is broadly similar across vertebrate taxa but is modified by species-specific factors. In terrestrial mammals, mucosal sloughing progresses from stomach through small intestine to colon over the first 24 to 48 hours at ambient temperature. In birds, autolysis is accelerated by the higher normal body temperature. In reptiles and amphibians, autolysis is slower at ambient temperature but progresses rapidly when the carcass is warmed. In marine mammals, autolysis is modified by the insulating blubber layer, which slows heat loss and accelerates deep tissue autolysis relative to terrestrial mammals of similar body size.

Diagnostic Anchor: Vital reaction at any lesion margin distinguishes antemortem from postmortem change. Fibrin deposition, inflammatory cell infiltrate, and hemorrhage with intact red blood cell integrity constitute vital reaction; postmortem hemoglobin imbibition of tissue does not.

Trap Logic: The look-alike for autolytic mucosal sloughing is severe antemortem enteritis with mucosal necrosis. Discrimination: antemortem necrotic enteritis is bordered by inflammatory response on histopathology; autolytic sloughing is not. The look-alike for autolytic hepatic softening is antemortem hepatic necrosis. Discrimination: antemortem hepatic necrosis demonstrates loss of hepatocyte architecture with inflammatory response; autolytic change demonstrates loss of hepatocyte architecture without response.

Zoonotic/Reportable Flag: Decomposed carcass status does not exclude zoonotic pathogen presence and may complicate biosafety assessment. Personal protective equipment appropriate to the anticipated pathogen risk (respiratory protection for HPAI-suspect avian carcasses, gloves and eye protection for rabies-suspect mammals, containment garments for TB-suspect ungulates) is maintained regardless of postmortem interval.

Taxonomic Group	Primary Positioning	First Substantive Access Step	Species-Specific Anatomic Priority	Common Technical Pitfall
Small and medium terrestrial mammals	Dorsal recumbency	Ventral midline skin incision	Standard pluck removal sequence	Insufficient in-situ examination before pluck removal
Large mammals and megavertebrates	Lateral recumbency	Paracostal incision after limb removal	Standardized site sampling within intact organs	Failure to document sample sites for later histologic reference

Cetaceans	Lateral recumbency in field or dorsal in facility	Flensing pattern parallel incisions	Blubber layer preservation for interpretive value	Loss of blubber orientation during removal
Birds	Dorsal recumbency	Ventral coelomic incision with keel removal	Air sac wall preservation before organ displacement	Air sac disruption before wet-mount or histologic sampling
Chelonians	Dorsal recumbency	Plastron removal via bridge incision	Faveolar lung access after coelomic viscera removal	Cardiac laceration during plastron separation
Squamates	Ventral or dorsal recumbency	Ventral midline incision	Caudal-to-cranial systematic access in snakes	Failure to examine venom glands in venomous species
Anurans and caudates	Ventral recumbency	Ventral midline incision under magnification	Skin preservation for chytridiomycosis assessment	Cutaneous disruption before histologic sampling
Teleosts	Right lateral recumbency	Ventral midline plus dorsal-lateral incision	Wet-mount gill and skin scrape before dissection	Coelomic contamination of gill and skin samples
Elasmobranchs	Ventral recumbency	Ventral midline incision	Spiral valve intestine and rectal gland examination	Failure to sample cartilaginous vertebrae for skeletal disease

CLINICAL PEARL: The field-necropsy pathologist collects samples for the anticipated diagnostic questions and for the unanticipated ones. A representative panel of formalin-fixed tissue from every organ system, a fresh-frozen tissue panel from liver, kidney, spleen, and lung, and appropriate microbiologic samples permit downstream workup of nearly any diagnostic hypothesis that emerges after the field visit has ended. Sample capacity is finite; the discipline of collecting representative panels rather than lesion-focused samples pays back on every case in which the initial gross impression proves incorrect.

Multifocal Organ Involvement Recognized During Systematic Necropsy: Concurrent lesions across three or more organs identified during in-situ survey. Anchor: explicit noting of multifocal distribution in the report and expanded ancillary workup. Trap: autolytic pseudo-multifocal pallor discriminated by absent inflammatory response. Flag: multifocal patterns disproportionately reflect zoonotic agents.

Fatal Trauma Pattern Recognition in Free-Ranging Mammals: Concurrent skeletal, soft tissue, and organ injury consistent with a defined mechanism. Anchor: vital reaction at wound sites distinguishes antemortem from postmortem. Trap: postmortem scavenger predation superimposed on antemortem disease. Flag: federally protected species require law enforcement notification.

Air Sacculitis Pattern in Avian Necropsy Across Orders: Air sac wall thickening or exudate on in-situ examination before organ displacement. Anchor: air sac sampling before coelomic disruption. Trap: postmortem air sac desiccation discriminated by absent inflammatory infiltrate. Flag: air sacculitis during HPAI outbreak requires biosafety escalation.

Multifocal Hepatic and Splenic Necrosis Signaling Ranavirus in Chelonians and Anurans: Multifocal necrosis with intracytoplasmic viral inclusions across ectothermic vertebrates. Anchor: PCR for ranavirus major capsid protein gene. Trap: chelonian herpesvirus discriminated by intranuclear inclusions. Flag: WOAH-notifiable amphibian disease.

Gill Pathology Pattern in Teleost Necropsy Interpretation: Lamellar hyperplasia, clubbing, or necrosis with distribution informing etiology. Anchor: wet-mount microscopy before formalin fixation. Trap: postmortem gill autolysis discriminated by preserved architecture without response. Flag: several viral gill pathogens are WOAH-notifiable.

Postmortem Interval Interpretation Across Necropsy Findings: Autolysis progression across organ systems to date postmortem interval and distinguish antemortem lesions from postmortem change. Anchor: vital reaction at lesion margins. Trap: autolytic mucosal sloughing discriminated from antemortem enteritis by inflammatory response. Flag: decomposed status does not exclude zoonotic pathogen presence.

Summary and Key Concepts

The systematic necropsy is the primary tool of wildlife and zoo pathology; general principles of external examination, in-situ organ survey, systematic removal, and standardized tissue collection apply across taxonomic groups with species-specific modifications.

Mammalian necropsy technique adapts to body size, from standard dorsal-recumbent pluck removal in small and medium mammals through lateral-recumbency paracostal approach in megavertebrates to flensing-pattern approach in cetaceans preserving blubber orientation.

Avian necropsy requires keel removal, in-situ air sac examination before organ displacement, and syrinx and pneumatized skeleton examination as species-specific interpretive channels absent from mammalian technique.

Reptile and amphibian necropsy varies substantially across chelonian, squamate, crocodilian, anuran, and caudate approaches, with chelonian plastron removal, snake caudal-to-cranial systematic access, and amphibian cutaneous preservation for chytridiomycosis assessment as recurring technical requirements.

Fish and aquatic invertebrate necropsy requires wet-mount microscopy of gill and skin samples before dissection, attention to species-specific organ systems including swim bladder, anterior kidney, and rectal gland, and specialized approaches for cephalopods and cnidarians.

Field necropsy and decomposed carcass interpretation retain diagnostic value with explicit acknowledgment of interpretive limitations; bone marrow, vitreous humor, and deep parenchymal tissue are the tissues most likely to retain interpretive weight in compromised carcasses.

CHAPTER 3: SPECIMEN HANDLING, ANCILLARY TESTING, AND BIOSAFETY

Learning Objectives

1. Apply appropriate tissue fixation, preservation, and shipping technique to non-domestic species specimens.
2. Select ancillary diagnostics — cytology, microbiology, molecular, and toxicology — appropriate to the case differential and species.
3. Recognize biosafety escalation triggers at case receipt and apply appropriate personal protective equipment during necropsy.
4. Prepare and submit samples meeting regulatory requirements, including chain-of-custody documentation for investigative cases.
5. Distinguish fixation artifact, sample contamination, and species-specific technical issues from antemortem disease findings.
6. Coordinate submission with reference laboratories accepting non-domestic species samples.

Ancillary testing extends the interpretive reach of the necropsy beyond what gross and histopathologic examination alone can provide. A well-designed ancillary panel confirms an infectious etiology suggested by lesion morphology, identifies a toxicant when clinical history is silent, characterizes an unusual cell population beyond what light microscopy can resolve, and detects agents present at concentrations below the histopathologic detection threshold. A poorly designed ancillary panel produces uninterpretable results, wastes limited fresh tissue, and generates false-negative findings that may be misread as ruling out an etiology that was in fact present. The pathologist working in wildlife and zoo species carries a disproportionate ancillary-testing burden because species-specific validation of many diagnostic assays does not exist, and interpretive weight granted to a test result depends on the pathologist's judgment about the assay's likely performance in the species.

This chapter organizes specimen handling and ancillary testing into four operational domains: tissue fixation and preservation with the shipping considerations that follow, the selection and interpretation of ancillary diagnostics across cytology, microbiology, molecular, and toxicology categories, the biosafety framework applied to non-domestic species necropsy, and the regulatory sample submission and chain-of-custody requirements applicable to investigative and reportable cases. Each domain carries recurring pitfalls that generate diagnostic error more frequently than any specific disease misinterpretation; recognition of the pitfalls is what distinguishes competent from expert practice.

Tissue Fixation, Preservation, and Shipping

Formalin Fixation Principles

Formalin fixation is the reference standard for histopathologic preservation and works by crosslinking cellular proteins to arrest autolysis and preserve cellular architecture. Ten percent neutral buffered formalin is the standard fixative for veterinary histopathology and is compatible with most immunohistochemistry, most molecular diagnostics performed on formalin-fixed paraffin-embedded tissue, and long-term storage. The tissue-to-fixative ratio of at least one to ten by volume is required for adequate penetration; tissue submerged in inadequate fixative volume will fix peripherally while the center undergoes continued autolysis, producing a characteristic pattern of well-preserved surface architecture with autolytic parenchymal change centrally. Tissue thickness is the second determinant of fixation quality: formalin penetrates approximately 3 to 5 mm per 24 hours, so tissue sections thicker than 5 mm will fix inadequately at the center regardless of duration. Tissue is trimmed to appropriate thickness at the time of collection rather than at trim-in, because thick tissue submerged in fixative for shipping will not fix during transit.

Alternative Fixatives and Their Applications

Alternative fixatives are applied when specific diagnostic requirements exceed formalin's capabilities. Bouin fixative preserves nuclear detail more sharply than formalin and is used historically for reproductive tract and gastrointestinal biopsy interpretation; the picric acid component stains tissue yellow and requires extended washing before some downstream applications. Glutaraldehyde is the fixative of choice for electron microscopic examination because it crosslinks membrane proteins more completely than formalin and preserves ultrastructural detail; glutaraldehyde-fixed tissue is post-fixed in osmium tetroxide before embedding in epoxy resin. Ethanol fixation preserves nucleic acid integrity for some molecular applications but disrupts membrane architecture and is unsuitable for most histopathologic interpretation. RNAlater and equivalent stabilizing solutions preserve RNA for downstream molecular diagnostics without formalin's crosslinking effect, and are the fixative of choice for transcriptomic and viral load applications where fresh-frozen collection is not feasible.

Fresh Tissue Preservation and Cold Chain

Fresh tissue preservation is required for viral isolation, some polymerase chain reaction applications, most toxicological analyses, most microbiologic culture, and several molecular diagnostics. Fresh tissue is collected into sterile containers immediately after removal from the carcass and transferred to appropriate cold storage without delay. Refrigeration at 4 degrees Celsius is adequate for short-term storage before shipping. Freezing at negative 20 degrees Celsius is adequate for polymerase chain reaction and most toxicology applications for storage intervals of days to weeks. Ultra-low storage at negative 80 degrees Celsius is required for viral isolation, for long-term archival, and for tissues destined for downstream applications with unknown storage requirements. Liquid nitrogen storage at negative 196 degrees Celsius is required for cell viability applications and for cryopreservation of germplasm or diagnostic reference material. Freeze-thaw cycles compromise nucleic acid integrity and viral viability; aliquoting samples at the time of freezing prevents the need to thaw an entire sample for each downstream application.

Shipping Regulations and Diagnostic Sample Categories

Shipping regulations for diagnostic samples are governed by international and national air transport regulations and by biosafety category. Category A infectious substances (defined by International Air Transport Association Dangerous Goods Regulations as substances capable of causing permanent disability, life-threatening, or fatal disease in humans) require UN 2814 shipping, triple packaging, and specific labeling. Category B biological substances (all other infectious substances) require UN 3373 shipping with less restrictive packaging. Formalin-fixed tissue is subject to formaldehyde shipping regulations separately from the biosafety category and requires appropriate labeling as a hazardous chemical. Dry-ice shipments require UN 1845 classification and quantity notation. Non-domestic species samples may additionally require permits under Convention on International Trade in Endangered Species regulations if the species is CITES-listed; permits are obtained before the specimen is collected, not after.

THE COMPARATIVE NECROPSY PATTERN SYSTEM — Fixation-Artifact Pattern Masking Multifocal Necrosis

---

The Pattern: Central autolytic change with well-preserved peripheral architecture on histopathologic sections, producing an appearance of central pallor and cellular dropout that mimics multifocal necrosis on the gross specimen.

Cross-Taxa Signature: Recognized across every taxonomic group when tissue-to-fixative ratio was inadequate or when tissue thickness at collection exceeded 5 mm. The pattern is characteristic: the central artifact is symmetric within each tissue section, is distributed uniformly across all sections regardless of anatomic location, and lacks the inflammatory response expected at the margins of true necrotic foci. The pattern is more prominent in tissues with high metabolic autolysis rates (liver, kidney, pancreas) and in animals with high antemortem body temperature (birds relative to reptiles).

Diagnostic Anchor: Recognition of the artifact on histopathology triggers review of the fixation history (tissue thickness at collection, fixative volume, delay to fixation). Confirmation is by re-examination of remaining fresh-frozen tissue if available, or by acceptance of the fixation limitation and appropriate interpretive caveat in the report.

Trap Logic: The look-alike is true multifocal hepatic or renal necrosis of infectious or toxicologic etiology. Discrimination: true multifocal necrosis demonstrates variable size and shape of necrotic foci across sections, inflammatory response at foci margins, and, in infectious causes, agents detectable by staining or molecular methods. Fixation artifact is uniformly symmetric, lacks inflammatory response, and lacks demonstrable agent.

Zoonotic/Reportable Flag: The fixation-artifact pattern is not itself infectious. Its recognition matters because misinterpretation as true multifocal necrosis may trigger inappropriate infectious disease workup, false reporting to regulatory authorities, or false institutional biosafety response.

Figure 3.1: Fixation Artifact Versus Multifocal Necrosis: Comparison at 10× Magnification

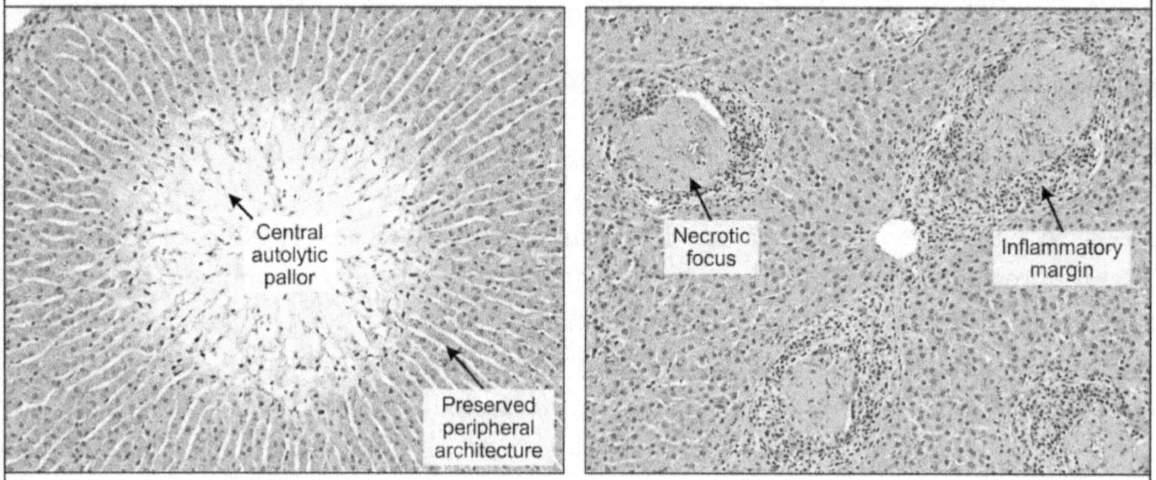

CAUTION: Tissue thickness at collection is the single most common determinant of fixation quality. Sections trimmed to 3 to 5 mm thickness fix reliably; sections trimmed to 10 mm or thicker will demonstrate central autolytic artifact regardless of fixative volume or fixation duration. Trim tissue at the necropsy bench, not at histology trim-in.

Ancillary Diagnostics: Cytology, Microbiology, Molecular, Toxicology

Cytology From Impression Smears and Aspirates

Cytology from postmortem impression smears and fine-needle aspirates provides rapid interpretive information that precedes histopathology by days to weeks and can direct ancillary sample submission on the same day as necropsy. Impression smears of cut surfaces of solid organs are made by gently touching a clean glass slide to the cut surface without smearing; the resulting monolayer preserves cellular morphology adequately for cytologic interpretation. Fine-needle aspirates of discrete masses or fluid collections provide cellular material that is smeared onto slides using standard cytology technique. Cytology preparations are air-dried, fixed briefly in methanol, and stained with Romanowsky-type stains (Diff-Quik, Wright, May-Grünwald-Giemsa) for routine interpretation. Cytology has interpretive limitations distinct from histopathology: architectural information is absent, and the population of cells sampled may not represent the whole lesion. Cytology adds value when it provides rapid direction rather than definitive diagnosis.

Microbiologic Culture and Special Stains

Microbiologic culture of fresh tissue is the reference standard for identification and characterization of bacterial pathogens. Aerobic and anaerobic bacterial culture require distinct transport and incubation conditions; the pathologist selects culture requests based on the anticipated differential rather than by reflex. Mycobacterial culture requires specialized media (Löwenstein-Jensen, Middlebrook 7H10) and prolonged incubation of up to 12 weeks; a suspicion of mycobacterial disease at necropsy is communicated to the microbiology laboratory before sample submission because standard bacterial workup does not detect mycobacterial growth. Mycologic culture uses Sabouraud dextrose agar and related media; identification of fungal isolates is by colony morphology, microscopy, and molecular methods. Special histopathologic stains (Gram, Grocott-Gomori methenamine silver, Ziehl-Neelsen, Warthin-Starry, Giemsa) demonstrate agents in tissue sections when culture is unavailable or unrewarding; special stains are ordered by the pathologist based on histopathologic differential rather than reflexively.

Molecular Diagnostics and Species-Specific Validation

Molecular diagnostics, primarily polymerase chain reaction and its variants, extend detection sensitivity below the histopathologic threshold and permit agent identification in cases where culture is impractical or unrewarding. The interpretive limitation in non-domestic species is species-specific validation: a polymerase chain reaction assay validated in one species may perform differently in another because primer target sequences may differ, host cellular background may differ, and internal controls may not amplify. The pathologist working an assay of unknown species-specific performance interprets the result with appropriate caveat: a positive result from a validated primer set on a well-preserved sample is interpretable; a negative result may reflect true absence or assay failure. Next-generation sequencing approaches, including metagenomic sequencing, are increasingly available for cases where the target agent is unknown; interpretive weight requires consideration of environmental contamination and of the bioinformatic pipeline used.

Toxicology and Species-Appropriate Sample Selection

Toxicology sample selection is driven by the anticipated toxicant class and by species-specific pharmacokinetics. Heavy metal analysis on liver and kidney is the workhorse test for lead, mercury, cadmium, and related metals; species-specific reference ranges are limited but comparative ranges permit interpretation. Anticoagulant rodenticide analysis requires whole blood or serum in most protocols; second-generation anticoagulant rodenticides are recognized by liver residue analysis. Organophosphate and carbamate pesticide analysis relies on cholinesterase activity measurement in brain or blood plasma, with characteristic dose-response depression permitting diagnosis. Organochlorine and persistent organic pollutant analysis requires adipose tissue in sufficient volume; the volume requirement often precludes analysis in small species. Marine biotoxin analysis on gastrointestinal contents identifies domoic acid, saxitoxin, and brevetoxin exposures in marine mammals and seabirds. Species-appropriate laboratory selection is critical because the receiving laboratory must have method validation appropriate to the species matrix being submitted.

Applied Case: Ancillary Sample Strategy for a Suspected Anticoagulant Rodenticide Case

A mature female bald eagle (Haliaeetus leucocephalus) was received for necropsy from a state wildlife rehabilitator who had recovered the bird alive four days earlier with severe lethargy, pale mucous membranes, and evidence of subcutaneous hemorrhage over the pectoral musculature. The bird had died in care despite supportive treatment. The submission form noted a suspected diagnosis of anticoagulant rodenticide toxicosis and requested toxicological workup. The eagle had been recovered near a residential-agricultural interface with documented rodenticide use in nearby structures. Federal protection under the Bald and Golden Eagle Protection Act triggered chain of custody initiation at case receipt with notification of the US Fish and Wildlife Service law enforcement agent for the region.

External examination confirmed the antemortem observations: pale mucous membranes, marked subcutaneous ecchymotic hemorrhage over the pectoral and axillary regions, and blood-tinged fluid in the cloaca. Body condition was fair, reflecting the four days of supportive care between capture and death. The plumage was intact. No traumatic external injuries were identified. Photographic documentation preceded the coelomic incision as required for chain-of-custody cases.

Coelomic necropsy demonstrated extensive hemorrhage in multiple anatomic compartments. Subcutaneous hemorrhage extended along the fascial planes of the pectoral musculature bilaterally. The coelomic cavity contained approximately 40 milliliters of unclotted blood mixed with clotted material at the periphery. The pericardium contained a moderate volume of unclotted blood. The lungs demonstrated multifocal hemorrhage on the parenchymal surface with continued oozing at cut surface. The liver was congested and appeared normal in size and color. The spleen was enlarged and dark. The gastrointestinal tract contained partially digested prey material and no gross evidence of dietary anticoagulant source. The renal parenchyma appeared unremarkable. The brain demonstrated no gross lesions.

The ancillary sample strategy was driven by the clinical differential and by regulatory requirements. Toxicology sampling was primary. Liver was collected fresh-frozen into a 50-milliliter cryotube for anticoagulant rodenticide residue analysis at a reference toxicology laboratory with validated methods for avian tissue matrix; the sample size exceeded the minimum required for both first-generation and second-generation anticoagulant screens. Whole blood was collected from the pericardial and coelomic hemorrhage into a lithium-heparin tube for parallel toxicological analysis, providing a secondary matrix that would confirm the liver residue interpretation. Kidney was collected fresh-frozen into a separate cryotube for heavy metal analysis given the possibility of lead exposure in a bird of prey feeding on shot mammal or bird carrion, a coincident cause of hemorrhage in raptors that must be excluded before an anticoagulant diagnosis is issued. Bone (femur) was collected for potential chronic lead exposure analysis if acute lead was not identified.

Histopathologic sampling followed the standard panel with attention to hemorrhage-affected tissues: liver, spleen, kidney, heart with pericardium, lung, brain, gastrointestinal tract at three levels, adrenal, and bone marrow from the femur. Formalin-fixed samples were placed into 10 percent neutral buffered formalin at greater than one-to-ten tissue-to-fixative ratio with tissue sections trimmed to 4 millimeter thickness at the necropsy bench. Microbiologic sampling was limited because the gross findings were consistent with a toxicological process and no exudate or abscessation warranted culture; a fresh-frozen liver and spleen were archived for potential downstream microbiologic testing if toxicology returned negative.

Chain of custody documentation captured every transfer. The initial receipt log recorded the specimen identification, submitting party, date and time of receipt, and receiving pathologist. Photographic documentation was retained in the case file. Each sample transferred from necropsy to storage was logged; each shipment to reference laboratory was logged with tracking number, receiving personnel signature, and shipping condition. The toxicology reference laboratory confirmed sample receipt and returned interim results within eight business days. Second-generation anticoagulant rodenticide residue in liver measured 0.42 micrograms per gram, above the threshold for clinically significant exposure; brodifacoum was the specific compound identified. Whole blood confirmed the finding. Kidney lead residue was below detection limit, excluding coincident lead exposure. The final morphologic diagnosis was multifocal internal hemorrhage secondary to brodifacoum-induced coagulopathy; the etiologic diagnosis was second-generation anticoagulant rodenticide toxicosis.

The case demonstrated the sample strategy principles articulated in the preceding subsections. Toxicology sample selection was matched to the anticipated compound class and to species-appropriate laboratory validation. Parallel-matrix collection (liver plus whole blood) provided confirmation. Coincident-cause exclusion (heavy metal analysis) prevented a diagnostic tunnel-vision error. Standard histopathology panel supported downstream interpretation regardless of the toxicology outcome. Chain of custody was maintained from receipt through disposition supporting the case's investigative use by federal law enforcement. The final report was distributed to the state wildlife health veterinarian, the US Fish and Wildlife Service law enforcement agent, and the submitting rehabilitator with distribution to the institutional pathology archive.

THE COMPARATIVE NECROPSY PATTERN SYSTEM — Systemic Inflammatory Response Pattern on Impression Smear Cytology

The Pattern: Cytologic evidence of degenerate neutrophils, karyorrhectic nuclear debris, and reactive lymphocyte populations on impression smears of multiple solid organs (liver, spleen, lymph node) taken at necropsy, indicating systemic inflammatory response before histopathology is available.

Cross-Taxa Signature: Recognized across mammalian, avian, and reptile taxa. The cytologic hallmarks — degenerate neutrophils with karyorrhexis, activated macrophage populations, reactive lymphocytes — are broadly comparable across taxonomic groups despite species-specific cell morphology differences. In birds, the equivalent of the mammalian neutrophil is the heterophil, which demonstrates characteristic degeneration with rod-shaped granule dissolution and karyorrhexis. In reptiles, the equivalent inflammatory cell populations demonstrate similar degenerative signatures under systemic inflammation. Recognition of the pattern on same-day cytology directs urgent microbiologic culture, molecular sampling, and biosafety escalation before histopathologic confirmation is available.

Diagnostic Anchor: Impression smear cytology of liver, spleen, and one or two lymph nodes at necropsy provides the same-day interpretive channel. Presence of degenerate inflammatory cells with bacterial rods or cocci visible on cytology is diagnostic anchor for bacterial septicemia and triggers appropriate downstream workup and biosafety response.

Trap Logic: The look-alike is postmortem cytologic degeneration of tissue-resident inflammatory cells in a carcass with prolonged postmortem interval, which produces cellular degenerative appearance without antemortem systemic disease. Discrimination: postmortem degenerative change affects all cell populations symmetrically and lacks the reactive lymphocyte population that accompanies true antemortem inflammation. Presence of extracellular bacterial rods in a carcass with prolonged postmortem interval reflects postmortem bacterial overgrowth rather than antemortem septicemia and must be interpreted accordingly.

Zoonotic/Reportable Flag: Cytologic identification of systemic inflammatory response with visible bacterial rods triggers biosafety escalation for the remainder of the necropsy. Confirmation of specific agent (Bacillus anthracis, Francisella tularensis, Yersinia pestis, Brucella species) may require immediate regulatory notification depending on the identified organism.

Biosafety and Personal Protective Equipment for Non-Domestic Species Necropsy

Biosafety Level Assignment at Case Receipt

Biosafety level assignment for a wildlife or zoo case begins at case receipt, before the carcass is placed on the necropsy table. The submission history, species, geographic origin, and clinical presentation together permit initial assessment of the anticipated pathogen risk. Cases without specific risk indicators are managed at Biosafety Level 2 practices, which is the routine baseline for veterinary diagnostic necropsy. Cases with specific risk indicators — a psittacine received during an active regional highly pathogenic avian influenza outbreak, a wild carnivore with neurologic clinical signs, a nonhuman primate of unknown health history, a bat submitted for rabies testing — are escalated to Biosafety Level 3 practices. Cases with potential exposure to select agents (Bacillus anthracis, Francisella tularensis, Yersinia pestis, viral hemorrhagic fever agents) require Biosafety Level 3 or higher and coordination with institutional biosafety and public health authorities. Biosafety Level 4 pathogens (Marburg, Ebola, Nipah, Hendra) are not necropsied outside of specifically designated high-containment facilities.

Personal Protective Equipment Selection and Use

Personal protective equipment for non-domestic species necropsy varies by biosafety level and by anticipated pathogen exposure route. Baseline BSL-2 practice includes dedicated laboratory coat, disposable outer gown, cut-resistant gloves under nitrile examination gloves, eye protection or face shield, and closed-toe footwear. BSL-3 practice adds N95 or higher respiratory protection, powered air-purifying respirator for cases with high aerosol generation potential, disposable coveralls, and containment technique that minimizes aerosol generation during dissection. Sharps management is a nontrivial component of biosafety practice: scalpel blades are removed with forceps rather than by hand, cut-resistant gloves are worn beneath examination gloves at all times, and sharps disposal containers are within immediate reach of the necropsy table. Aerosol-generating steps (bone cutting, high-pressure water rinsing, opening pressurized cavities) are performed with additional respiratory protection and, where feasible, within downdraft or Class I biological safety cabinet containment.

Hard-Stop Zoonotic Recognition

Certain zoonotic patterns require immediate cessation of the necropsy pending biosafety consultation. Herpes B disease in a macaque (mucocutaneous vesicles, oral ulceration, or a macaque of unknown health history) is a hard-stop because human infection has a substantial fatal encephalitis probability. Rabies suspect in a carnivore or bat (behavioral abnormalities antemortem, prolonged prodromal illness) triggers hard-stop because unprotected exposure carries prophylaxis requirements. Anthrax suspect in an ungulate (peracute death, splenomegaly, dark unclotted blood from natural orifices) triggers hard-stop because spore aerosolization risk is high and the carcass should not be opened. Highly pathogenic avian influenza suspect in an exposed mammal during an active regional outbreak triggers biosafety escalation before continued dissection. The pathologist's obligation is to recognize the pattern from initial gross observation and to escalate before continuing rather than to complete the necropsy and manage the exposure retrospectively.

THE COMPARATIVE NECROPSY PATTERN SYSTEM — Zoonotic-Signature Pattern at Necropsy Case Receipt

---

The Pattern: Recognition of a species-and-signal combination at case receipt that triggers biosafety escalation before the necropsy begins.

Cross-Taxa Signature: The recurring signatures cross taxa but cluster by species and epidemiologic context. In macaques: any submission with mucocutaneous vesicles or oral ulceration, or of unknown health history, is treated as herpes B suspect. In wild or unknown-health-history carnivores: neurologic clinical signs are treated as rabies suspect. In ungulates found dead in warm season with splenomegaly and dark unclotted blood: anthrax suspect. In mammalian carnivores or mustelids received during active regional highly pathogenic avian influenza outbreak: HPAI spillover suspect. In bats: any bat submitted for necropsy is treated as rabies suspect regardless of clinical history.

Diagnostic Anchor: The anchor is the pattern of recognition itself and the associated protocol activation. Escalation to appropriate biosafety level, notification of institutional biosafety officer, coordination with public health authorities where applicable, and modification of the necropsy plan to minimize aerosol generation and personnel exposure precede continued dissection.

Trap Logic: The look-alike is a case that lacks obvious risk signals at receipt but harbors a zoonotic agent revealed during dissection. Discrimination: the biosafety-conservative default of BSL-2 practice on every wildlife case, with escalation triggered by any risk signal discovered during dissection, mitigates the risk. A case without initial risk indicators can be escalated mid-necropsy if findings warrant.

Zoonotic/Reportable Flag: Hard-stop conditions include herpes B in macaques, rabies in carnivores and bats, anthrax in ungulates, and HPAI in spillover-suspect mammals. Each triggers specific reporting pathway to institutional biosafety, state or federal animal health authority, and, in humans-exposed cases, occupational health and public health authorities.

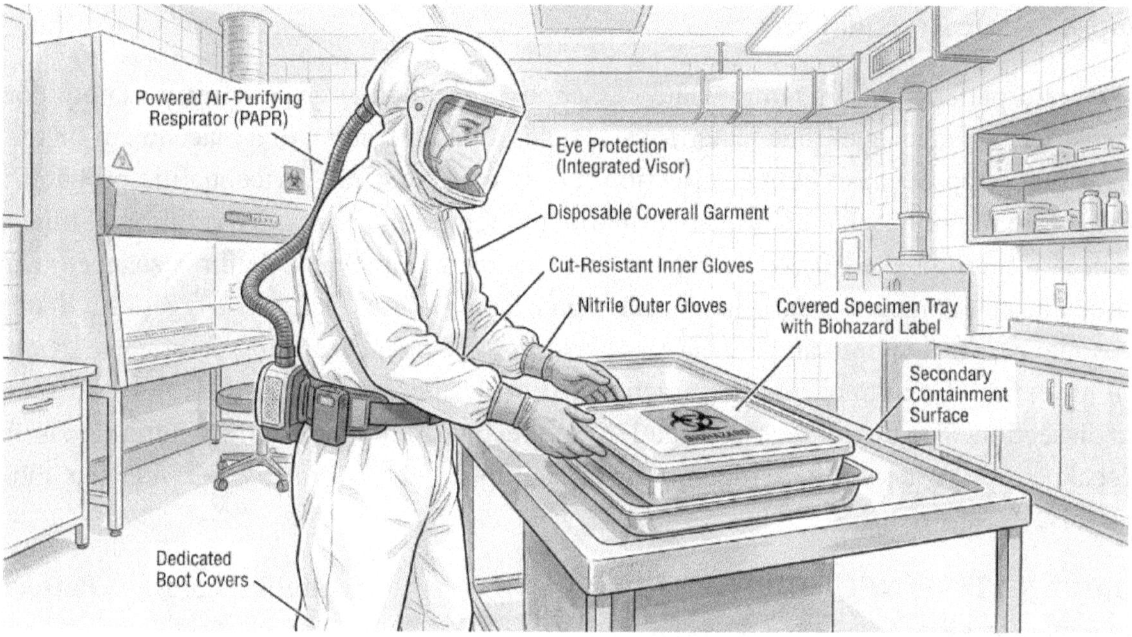

Regulatory Sample Submission and Chain of Custody

Regulatory Reporting Pathways for Wildlife Cases

Regulatory reporting pathways for wildlife cases follow jurisdiction-specific requirements that must be known before a case with reportable-disease potential is opened. Federally reportable diseases in the United States include highly pathogenic avian influenza, foot-and-mouth disease, chronic wasting disease, bovine tuberculosis, brucellosis, and several others, with pathways coordinated through USDA APHIS Veterinary Services. State-reportable diseases vary by jurisdiction; the state animal health official and the state wildlife health veterinarian are the appropriate contacts. Marine mammal cases with unusual mortality event potential require coordination with NOAA Fisheries Marine Mammal Health and Stranding Response Program. Federally protected species (bald and golden eagles, migratory birds, endangered species) with unusual mortality require US Fish and Wildlife Service notification. Institutional reporting at accredited zoos follows Association of Zoos and Aquariums protocols and Species Survival Plan coordinator communication.

Sample Preparation for Reference Laboratory Submission

Sample preparation for reference laboratory submission follows the receiving laboratory's specific requirements and forms. Sample identification with unique case number, species, tissue type, preservative, and collection date is a minimum standard; some laboratories require additional fields including submitting pathologist contact information, purpose of testing, and expected turnaround. Sample volume must meet the receiving laboratory's requirements as noted; a submission with inadequate volume may not be flagged until weeks later. Shipping method depends on sample type: formalin-fixed tissue in leak-proof containers with UN 3373 or Category A packaging as appropriate; fresh-frozen tissue in dry-ice shipments with UN 1845 classification; microbiologic samples in appropriate transport media. Submission timing considers laboratory hours, holidays, and weekend receipt to avoid samples sitting on loading docks. Communication with the reference laboratory before submission is a standard step for non-routine cases; the laboratory may adjust processing protocols based on the anticipated diagnostic question.

Chain of Custody in Investigative Cases

Chain of custody in investigative cases documents the movement and control of the specimen from receipt through disposition, and is required when the case may enter legal or law-enforcement proceedings. The chain-of-custody record begins at case receipt with documented identification, timestamp, and receiving personnel. Every subsequent transfer of physical control of the specimen — from receipt to necropsy, from necropsy to storage, from storage to shipping to reference laboratory, from reference laboratory to disposition — is documented with timestamp, transferring personnel, and receiving personnel. The specimen is stored in secured containment (locked freezer or refrigerator with limited access) throughout. Sample archives from investigative cases are held indefinitely pending resolution of the underlying investigation; premature disposal of tissue from an investigative case may compromise prosecution. Communication with the coordinating law-enforcement agency (US Fish and Wildlife Service Office of Law Enforcement, NOAA Fisheries Office of Law Enforcement, state wildlife agency law enforcement) is initiated at case receipt and continues through case closure.

Documentation Standards for Institutional Records

Documentation standards for institutional records extend beyond individual case reports to include archival storage of gross photographs, histopathologic slides, wet tissue archives, and paraffin blocks. Standards vary by institution but generally require retention of paraffin blocks for at least 10 years, of slides for at least 10 years, and of gross photographs for the same interval; regulatory-relevant cases and investigative cases are retained indefinitely. Digital archiving of gross photographs, slide scans, and case reports supports downstream research, teaching, and reference. The pathologist working in a zoo or wildlife context is a source of longitudinal population-level pathology data; well-organized institutional archives permit retrospective analysis of population trends, unusual mortality event characterization, and reference for future case interpretation.

THE COMPARATIVE NECROPSY PATTERN SYSTEM — Chain-of-Custody Documentation Pattern for Investigative Wildlife Cases

---

The Pattern: A standardized documentation trail from case receipt through disposition that establishes control of the specimen and supports downstream investigative use of pathology findings.

Cross-Taxa Signature: The documentation requirements apply across taxa but the specific investigative context varies. Federally protected raptor mortality (bald eagle, golden eagle) commonly enters US Fish and Wildlife Service investigative proceedings and requires coordinated chain of custody. Marine mammal mortality of federally protected species enters NOAA Fisheries proceedings. Endangered species mortality requires Endangered Species Act-associated documentation. Livestock-wildlife interface cases (bovine tuberculosis in cervids, brucellosis in ungulates) may enter USDA APHIS investigative proceedings. The pattern of documentation is consistent; the specific coordinating agency depends on the affected species.

Diagnostic Anchor: The anchor is documented control at every transfer point. A case with intact chain of custody supports downstream investigative use; a case with a documented gap in chain of custody may be excluded from proceedings.

Trap Logic: The look-alike is a case that appeared routine at receipt but became investigative during workup, with chain of custody not initiated at receipt. Discrimination: the biosafety-conservative default of chain-of-custody initiation on any case with federally protected species status, unusual mortality potential, or suspicious circumstances mitigates the risk. Retrospective chain-of-custody construction is possible but reduces the interpretive weight the documentation carries.

Zoonotic/Reportable Flag: Investigative cases involving federally protected species (Migratory Bird Treaty Act, Bald and Golden Eagle Protection Act, Marine Mammal Protection Act, Endangered Species Act) require coordination with federal law enforcement. Chain of custody is initiated at receipt and maintained through case closure regardless of the pathology findings.

Figure 3.3: Systemic Inflammatory Response on Impression Smear: Splenic Cytology from Suspected Septicemia.

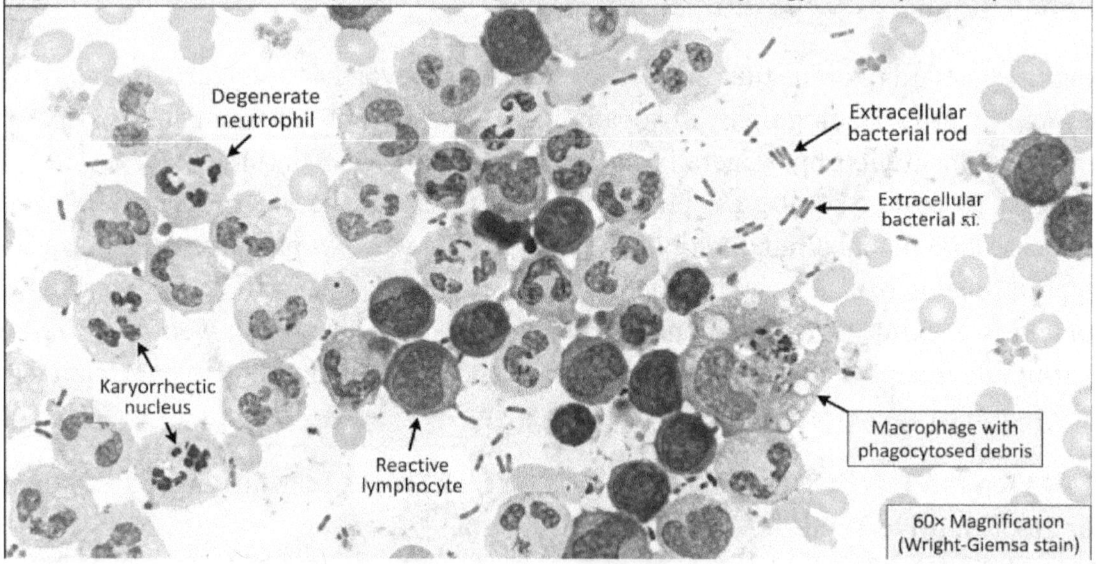

Ancillary Test Category	Sample Type Required	Preservation Method	Species-Specific Consideration	Common Interpretive Pitfall
Aerobic bacterial culture	Fresh sterile tissue or swab in transport medium	Refrigeration; ship within 24 hours	Species-specific normal flora affects contamination assessment	Postmortem bacterial overgrowth misinterpreted as antemortem infection

Mycobacterial culture	Fresh tissue or lymph node in sterile container	Refrigeration; specialty laboratory notification required	Prolonged incubation (up to 12 weeks) required	Standard bacterial culture will not detect mycobacterial growth
Polymerase chain reaction	Fresh-frozen tissue or FFPE tissue	Negative 80 or negative 20 Celsius; RNAlater as alternative	Species-specific primer validation may not exist	Negative result may reflect assay failure rather than agent absence
Heavy metal analysis	Liver, kidney, or bone in metal-free container	Refrigeration or freezing; avoid metal instruments	Species-specific reference ranges limited	Comparative reference required for interpretation
Anticoagulant rodenticide	Liver in cryotube	Freezing at negative 20 or lower	Second-generation compounds recognized in liver residue	Whole blood alternative for acute cases
Cholinesterase activity	Brain or whole blood in cryotube	Frozen shipment	Species-specific baseline activity varies	Chilled specimens preferred over refrigeration for shorter transit
Viral isolation	Fresh-frozen tissue in cryotube	Negative 80 Celsius; liquid nitrogen if long transit	Species-specific cell line availability varies	Freeze-thaw cycles compromise viral viability
Marine biotoxin analysis	Gastrointestinal contents in cryotube	Frozen shipment	Domoic acid, saxitoxin, brevetoxin panels selected by clinical context	Volume requirements may exceed small-species sample capacity

CLINICAL PEARL: The most common reason for uninterpretable ancillary test results is inadequate sample quality at collection. The pathologist who spends 30 seconds ensuring appropriate tissue thickness, fresh-frozen collection into an appropriate container, and sterile technique at collection prevents weeks of downstream troubleshooting when the assay result is compromised.

EVIDENCE: Species-specific validation of molecular diagnostic assays is limited across non-domestic species. Assay performance data from the receiving reference laboratory should be requested before interpretive weight is assigned to a novel result, and interpretive comments in the report should acknowledge the validation status of the assay in the species.

THE COMPARATIVE NECROPSY PATTERN SYSTEM — Chapter 3 Specimen Handling Patterns

Fixation-Artifact Pattern Masking Multifocal Necrosis: Central autolytic change with symmetric peripheral preservation on histopathology, mimicking multifocal necrosis. Anchor: recognition of the artifact pattern with fixation history review. Trap: true multifocal necrosis discriminated by variable focus size and inflammatory response. Flag: misinterpretation may trigger inappropriate infectious disease workup and false reporting.

Systemic Inflammatory Response Pattern on Impression Smear Cytology: Degenerate inflammatory cells and reactive lymphocytes on organ impression smears indicating systemic inflammation before histopathology. Anchor: same-day cytology directing microbiologic and molecular workup. Trap: postmortem cytologic degeneration discriminated by symmetric change without reactive lymphocyte population. Flag: cytologic bacterial rods trigger biosafety escalation.

Zoonotic-Signature Pattern at Necropsy Case Receipt: Species-and-signal combinations requiring biosafety escalation before necropsy begins (macaque with vesicles, carnivore with neurologic signs, ungulate with peracute death and splenomegaly, HPAI-exposed mammal). Anchor: pattern-of-recognition with protocol activation. Trap: case without initial risk signals discovered mid-necropsy discriminated by escalation trigger built into workflow. Flag: hard-stop conditions require reporting to biosafety, animal health, and public health authorities.

Chain-of-Custody Documentation Pattern for Investigative Wildlife Cases: Standardized documentation trail from receipt through disposition supporting downstream investigative use. Anchor: documented control at every transfer point. Trap: retrospective chain-of-custody construction discriminated by intact original documentation. Flag: federally protected species and unusual mortality events require federal law enforcement coordination.

Summary and Key Concepts

Formalin fixation at appropriate tissue-to-fixative ratio and tissue thickness is the reference standard for histopathologic preservation; fixation artifact from inadequate fixation mimics multifocal necrosis on histopathology and is a recurring source of diagnostic error.

Fresh tissue preservation for viral isolation, molecular diagnostics, and toxicology requires appropriate cold-chain management; freeze-thaw cycles compromise nucleic acid integrity and viral viability, and aliquoting at time of freezing prevents downstream sample loss.

Ancillary diagnostics across cytology, microbiology, molecular, and toxicology categories are selected based on anticipated differential and species-specific assay validation; a poorly designed panel wastes fresh tissue and produces uninterpretable results.

Biosafety level assignment begins at case receipt and escalates based on species-and-signal combinations; hard-stop zoonotic patterns (herpes B in macaques, rabies in carnivores and bats, anthrax in ungulates, HPAI in spillover-suspect mammals) require immediate cessation and biosafety consultation.

Regulatory reporting pathways for wildlife cases follow jurisdiction-specific requirements coordinated through USDA APHIS, state animal health and wildlife health authorities, NOAA Fisheries, US Fish and Wildlife Service, and institutional biosafety programs.

Chain of custody in investigative cases is initiated at receipt on any case with federally protected species status, unusual mortality potential, or suspicious circumstances, and maintained through case closure with coordination with federal law enforcement partners.

CHAPTER 4: CARDIOVASCULAR PATHOLOGY ACROSS TAXA

Learning Objectives

1. Interpret comparative cardiac anatomic variation across mammals, birds, reptiles, amphibians, and fish as it modifies lesion interpretation.
2. Recognize the major cardiomyopathy patterns in non-domestic species and their species-specific predispositions.
3. Identify vascular disease patterns including mineralization, atherosclerosis, and vasculitis across taxa.
4. Interpret pericardial and endocardial pathology in the context of infectious, degenerative, and neoplastic differentials.
5. Apply the Comparative Necropsy Pattern callout structure to cardiovascular lesion recognition across unfamiliar species.
6. Coordinate ancillary cardiac testing including cardiac biomarker analysis and cardiac molecular diagnostics in wildlife and zoo cases.

Cardiovascular pathology in wildlife and zoo species requires the pathologist to hold comparative anatomic knowledge in mind before applying pathologic reasoning. The four-chambered mammalian heart is one solution among several that vertebrate evolution has produced, and lesion interpretation depends first on recognizing which anatomic frame the species belongs to. A three-chambered heart in a snake is not diseased because it lacks complete ventricular septation; a two-chambered heart in a teleost fish is anatomically correct; a partially septated ventricle in a crocodilian reflects lineage-specific anatomy rather than pathology. Once the anatomic frame is recognized, the pathologic interpretation is transportable: the cardiomyopathies, vascular diseases, and pericardial diseases that affect mammals also affect other vertebrate classes, with species-specific etiologic profiles and species-specific gross and histopathologic manifestations.

This chapter organizes cardiovascular pathology into four operational domains. Comparative cardiac anatomy provides the interpretive frame within which lesions are read. Cardiomyopathies are considered by primary pathologic process rather than by taxonomic origin because the underlying mechanisms of dilated, hypertrophic, restrictive, and arrhythmogenic cardiomyopathy have taxonomic distributions that recur across evolutionary distance. Vascular disease across taxa addresses the disorders of large vessels, medium and small vessels, and microvasculature, with attention to the mineralization, atherosclerotic, and vasculitic patterns that recur in non-domestic species. Pericardial and endocardial pathology completes the cardiovascular chapter with attention to infectious, degenerative, and neoplastic pericardial and endocardial disease across taxa.

Comparative Cardiac Anatomy Relevant to Pathology

The Mammalian Four-Chambered Heart and Species-Specific Variation

The mammalian four-chambered heart is the anatomic reference against which the pathologist trained in domestic species reads cardiac lesions. Two atria and two ventricles are separated by complete septation; systemic and pulmonary circulations are functionally isolated. Species-specific variation exists within the mammalian frame: relative ventricular wall thickness differs across species based on the pressure workload each ventricle sustains, and the ratio of left to right ventricular wall thickness varies more than is often appreciated. In cetaceans and pinnipeds, the right ventricular wall is proportionately thicker than in terrestrial mammals because of the demands of diving physiology on the pulmonary circulation. In ratite birds and megaherbivores, the left ventricular wall is proportionately thicker because of the pressure workload of sustaining perfusion at high body mass. Aortic and pulmonary outflow tract anatomy varies across mammals in specific and interpretable ways; the pathologist working an unfamiliar mammalian species considers comparative reference to closely related domestic species when interpreting the outflow tracts.

Avian Cardiac Anatomy and Species-Specific Interpretation

Avian cardiac anatomy resembles mammalian anatomy in the four-chambered plan but differs in several interpretively important ways. The right atrioventricular valve is a single muscular flap rather than a leaflet system, and disease processes that produce leaflet degeneration in mammals present differently in birds. The pulmonary arterial system connects to a countercurrent bronchial vascular arrangement that supports the avian air sac respiratory physiology; disease processes involving the pulmonary vasculature must be interpreted with this arrangement in mind. Avian cardiac reserve and cardiac response to stress differ from mammalian reserve; captive avian species are prone to acute cardiac decompensation under handling or capture stress, and terminal event cardiac lesions in birds must be interpreted in the context of any recent handling.

Reptile and Amphibian Cardiac Anatomy

Reptile cardiac anatomy varies substantially across lineages. Chelonians, squamates, and most non-crocodilian reptiles have a functionally three-chambered heart with two atria and a single ventricle that is partially subdivided by intraventricular structures (the muscular ridge in chelonians, the vertical septum in varanids and pythons). Crocodilians have a complete ventricular septation and a four-chambered heart with a specialized foramen of Panizza connecting the aortae. Amphibians have a three-chambered heart with an incompletely septated bulbus arteriosus. In each lineage, the anatomic arrangement is a normal adaptation to physiologic function; lesion interpretation requires the pathologist to know the species-appropriate anatomic frame before assessing whether an observed structure is diseased. Failure to recognize the intraventricular muscular ridge in chelonians as a normal anatomic structure has produced misinterpretation as ventricular mass in the historic pathology literature.

Fish Cardiac Anatomy

Teleost cardiac anatomy is a two-chambered arrangement with a single atrium and single ventricle serving the systemic circulation through a muscular bulbus arteriosus. The gills provide oxygenation between the ventricular outflow and the systemic circulation. Elasmobranchs have similar single-atrium single-ventricle anatomy with a muscular conus arteriosus. In both groups, the ventricular wall consists of a compact outer layer and a spongy inner layer with variable proportions across species. Species with high-performance swimming (tunas, sharks with active predation strategies) have thicker compact ventricular walls relative to species with lower activity. Cardiac disease in teleosts and elasmobranchs is interpreted against this two-chambered frame; assessment of ventricular wall structure requires species-appropriate reference.

Cardiac Reserve and Physiologic Response to Stress Across Taxa

Cardiac reserve — the capacity of the heart to increase output above baseline in response to physiologic demand — varies across taxa in ways that modify lesion interpretation. Endothermic species maintain higher baseline cardiac output than ectothermic species and demonstrate correspondingly higher metabolic reserve; the mammalian and avian heart operates at higher baseline heart rate and stroke volume than the reptilian heart, and the acute cardiovascular response to stress produces different physiologic and histopathologic consequences. Capture-related cardiac injury is a documented phenomenon in wildlife species handled for management or research; the histopathologic hallmark is myofiber contraction band necrosis, most prominent in the left ventricular free wall, produced by catecholamine-induced coronary vasospasm and myocardial ischemia during peak sympathetic activation. The lesion pattern is recognized across ungulates, carnivores, primates, and some avian species subjected to capture stress. Terminal event capture myopathy findings must be distinguished from primary myocardial disease when interpreting cardiac lesions in a recently captured animal.

Cardiac Biomarkers in Non-Domestic Species Diagnosis

Cardiac troponin I and cardiac troponin T are conserved across vertebrate classes and provide interpretive information when cross-reactive assays are used on postmortem or perimortem serum samples. Elevated cardiac troponin in a serum or pericardial fluid sample from a non-domestic species case supports a diagnosis of acute myocardial injury regardless of specific etiology and complements the histopathologic assessment. Species-specific reference ranges for cardiac troponin are limited but the direction and magnitude of elevation are interpretable across taxa. Natriuretic peptides (BNP, NT-proBNP) similarly have cross-reactive assays available and provide information about chronic myocardial stretch and dysfunction. Cardiac biomarker collection at necropsy from pericardial fluid or perimortem serum is a standard step in cardiac cases and provides same-day interpretive direction before histopathology is available.

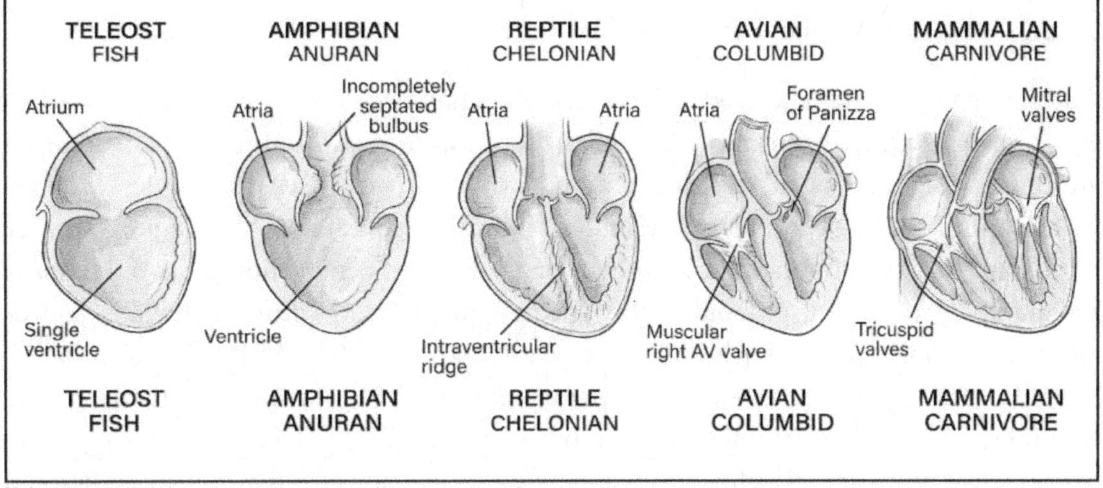

Figure 4.1: Comparative Vertebrate Cardiac Anatomy: Chamber Arrangement Across Five Taxonomic Groups.

THE COMPARATIVE NECROPSY PATTERN SYSTEM — Ventricular Wall Thickness Pattern Recognition Across Endothermic and Ectothermic Taxa

---

The Pattern: Interpretation of ventricular wall thickness relative to species-appropriate reference, distinguishing physiologic hypertrophy from pathologic hypertrophy, and physiologic thinness from pathologic dilation.

Cross-Taxa Signature: Ventricular wall thickness reference varies across taxa but the interpretive principle is transportable. In mammals, left ventricular wall thickness proportionate to right is expected; asymmetric thickening suggests pathologic hypertrophy secondary to systemic hypertension, valvular disease, or infiltrative process. In birds, the same principle applies with species-specific reference thickness data limited. In reptiles, the intraventricular muscular arrangements must be recognized as normal before wall thickness is assessed. In fish, compact-versus-spongy layer proportion is the species-appropriate assessment rather than absolute wall thickness.

Diagnostic Anchor: Comparative reference to closest available taxonomic relative with published wall thickness data, combined with clinical context (age, body condition, terminal event), constitutes the anchor for interpretation. Explicit acknowledgment of extrapolation is included in the report.

Trap Logic: The look-alike is normal species-specific variation misinterpreted as pathology. Chelonian intraventricular muscular ridge misread as ventricular mass, cetacean right ventricular thickness misread as pulmonary hypertension, and reptile species-specific ventricular arrangement misread as ventricular septal defect are the recurring errors. Discrimination: species-specific anatomic reference must be established before pathologic interpretation is applied.

Zoonotic/Reportable Flag: Cardiac anatomic variation is not itself infectious or reportable. Recognition matters because misinterpretation may propagate through case reports and populate downstream reference material with anatomically incorrect claims.

Cardiomyopathies in Non-Domestic Species

Dilated Cardiomyopathy Across Taxa

Dilated cardiomyopathy is characterized by biventricular chamber dilation with thinned ventricular walls, reduced myocardial contractility, and progressive congestive heart failure. In non-domestic species, dilated cardiomyopathy has been documented in nonhuman primates (particularly captive gorillas, orangutans, and chimpanzees), in captive felids (including large cats such as jaguars and cheetahs), in psittacines, in some captive ungulates, and in cetaceans. The gross morphology is remarkably consistent across taxa: markedly enlarged, globoid, flabby heart with thinned ventricular walls and dilated atria. Histopathology demonstrates myocardial fiber attenuation, interstitial fibrosis, and occasional lymphocytic infiltrate in cases with an inflammatory etiology. Etiologies include taurine deficiency in some captive felids (where dietary reformulation has substantially reduced incidence), genetic factors in nonhuman primates (with lineage clustering documented in captive great ape populations), and viral myocarditis progression in other species.

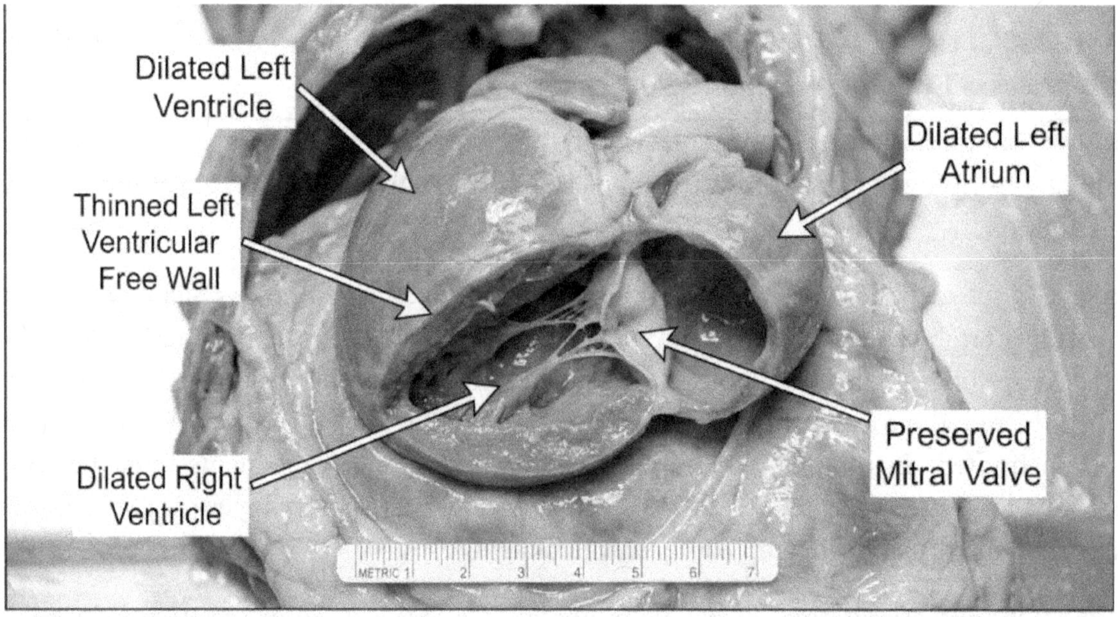

Figure 4.2: Dilated Cardiomyopathy in a Captive Jaguar: Gross Morphology at Necropsy.

Hypertrophic Cardiomyopathy

Hypertrophic cardiomyopathy is characterized by asymmetric or concentric ventricular wall thickening without an identified pressure-load explanation, producing diastolic dysfunction and progressive myocardial disease. In captive felids, hypertrophic cardiomyopathy has been documented across multiple genera and represents an important cause of morbidity and mortality in captive large cats. The lesion pattern includes left ventricular concentric hypertrophy, papillary muscle hypertrophy, and characteristic left atrial dilation secondary to diastolic dysfunction. Histopathologic hallmarks include myocardial fiber disarray, interstitial fibrosis, and occasional intramural coronary vessel wall thickening. The lesion pattern is transportable across taxa; a young or middle-aged captive felid with concentric ventricular hypertrophy without a systemic hypertension explanation, without renal disease, and without evidence of infiltrative process demonstrates hypertrophic cardiomyopathy until an alternative explanation is identified.

Restrictive and Arrhythmogenic Cardiomyopathies

Restrictive cardiomyopathy is characterized by ventricular walls of normal thickness with markedly restricted diastolic filling secondary to infiltrative or fibrotic myocardial disease. The lesion pattern includes marked biatrial dilation with relatively preserved ventricular chamber size and wall thickness. Histopathology demonstrates the infiltrative or fibrotic process responsible: amyloidosis, hemochromatosis-associated myocardial iron deposition, or endomyocardial fibrosis. Restrictive cardiomyopathy has been documented in captive nonhuman primates and in cetaceans. Arrhythmogenic cardiomyopathy is characterized by fibrofatty replacement of ventricular myocardium, most prominently the right ventricular free wall, producing arrhythmia-mediated sudden death. Documented in domestic species with a growing literature in non-domestic species, arrhythmogenic cardiomyopathy is recognized by histopathologic demonstration of fibrofatty replacement in a distribution consistent with the disease process.

Applied Case: Hypertrophic Cardiomyopathy in a Captive Snow Leopard

A 12-year-old female snow leopard (Panthera uncia), part of a Species Survival Plan managed collection, was found deceased in her habitat in the early morning. Antemortem history included two brief syncopal episodes over the preceding three months, mild but progressive weight loss over the preceding year, and reduced activity relative to conspecific individuals in the collection. Antemortem cardiac assessment had been limited because the animal did not consistently accept the transport crate required for radiographic or echocardiographic imaging; a single planned imaging session had been cancelled six weeks before death after the animal declined to enter the transport crate. The collection veterinarian's differential at last recorded assessment included primary cardiac disease, chronic renal disease with cardiovascular consequence, and endocrinopathy.

Necropsy was performed within four hours of discovery. External examination confirmed the antemortem observation of thin body condition; the coat was in appropriate seasonal condition and no external trauma was identified. Coelomic examination demonstrated no ascitic fluid and no gross evidence of hepatic congestion. Thoracic examination demonstrated a moderately enlarged cardiac silhouette with the heart occupying an increased proportion of the thoracic cavity. Pericardial fluid volume was mildly increased at approximately 25 milliliters of clear straw-colored fluid. Cytology of the pericardial fluid was submitted at necropsy and returned a low-cellularity transudate with rare mesothelial cells and no inflammatory cell infiltrate.

The heart weighed 340 grams, which was moderately elevated for the animal's body weight when compared with published felid reference data corrected for body size. Gross examination of the heart demonstrated concentric left ventricular wall thickening with the left ventricular free wall measuring 22 millimeters and the interventricular septum measuring 19 millimeters at the mid-ventricular level. The left atrium was markedly dilated with the atrial appendage extending well beyond expected anatomic position.

The papillary muscles were prominently hypertrophied and encroached on the ventricular chamber. The mitral and tricuspid valves demonstrated no gross vegetations, thickening, or perforations. The great vessels were unremarkable. The coronary arteries were grossly patent. The right ventricular wall was of appropriate thickness relative to the left. No regional wall thinning suggesting ischemic cardiomyopathy was identified.

Same-day cytology of an impression smear from the cut surface of the left ventricular free wall was uninformative for a specific etiology but demonstrated cardiomyocytes without prominent inflammatory infiltrate, consistent with a chronic non-inflammatory cardiomyopathy. Cardiac troponin I on perimortem serum was substantially elevated at a concentration exceeding the reference range extrapolated from domestic felid data by more than tenfold, supporting acute myocardial injury as part of the terminal event. Same-day interpretive impression was primary hypertrophic cardiomyopathy with acute terminal event; alternative differentials included concentric hypertrophy secondary to systemic hypertension (excluded by absent renal or vascular pathology on gross examination), infiltrative cardiomyopathy (unlikely given the concentric hypertrophic morphology), and hypertrophic response to chronic outflow obstruction (excluded by absent outflow tract pathology).

Histopathology confirmed the gross impression. Multiple ventricular myocardial sections demonstrated pronounced myocardial fiber disarray with cardiomyocytes oriented in short, disorganized arrays rather than the parallel arrangement of normal myocardium. Interstitial fibrosis was moderate to marked and highlighted by Masson trichrome stain. Small intramural coronary arteries demonstrated medial wall thickening consistent with the small-vessel disease documented in hypertrophic cardiomyopathy. No inflammatory infiltrate, no viral inclusion bodies, and no infiltrative process (amyloid, iron) were identified. The final morphologic diagnosis was severe left ventricular concentric hypertrophy with prominent myocardial fiber disarray, marked interstitial fibrosis, and small intramural coronary arteriopathy consistent with hypertrophic cardiomyopathy.

Ancillary molecular workup was undertaken given the SSP relevance of the case. Fresh-frozen ventricular myocardium was submitted to a reference laboratory with validated methodologies for sequencing the sarcomeric protein genes known to harbor hypertrophic cardiomyopathy-associated variants in domestic and non-domestic felids. Results returned an MYBPC3 gene variant identified in the animal's genome; the variant had been documented in one prior captive snow leopard from an unrelated collection with hypertrophic cardiomyopathy. The finding supported a genetic contribution to the phenotype and had implications for management of the collection's ongoing breeding program.

The institutional report was structured as gross findings, histopathologic findings, ancillary results, morphologic and etiologic diagnoses, and interpretive comments. Distribution included the collection veterinarian, the SSP coordinator for snow leopards, the collection director, and the pathology archive. The SSP coordinator communicated the finding to participating institutions with breeding-relevant animals from related lineages; genetic screening was discussed as a management tool for the population. The case illustrated cardiovascular pathology's translational function at the population level: an individual necropsy finding shaped population-level management decisions across multiple institutions through the

SSP structure. Comparative reasoning drove the case throughout: the gross hypertrophic pattern was recognized against domestic felid HCM reference; the histopathologic hallmarks of fiber disarray, interstitial fibrosis, and small-vessel disease were transportable across felid species; the molecular genetic assay was interpretable in the snow leopard because the sarcomeric protein genes are conserved across felid lineages. Species-specific extrapolation was flagged explicitly in the report because reference thresholds for cardiac troponin and for heart weight normalization in snow leopards had been derived from comparative felid data rather than snow-leopard-specific reference.

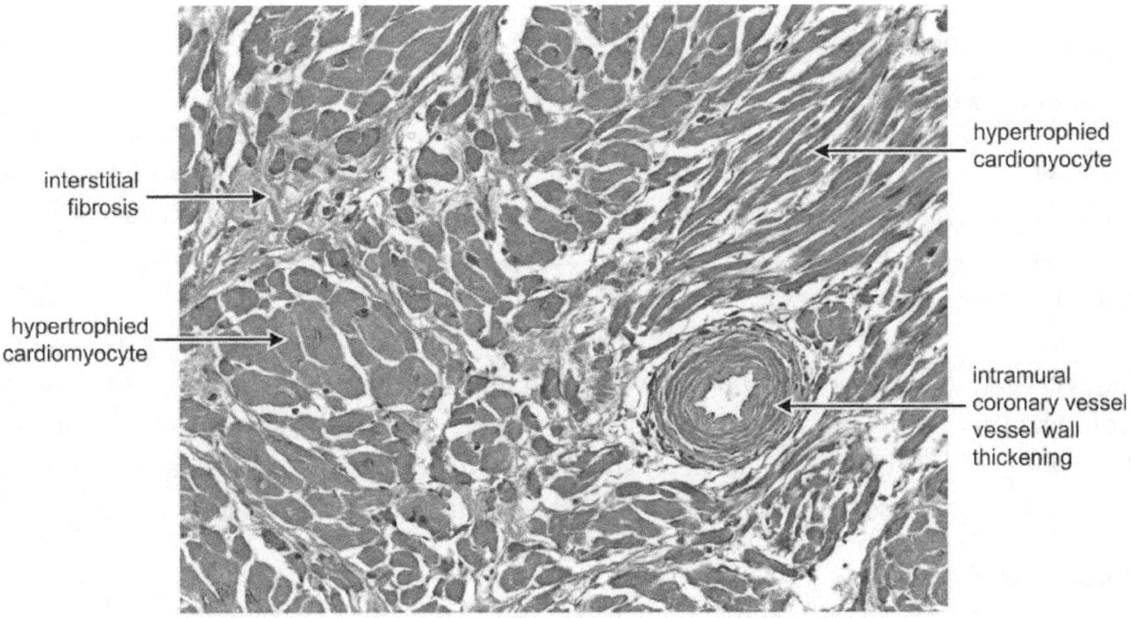

Figure 4.3. Myocardial fibrosis in hypertrophic cardiomyopathy in ventricular myocardium of a captive large felid. (10×).

THE COMPARATIVE NECROPSY PATTERN SYSTEM — Dilated Cardiomyopathy Pattern Across Nonhuman Primates and Captive Felids

The Pattern: Markedly enlarged, globoid, flabby heart with thinned ventricular walls, dilated atria, and reduced myocardial contractility during antemortem imaging when available, with histopathologic evidence of myocardial fiber attenuation and interstitial fibrosis.

Cross-Taxa Signature: Recognized in nonhuman primates (particularly gorillas, orangutans, and chimpanzees), captive felids (particularly jaguars and cheetahs), psittacines, some captive ungulates, and cetaceans. The gross morphology is consistent across taxa; the etiologic profile varies. Captive great ape lineage-clustered cases point toward genetic factors; historical taurine-deficiency cases in captive felids have been largely mitigated by dietary reformulation; viral myocarditis progression may account for cases in other species.

Diagnostic Anchor: Documentation of the globoid, flabby, thin-walled morphology on gross examination with corresponding histopathologic findings of myocardial fiber attenuation and interstitial fibrosis. Antemortem imaging findings of reduced contractility support the diagnosis when available.

Trap Logic: The look-alike is severe volume overload from valvular insufficiency, which produces secondary chamber dilation and wall thinning without primary myocardial disease. Discrimination: valvular disease demonstrates identifiable valvular lesions on gross examination; primary dilated cardiomyopathy demonstrates preserved valvular architecture with primary myocardial fiber attenuation.

Zoonotic/Reportable Flag: Not zoonotic. Institutionally reportable at Species Survival Plan facilities for lineage documentation and for population-level management of the disease, particularly in captive great ape populations where genetic contribution is documented.

Vascular Disease Across Taxa

Vascular Mineralization and Atherosclerosis

Vascular mineralization is characterized by mineral deposition within the walls of large and medium vessels, producing loss of vascular compliance and, in advanced cases, luminal narrowing. In captive psittacines, aortic and coronary artery mineralization is common and is associated with chronic dyslipidemia, chronic dietary excess of high-fat commercial pelleted diets, and species-specific predisposition. In aged captive non-domestic mammals, aortic mineralization is a recurring incidental finding at necropsy that may or may not have contributed to the terminal event. Atherosclerosis with cholesterol-laden intimal plaques is documented in captive psittacines, in captive nonhuman primates (particularly with chronic dietary imbalance), and in captive cetaceans. The lesion pattern is remarkably consistent with domestic species atherosclerosis, and the pathologic interpretation is transportable.

Vasculitis Across Taxa

Vasculitis in non-domestic species is most commonly infectious in etiology. Herpesvirus disease in elephants (elephant endotheliotropic herpesvirus) produces prominent vascular endothelial involvement with hemorrhage, and the disease is characterized histopathologically by endothelial cell viral inclusion bodies with associated vasculitis. Ranavirus disease in chelonians and anurans produces vasculitis as part of the systemic disease presentation. Fungal vasculitis with vessel wall invasion is documented in aspergillosis of psittacines and marine mammals. Bacterial vasculitis is documented in salmonellosis of reptiles and birds. The lesion pattern of vasculitis (vessel wall inflammation with medial and adventitial infiltrate, possible mural thrombosis, and perivascular tissue reaction) is transportable across taxa; the etiologic profile requires species-specific ancillary workup.

Species-Specific Vascular Predispositions

Species-specific vascular predispositions include the aortic dissection and rupture recognized in captive cheetahs and some other large felids, which produces sudden death without antemortem clinical warning and is recognized at necropsy by aortic wall dissection with pericardial or thoracic hemorrhage. Aortic body tumors are documented in captive nonhuman primates and psittacines. Pulmonary artery mineralization with associated pulmonary hypertension is documented in captive psittacines, particularly African grey parrots. Peripheral arterial disease with distal extremity ischemia is documented in captive avian species and in some captive nonhuman primates.

Applied Case: Sudden Death From Aortic Dissection in a Captive Cheetah

A 6-year-old male cheetah (Acinonyx jubatus), housed in a Species Survival Plan managed collection, was found deceased in his outdoor enclosure with no antemortem clinical warning. Keepers had observed the animal at afternoon feeding approximately 90 minutes before discovery; the animal had been active and had consumed his diet. Post-discovery examination by the collection veterinarian noted no evidence of external trauma. The submission form recorded sudden death without antemortem clinical signs and requested comprehensive necropsy with attention to cardiovascular pathology given the species predisposition.

External examination was unremarkable. Body condition was appropriate. The coat was in appropriate seasonal condition. No wounds, no external hemorrhage, and no evidence of struggle were identified. Coelomic entry demonstrated a substantial volume of unclotted blood mixed with clotted material in the mediastinum and thoracic cavity, approximating 400 milliliters. The pericardial sac was distended with hemorrhagic fluid; upon opening, approximately 200 milliliters of frank hemorrhage was released. The heart itself demonstrated no primary myocardial lesions on gross inspection; the ventricular wall thickness was appropriate, the atria were of normal size, and the valvular structures were intact.

The source of hemorrhage was identified during systematic examination of the great vessels. The ascending aorta demonstrated a longitudinal tear approximately 8 millimeters in length located approximately 2 centimeters distal to the aortic valve, with dissection of the aortic wall extending from the intimal tear circumferentially and distally along the aortic arch to the level of the brachiocephalic trunk. Blood had escaped through the intimal tear into the medial and adventitial layers of the aorta, tracked distally along the dissection plane, and ultimately ruptured through the adventitia into the pericardial sac at the level of the aortic arch. The pattern of hemorrhage — pericardial tamponade with adventitial rupture at the aortic arch — was the definitive cardiovascular event responsible for the sudden death.

Cross-taxa reasoning at case interpretation was straightforward: aortic dissection with pericardial tamponade in a young to middle-aged captive cheetah is a documented species predisposition, and the gross pattern was consistent with published case series. The lesion pattern is comparable to dissecting aortic aneurysm in humans with underlying connective tissue disorders and in some domestic canine populations with genetic predisposition; the underlying pathophysiology involves medial degeneration with loss of elastic tissue integrity, and the cheetah species is documented to have a genetic predisposition producing similar aortic medial pathology. Comparable dissection events have been documented in other captive large felids at lower frequency but without the population-level prominence seen in cheetahs.

Histopathologic characterization of the aortic wall demonstrated marked disruption of the medial elastic lamellae with loss of normal elastic tissue architecture, mucoid degeneration of the medial ground substance, and cystic medial change consistent with medial degeneration. Adjacent unaffected aortic segments demonstrated similar medial pathology of lesser severity, suggesting the medial degeneration was a systemic aortic wall abnormality with acute superimposed dissection at the site of intimal tear.

Verhoeff-Van Gieson staining highlighted the elastic tissue disruption. Histopathology of other vascular beds (pulmonary artery, coronary arteries, mesenteric arteries) demonstrated less severe but similar medial pathology, supporting a systemic vascular process rather than an isolated aortic lesion.

The final morphologic diagnosis was acute ascending aortic dissection with pericardial tamponade secondary to systemic aortic medial degeneration. Ancillary molecular workup with fresh-frozen aortic tissue targeting collagen and elastic tissue-related genes was initiated for population-level relevance to the SSP; results were pending at the time of report distribution but would inform breeding management decisions for the species. Institutional reporting followed the standard SSP pathway. The case reinforced the species-specific vascular predisposition documented in captive cheetahs and contributed to the ongoing population-level surveillance for cardiovascular disease in the species. Comparative reasoning was again the interpretive bridge: the aortic dissection pattern was recognizable against domestic and human vascular disease reference; the histopathologic hallmarks of medial degeneration were transportable across species; and the population-level management implications were addressed through the SSP structure that coordinates captive cheetah conservation.

THE COMPARATIVE NECROPSY PATTERN SYSTEM — Vascular Mineralization Pattern in Captive Psittacines and Aged Non-Domestic Mammals

The Pattern: Mineral deposition within the walls of the aorta, coronary arteries, and other large and medium vessels, producing loss of vascular compliance and, in advanced cases, luminal narrowing with associated end-organ ischemic changes.

Cross-Taxa Signature: Recognized in captive psittacines (particularly African grey parrots, Amazon parrots, and cockatoos) as a common necropsy finding with a strong association with dietary composition and chronic dyslipidemia. Documented in aged captive non-domestic mammals as an age-associated finding that may or may not have contributed to terminal event. Documented in captive cetaceans with variable clinical relevance. In each taxonomic group, the gross appearance is similar: yellow-white, gritty, mineralized foci within vessel walls detected as rough texture on gross examination and confirmed by histopathology.

Diagnostic Anchor: Gross detection of vascular mineralization is confirmed by histopathology demonstrating medial mineral deposition, and by von Kossa staining when specific characterization is needed. Chronic dietary history in captive psittacines contextualizes the finding.

Trap Logic: The look-alike is postmortem mineralization artifact in vessels affected by prolonged formalin fixation with calcium salts precipitating from the tissue-fixative interaction. Discrimination: postmortem artifact affects the outer vessel wall predominantly and lacks the medial concentric distribution of true dystrophic mineralization; von Kossa staining is diagnostic for true mineral deposition.

Zoonotic/Reportable Flag: Not zoonotic. Institutionally reportable at Species Survival Plan facilities managing psittacine populations for dietary reformulation and population-level management.

Pericardial and Endocardial Pathology

Pericardial Effusion and Pericarditis

Pericardial effusion in non-domestic species reflects the same range of underlying processes as in domestic species: cardiac disease with congestive failure, infectious pericarditis, neoplastic pericardial disease, uremic pericarditis, traumatic pericardial disease, and idiopathic pericardial effusion. Grossly, pericardial effusion is characterized by fluid volume, color, and clarity, with each parameter carrying interpretive weight. Serous fluid suggests a low-inflammation etiology such as congestive heart failure or idiopathic disease. Hemorrhagic fluid suggests traumatic or neoplastic disease. Fibrinous or purulent fluid suggests infectious pericarditis. Cytologic examination of pericardial fluid at necropsy provides same-day interpretive direction and is a standard step in cardiac cases with pericardial effusion.

Endocarditis and Valvular Disease

Endocarditis in non-domestic species is most commonly bacterial in etiology, with vegetative lesions on cardiac valves producing valvular dysfunction and, in cases with lesion embolization, distant organ involvement. The lesion pattern is recognizable across taxa: raised, granular, friable material on valve leaflets with underlying fibrin deposition and inflammatory infiltrate. Histopathology demonstrates the fibrinocellular vegetation with embedded bacterial colonies. The pathologist working an endocarditis case samples the vegetative lesion for aerobic and anaerobic bacterial culture at necropsy because the vegetation may harbor viable organisms even in cases where systemic blood culture would be negative. Valvular degenerative disease in aged non-domestic species produces valvular thickening and, in advanced cases, valvular insufficiency; the lesion pattern is comparable to myxomatous valvular degeneration in domestic species.

Cardiac Neoplasia in Non-Domestic Species

Cardiac neoplasia in non-domestic species is uncommon but documented across taxa. Aortic body tumors and heart base tumors are recognized in captive psittacines and nonhuman primates. Cardiac hemangiosarcoma is documented in captive large mammals. Cardiac lymphoma with epicardial or myocardial infiltration is documented in captive nonhuman primates and in some captive avian species. Metastatic cardiac disease from primary neoplasms in other organs is documented across taxa. The pathologist encountering an unusual cardiac mass performs the standard mass workup: gross characterization, histopathology with immunohistochemistry as needed, and consideration of primary versus metastatic origin.

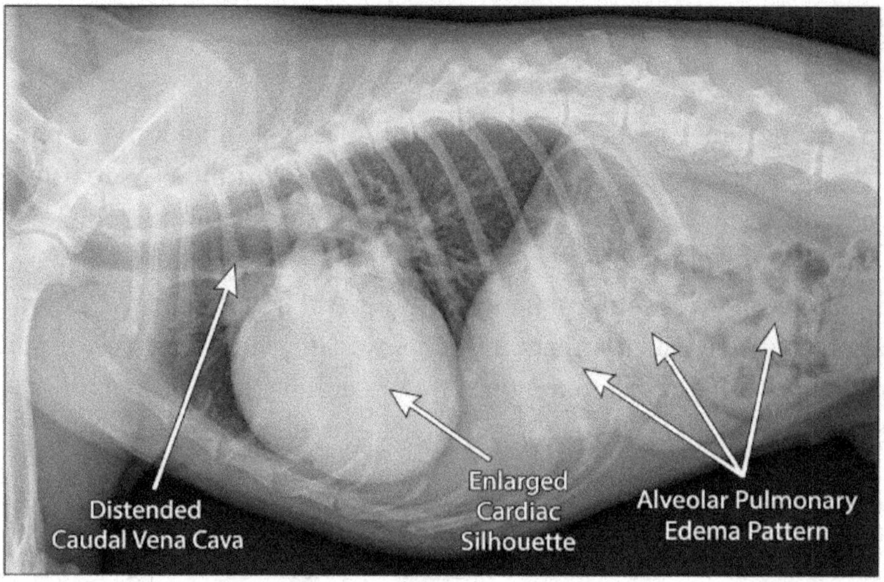

Figure 4.4: Cardiac Silhouette Enlargement on Post-Mortem Radiography: Cardiomyopathy in a Captive Nonhuman Primate.

THE COMPARATIVE NECROPSY PATTERN SYSTEM — Fibrinous Pericardial Effusion Pattern Signaling Septic Pericarditis Across Taxa

The Pattern: Fibrinous to fibrinopurulent pericardial effusion with associated pericardial visceral and parietal thickening, indicating septic pericarditis of infectious etiology.

Cross-Taxa Signature: Recognized across mammalian, avian, and reptile taxa. In ruminants and captive artiodactyls, septic pericarditis has classically been associated with traumatic reticulopericarditis from ingested metallic foreign body penetration; the pattern remains relevant in captive collections. In birds, septic pericarditis is documented as a complication of avian cholera in waterfowl, of colibacillosis in captive gallinaceous birds, and of chlamydiosis in psittacines. In reptiles, septic pericarditis is documented as a complication of systemic bacterial septicemia. The unifying gross appearance across taxa is a thickened, dull, sometimes shaggy pericardial surface with fibrinous exudate.

Diagnostic Anchor: Cytologic examination of pericardial fluid demonstrates degenerate neutrophils, karyorrhectic debris, and, often, visible bacterial organisms. Aerobic and anaerobic culture of pericardial fluid at necropsy establishes the etiologic organism. Histopathology of the pericardium confirms the fibrinous or fibrinopurulent character.

Trap Logic: The look-alike is hemorrhagic pericardial effusion secondary to cardiac trauma or ruptured atrial hemangiosarcoma, which produces gross fluid accumulation without infectious etiology. Discrimination: hemorrhagic effusion cytologically demonstrates predominantly erythrocytes and neoplastic cells if a mass is the source; septic effusion demonstrates the degenerate neutrophil population characteristic of infection.

Zoonotic/Reportable Flag: Septic pericarditis with Chlamydia or Chlamydophila organisms in psittacines is a zoonotic concern with occupational health implications; institutional biosafety notification and personnel exposure follow-up are activated. Septic pericarditis with Mycobacterium organisms similarly requires biosafety notification. Other bacterial etiologies are generally not zoonotic but may be institutionally reportable at collection facilities.

Cardiomyopathy Type	Gross Morphology	Histopathologic Hallmark	Species Predisposed	Key Discriminator
Dilated cardiomyopathy	Globoid, flabby, thin-walled biventricular dilation	Myocardial fiber attenuation and interstitial fibrosis	Captive great apes, captive large felids (historical taurine deficiency), captive psittacines, cetaceans	Preserved valvular architecture with primary myocardial fiber attenuation
Hypertrophic cardiomyopathy	Asymmetric or concentric ventricular wall thickening; papillary muscle hypertrophy; left atrial dilation	Myocardial fiber disarray and interstitial fibrosis	Captive large felids across multiple genera	Concentric hypertrophy without systemic hypertension or infiltrative process explanation
Restrictive cardiomyopathy	Marked biatrial dilation with normal ventricular wall thickness	Infiltrative or fibrotic myocardial disease (amyloid, iron, endomyocardial fibrosis)	Captive nonhuman primates and cetaceans	Preserved ventricular wall with severe atrial dilation reflecting diastolic dysfunction
Arrhythmogenic cardiomyopathy	Right ventricular free wall thinning with fibrofatty appearance	Fibrofatty myocardial replacement, predominantly right ventricular	Documented in domestic species; emerging in non-domestic literature	Fibrofatty replacement distribution on histopathology
Ischemic cardiomyopathy	Regional wall thinning corresponding to coronary vascular distribution	Myocardial fibrosis in coronary distribution with remote infarct areas	Aged captive mammals with vascular disease	Distribution mapping to coronary vascular anatomy

CLINICAL PEARL: The single most useful step in cardiac necropsy of an unfamiliar species is establishing the species-appropriate anatomic reference before applying pathologic interpretation. A pathologist reading a chelonian heart against a mammalian anatomic frame will find pathology that does not exist; the same pathologist reading against the chelonian anatomic frame will interpret correctly.

EVIDENCE: Historical documentation of taurine-deficiency dilated cardiomyopathy in captive large felids led to industry-wide dietary reformulation across zoological institutions, substantially reducing the incidence of the condition in modern captive populations. The example illustrates how zoo pathology contributes to population-level intervention: necropsy findings shaped the dietary standard, which shaped the captive population's cardiac disease burden.

THE COMPARATIVE NECROPSY PATTERN SYSTEM — Chapter 4 Cardiovascular Pattern Foundations

---

Ventricular Wall Thickness Pattern Recognition Across Endothermic and Ectothermic Taxa: Wall thickness interpretation against species-appropriate anatomic reference. Anchor: comparative reference to closest available taxonomic relative. Trap: chelonian intraventricular muscular ridge and reptile species-specific arrangements misread as pathology. Flag: recognition matters because misinterpretation propagates through case reports.

Dilated Cardiomyopathy Pattern Across Nonhuman Primates and Captive Felids: Globoid, flabby heart with thinned walls and dilated atria across taxa. Anchor: myocardial fiber attenuation with preserved valvular architecture on histopathology. Trap: volume overload from valvular disease discriminated by identifiable valvular lesions. Flag: institutionally reportable at SSP facilities for genetic contribution documentation.

Vascular Mineralization Pattern in Captive Psittacines and Aged Non-Domestic Mammals: Yellow-white gritty mineralization within vessel walls with medial concentric distribution. Anchor: histopathologic confirmation with von Kossa staining. Trap: postmortem mineralization artifact discriminated by outer wall predominance. Flag: institutionally reportable at SSP psittacine facilities for dietary reformulation.

Fibrinous Pericardial Effusion Pattern Signaling Septic Pericarditis Across Taxa: Fibrinous or fibrinopurulent pericardial exudate with pericardial thickening across mammals, birds, and reptiles. Anchor: cytologic examination of pericardial fluid with culture. Trap: hemorrhagic effusion from trauma or hemangiosarcoma discriminated by cellular content. Flag: chlamydial or mycobacterial etiology triggers biosafety and occupational health notification.

Summary and Key Concepts

Comparative cardiac anatomic knowledge is prerequisite to cardiovascular pathology interpretation in non-domestic species; species-specific anatomic reference must be established before pathologic interpretation is applied.

Dilated cardiomyopathy, hypertrophic cardiomyopathy, restrictive cardiomyopathy, and arrhythmogenic cardiomyopathy each demonstrate consistent gross and histopathologic patterns across taxa; species-specific etiologic profiles vary.

Vascular disease across taxa includes mineralization (prominent in captive psittacines and aged mammals), atherosclerosis, vasculitis (predominantly infectious in etiology), and species-specific predispositions such as aortic dissection in captive cheetahs.

Pericardial pathology across taxa reflects the range of processes documented in domestic species; cytologic examination of pericardial fluid at necropsy provides same-day interpretive direction and is a standard step.

Endocarditis in non-domestic species is most commonly bacterial with a lesion pattern transportable across taxa; sampling of vegetative lesions for culture at necropsy is required regardless of systemic blood culture status.

Zoo pathology cardiovascular findings have historically contributed to population-level intervention (dietary reformulation for taurine deficiency, dietary management for psittacine atherosclerosis) illustrating the discipline's translational function.

CHAPTER 5: RESPIRATORY PATHOLOGY ACROSS TAXA

Learning Objectives

1. Interpret comparative respiratory anatomic variation across taxa as it modifies lesion interpretation.
2. Recognize the major infectious pneumonia patterns in non-domestic species with their species-specific etiologic profiles.
3. Identify non-infectious respiratory disease including neoplasia, degenerative disease, and environmental injury across taxa.
4. Distinguish aspiration, traumatic pulmonary injury, and environmental lung injury from primary respiratory disease.
5. Apply the Comparative Necropsy Pattern callout structure to respiratory lesion recognition across unfamiliar species.
6. Coordinate ancillary respiratory diagnostics including bronchoalveolar or coelomic lavage cytology and molecular respiratory panels.

Respiratory pathology in non-domestic species requires the pathologist to recognize that the vertebrate respiratory system is more anatomically diverse than any other organ system except perhaps the reproductive tract. The mammalian alveolar lung, the avian air sac and parabronchial lung, the reptilian faveolar lung, the amphibian buccopharyngeal and cutaneous respiration, and the teleost gill each represent distinct evolutionary solutions to gas exchange, and each demands species-appropriate interpretive frames. A pathologist who reads a chelonian faveolar lung against the mammalian alveolar frame will misinterpret normal anatomy as pathology; a pathologist who reads an avian parabronchial lung against the mammalian frame will similarly fail. Comparative anatomic knowledge is prerequisite to comparative pathologic interpretation.

This chapter organizes respiratory pathology into four domains. Comparative respiratory anatomy provides the interpretive frame. Infectious pneumonias across taxa address the range of pneumonia patterns from suppurative bronchopneumonia through interstitial pneumonia through granulomatous pneumonia, with their species-specific etiologic profiles. Non-infectious respiratory disease covers neoplasia, degenerative disease, and other non-infectious processes. Aspiration, trauma, and environmental lung injury complete the chapter with attention to the recurring interpretive challenges of distinguishing primary respiratory disease from secondary injury.

Comparative Respiratory Anatomy: Air Sacs, Faveolar Lungs, Blowholes

The Avian Air Sac and Parabronchial Lung

Avian respiratory anatomy differs from mammalian anatomy in structural and functional ways that modify pathologic interpretation. Nine air sacs traverse the coelomic cavity and extend into the pneumatized skeleton, providing a bellows function that drives airflow through the paired lungs. The lungs themselves are relatively small, non-expansile, and dorsally adherent to the ribs and body wall. Airflow through the parabronchi is unidirectional across two respiratory cycles, producing continuous gas exchange rather than the tidal ventilation of mammals. This arrangement makes the air sac walls, rather than the alveolar surface, the primary site where infectious agents accumulate and where inflammatory response manifests. Air sacculitis is a recurring finding in avian respiratory disease and is often the first sign of infectious process before parenchymal lung involvement is evident. The pneumatized skeleton means that respiratory infection can extend contiguously into bone, producing osteomyelitis of the humerus, femur, and portions of the vertebral column.

The Reptile Faveolar Lung

Reptile lungs consist of an outer capsular layer and an inner faveolar surface with variable degrees of internal septation. In chelonians, the faveolar architecture is prominent with numerous large faveoli that resemble honeycomb structure on gross examination. In squamates, faveolar architecture varies from simple sac-like lungs in some snakes to more complex septated structures in monitors and iguanas. Crocodilian lungs are more complex with a multi-chambered architecture approaching mammalian complexity. Consolidation of a reptile faveolar lung produces gross findings distinct from mammalian pulmonary consolidation: the fluid or exudate fills the faveolar spaces rather than the alveoli, producing a firm, mucoid, sometimes friable consolidation pattern that differs from the classic hepatization of bacterial pneumonia in mammals. Histopathologic interpretation requires recognition of the normal faveolar architecture as the baseline reference.

Marine Mammal Respiratory Anatomy and the Blowhole Apparatus

Cetacean respiratory anatomy includes a blowhole with an elaborate muscular closure mechanism, reinforced tracheal cartilages that resist collapse under diving pressure, and lungs adapted to rapid inhalation and exhalation during surfacing. The reinforced trachea permits rapid tidal flow but modifies the interpretation of tracheal disease; the muscular blowhole apparatus is a distinct anatomic region that requires specific examination during marine mammal necropsy. Pinniped respiratory anatomy is closer to terrestrial mammalian anatomy but demonstrates modifications for diving physiology including bronchiolar constriction that redistributes blood flow during dives. Sirenian respiratory anatomy is intermediate, with adaptations for their exclusively aquatic habitat but without the diving specializations of cetaceans.

Amphibian and Fish Respiratory Anatomy

Amphibian respiration occurs across three surfaces: the buccopharyngeal mucosa, the skin, and the paired simple sac-like lungs. Cutaneous respiration is quantitatively significant in most amphibian species and requires intact epidermal integrity; any pathologic process disrupting the epidermis compromises respiratory function even if the lungs are unaffected. Fish gill anatomy consists of gill arches supporting numerous gill filaments each carrying multiple secondary lamellae that constitute the gas exchange surface. Gill pathology (lamellar hyperplasia, clubbing, fusion, necrosis) is the equivalent of mammalian pulmonary pathology and is interpreted against species-appropriate baseline gill architecture.

ure 5.1: Comparative Vertebrate Respiratory Anatomy: Five Structural Frames

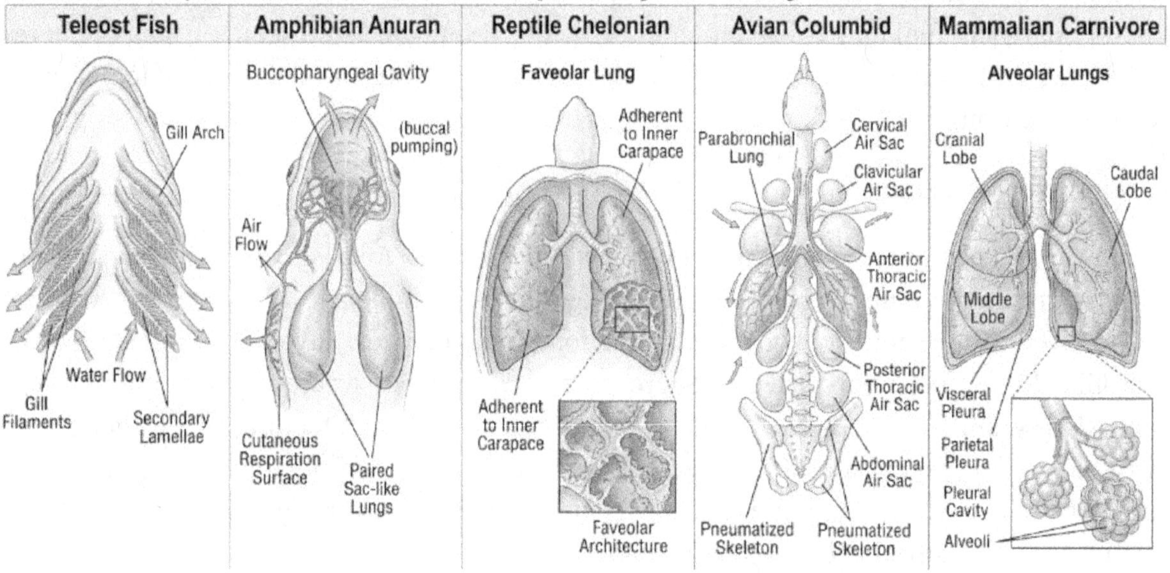

THE COMPARATIVE NECROPSY PATTERN SYSTEM — Faveolar Lung Consolidation Pattern in Reptiles Versus Alveolar Consolidation in Mammals

The Pattern: Firm, mucoid, sometimes friable consolidation filling the faveolar spaces of a reptile lung, distinct from the classic hepatization of mammalian bacterial pneumonia.

Cross-Taxa Signature: Recognized across chelonians, squamates, and crocodilians with prominent faveolar architecture. The gross appearance differs from mammalian bacterial pneumonia because the faveolar spaces fill with exudate rather than the alveolar surface being consolidated; the gross texture is mucoid to firm rather than the rubbery hepatization of mammals. Histopathology confirms the intraluminal accumulation of inflammatory cells and fibrin within the faveolar spaces with variable involvement of the septal walls.

Diagnostic Anchor: Recognition of the reptile-specific consolidation pattern with correlation to species-appropriate faveolar architecture. Sampling of the exudate for cytology and culture at necropsy identifies the etiologic agent.

Trap Logic: The look-alike is normal reptile faveolar architecture misread as consolidation, particularly in species with dense faveolar structure. Discrimination: true consolidation demonstrates loss of the normal faveolar organization with exudate filling; normal architecture demonstrates preserved spatial organization with air-filled spaces.

Zoonotic/Reportable Flag: Reptile pneumonias caused by Mycobacterium species are institutionally reportable and require biosafety precautions; salmonellosis is zoonotic and requires occupational health awareness.

Infectious Pneumonias Across Taxa

Bacterial Bronchopneumonia and Suppurative Pneumonia

Bacterial bronchopneumonia is characterized by cranioventral lung consolidation with prominent airway involvement, purulent exudate within airways and alveoli, and neutrophil-rich inflammatory response. In captive ungulates, bacterial bronchopneumonia is a recurring cause of morbidity and mortality, with Mannheimia haemolytica, Pasteurella multocida, and Mycoplasma species as common etiologic agents comparable to domestic ruminant respiratory disease. In captive nonhuman primates, Streptococcus pneumoniae, Klebsiella pneumoniae, and Bordetella bronchiseptica are recurring agents. In captive avian species, Escherichia coli, Bordetella avium, and species-specific agents produce bronchopneumonia patterns. In captive marine mammals, Streptococcus phocae and Brucella species produce systemic disease with prominent pulmonary involvement. The gross pattern of cranioventral consolidation with airway involvement is transportable across taxa; the etiologic profile varies by species and requires species-appropriate culture and molecular workup.

Interstitial and Viral Pneumonia

Interstitial pneumonia is characterized by involvement of the interstitial connective tissue with variable alveolar involvement, producing a diffuse pattern of pulmonary parenchymal thickening without the airway-centered consolidation of bacterial bronchopneumonia. Viral etiologies dominate the interstitial pneumonia differential across taxa. Morbilliviral pneumonia in cetaceans (cetacean morbillivirus with associated multinucleate giant cell formation and syncytia) is a documented cause of stranding events. Influenza virus in mammalian spillover produces interstitial pneumonia with characteristic necrotizing bronchiolitis. Herpesvirus pneumonia in captive species produces multifocal necrotizing pneumonia with characteristic inclusion bodies. Adenovirus pneumonia in psittacines and passerines produces intranuclear viral inclusion bodies within respiratory epithelium.

Granulomatous Pneumonia and Mycobacterial Disease

Granulomatous pneumonia is characterized by well-demarcated inflammatory foci with epithelioid macrophage cuffs, occasional multinucleate giant cells, and central necrosis in mature lesions. Mycobacterial disease is the recurring granulomatous pneumonia etiology across taxa. Mycobacterium bovis and M. tuberculosis in captive ungulates and nonhuman primates produce classical granulomatous pneumonia with cavitation in advanced cases. M. avium complex organisms in captive avian species, in psittacines, and in some captive mammals produce granulomatous respiratory disease with variable systemic involvement. Non-tuberculous mycobacteria of environmental origin (M. chelonae, M. abscessus, M. fortuitum) produce granulomatous disease in immunocompromised captive individuals and in some reptile species. Fungal granulomatous pneumonia (aspergillosis, cryptococcosis, coccidioidomycosis) produces overlapping gross morphology and is discriminated by histopathology and fungal culture.

Applied Case: Cetacean Morbillivirus in a Stranded Bottlenose Dolphin

An adult female bottlenose dolphin (Tursiops truncatus) was recovered dead from a beach on the mid-Atlantic coast during a period of elevated regional stranding activity. The stranding coordinator had documented an unusual mortality event declaration in the previous week based on stranding rates exceeding baseline. The carcass was recovered within an estimated 12 to 24 hours of death based on tissue condition and was transported refrigerated to a coordinating pathology laboratory participating in the NOAA Fisheries Marine Mammal Health and Stranding Response Program. The submission form recorded the unusual mortality event context and requested workup for morbillivirus among other differentials.

External examination demonstrated poor body condition with prominent axillary and lumbar concavity, moderately thin blubber layer (approximately 12 millimeters at the axillary standardized site, below reference for adult females in this population), and no evidence of net entanglement, projectile injury, or vessel strike. Superficial skin sloughing was consistent with the estimated postmortem interval. Blowhole examination demonstrated small volume of clear frothy fluid. Systematic necropsy proceeded by standard cetacean flensing approach with attention to preserving blubber orientation and to systematic organ examination.

Coelomic examination demonstrated moderate volume of clear serous fluid without pericardial or peritoneal exudate. The lungs were markedly heavy and firm with diffuse involvement of both lung fields rather than the cranioventral distribution of bacterial bronchopneumonia. Cut surface demonstrated diffuse parenchymal consolidation with a beefy red color and firm to rubbery texture; airways contained modest volume of blood-tinged foamy fluid. The tracheobronchial lymph nodes were moderately enlarged and edematous. The heart demonstrated no primary lesions. The liver demonstrated modest congestion consistent with terminal event but no primary hepatic disease. The kidneys were unremarkable on gross examination. The brain demonstrated no gross lesions but the meninges appeared moderately congested; a systematic examination of the ventricular system demonstrated modest ependymal reactivity.

Same-day cytology of an impression smear from cut lung surface demonstrated numerous multinucleate giant cells (syncytia) with prominent cytoplasmic and intranuclear inclusion bodies, and a mixed mononuclear inflammatory cell infiltrate. The finding was pathognomonic for morbilliviral pneumonia by cytology alone, with the syncytia and inclusion bodies together sufficient to establish the etiologic direction before histopathology was available. Biosafety practices during continued dissection were escalated to Biosafety Level 3 protocols with appropriate personal protective equipment because of the emerging concern about morbilliviral disease in stranded populations, and because of the unusual mortality event context that suggested active outbreak transmission.

Fresh tissue was collected for polymerase chain reaction targeting the cetacean morbillivirus phosphoprotein gene, for viral isolation on appropriate cell lines, and for the standard cetacean unusual mortality event tissue archive maintained by NOAA. Histopathology confirmed the cytologic impression: diffuse interstitial pneumonia with numerous multinucleate giant cells demonstrating intracytoplasmic and intranuclear eosinophilic viral inclusion bodies, alveolar epithelial hyperplasia, and mixed mononuclear inflammatory infiltrate. Additional sampling of brain confirmed the meningeal reactivity noted grossly and demonstrated multifocal nonsuppurative meningoencephalitis with occasional syncytial giant cells in the cortex. Polymerase chain reaction returned positive for cetacean morbillivirus within 48 hours of submission, confirming the diagnosis and triggering the unusual mortality event coordinating response.

The final morphologic diagnosis was severe diffuse interstitial giant cell pneumonia with multifocal nonsuppurative meningoencephalitis. The etiologic diagnosis was cetacean morbillivirus infection. Institutional and regulatory reporting followed the standard unusual mortality event pathway: findings were reported to the NOAA Fisheries regional coordinator, aggregated with concurrent stranding pathology from the coordinating network of laboratories, and contributed to the population-level surveillance data. The case illustrated cross-taxa reasoning applied to a marine mammal context: the interstitial pneumonia with syncytia pattern is recognized across morbillivirus disease in humans (measles), in ruminants (rinderpest, peste des petits ruminants), in carnivores (canine distemper), and in cetaceans (cetacean morbillivirus). The gross and histopathologic hallmarks were transportable across mammalian orders; the specific virus was cetacean-specific and required cetacean-validated molecular workup. The population-level implications flowed through the coordinated stranding network structure that permits marine mammal disease surveillance in the way that no single institution could accomplish.

THE COMPARATIVE NECROPSY PATTERN SYSTEM — Cross-Taxa Bronchopneumonia Pattern Signaling Bacterial Pneumonia

---

The Pattern: Cranioventral lung consolidation with prominent airway involvement, purulent exudate within airways and alveoli, and neutrophil-rich inflammatory response indicating bacterial bronchopneumonia.

Cross-Taxa Signature: Recognized across captive ungulates (Mannheimia and Pasteurella dominant), captive nonhuman primates (Streptococcus pneumoniae and Klebsiella dominant), captive avian species (Escherichia coli and Bordetella avium dominant in gallinaceous birds), and captive marine mammals (Streptococcus phocae and Brucella species). The gross pattern of cranioventral consolidation with airway involvement is transportable across taxa; the etiologic profile is species-specific and requires species-appropriate culture.

Diagnostic Anchor: Gross recognition of cranioventral consolidation with airway involvement, confirmed by histopathology demonstrating suppurative inflammation with airway centered distribution, and etiologic identification by aerobic bacterial culture from fresh lung tissue collected at necropsy.

Trap Logic: The look-alike is aspiration pneumonia, which produces cranioventral consolidation with foreign material within airways and characteristic inflammatory response including multinucleate foreign body giant cells. Discrimination: aspiration demonstrates identifiable foreign material or foreign-body inflammatory response; primary bacterial bronchopneumonia does not.

Zoonotic/Reportable Flag: Bacterial bronchopneumonia caused by Streptococcus zooepidemicus, some Klebsiella strains, and Brucella species carries occupational health implications. Marine mammal pneumonia with Brucella species requires notification of state animal health authority and occupational health follow-up for personnel.

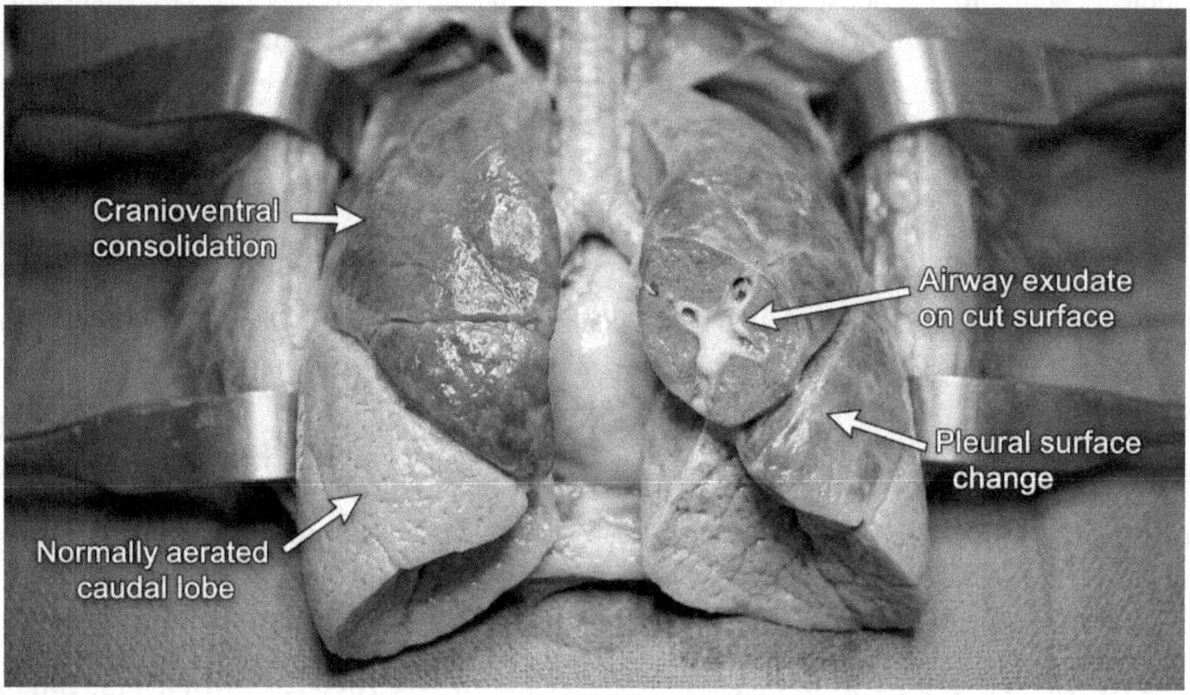

Non-Infectious Respiratory Disease

Pulmonary Neoplasia

Primary pulmonary neoplasia in non-domestic species includes bronchial and bronchiolar carcinomas, alveolar carcinomas, mesenchymal neoplasms, and, less commonly, primary pulmonary lymphoma. Metastatic pulmonary disease from distant primary neoplasms is documented across taxa. Aged captive nonhuman primates, captive large felids, and captive avian species demonstrate primary pulmonary neoplasia at rates comparable to domestic species. The gross pattern of pulmonary neoplasia includes discrete masses (primary carcinoma), multifocal nodular pattern (metastatic disease), and diffuse infiltrative pattern (lymphoma or diffuse alveolar carcinoma). Histopathologic characterization with immunohistochemistry as needed distinguishes primary from metastatic disease and refines the specific tumor type.

Pulmonary Mineralization and Fibrosis

Pulmonary mineralization in captive psittacines is a recurring necropsy finding associated with chronic hypercalcemia, hypervitaminosis D, and chronic dietary imbalance. The gross pattern includes multifocal small firm foci throughout the parenchyma, sometimes with vascular mineralization. Pulmonary fibrosis in aged captive species produces progressive interstitial thickening with restrictive lung function. Chronic hypersensitivity pneumonitis in captive avian species produces interstitial fibrosis with mixed cellular infiltrate and is documented in relation to environmental antigen exposure in exhibits with inadequate ventilation.

Air Sac Cystadenoma and Species-Specific Neoplasia

Air sac cystadenoma in captive psittacines is a species-specific neoplastic entity that presents as one or more cystic masses arising from the air sac wall. The lesion is often incidental at necropsy but can produce coelomic space-occupying effects. Species-specific pulmonary neoplasia in other taxa includes uterine leiomyoma-like pulmonary lesions in some captive rodent species and species-specific carcinoma patterns in captive amphibians. The pathologist encountering an unfamiliar pulmonary mass considers primary versus metastatic origin, characterizes the mass by standard histopathology, and consults the comparative literature for species-specific tumor entities.

Applied Case: Pulmonary Aspergillosis in a Captive African Grey Parrot

An adult male African grey parrot (Psittacus erithacus) housed in a mixed avian collection had been in declining condition for approximately three weeks before death. Antemortem clinical signs recorded by the collection veterinarian included progressive weight loss, tail-bobbing consistent with respiratory effort, and reduced vocalization. Imaging performed six days before death demonstrated multifocal pulmonary opacities and mild air sac opacification consistent with pulmonary aspergillosis, and antifungal therapy had been initiated with limited response. The animal was found deceased on the morning of the seventh day of therapy. The submission requested confirmation of the imaging-based clinical diagnosis and characterization of disease extent.

External examination demonstrated marked underweight body condition with keel prominence, dull plumage, and small volume of clear fluid in the choanal region. Coelomic necropsy by standard avian approach demonstrated the keel and pectoral musculature reflected to expose air sac architecture in situ before any organ displacement. The clavicular, cranial thoracic, and abdominal air sacs demonstrated marked wall thickening with white plaque-like exudate adherent to serosal surfaces and, in the abdominal air sac, several discrete raised firm nodules approximately 3 to 8 millimeters in diameter. The pulmonary parenchyma demonstrated multifocal firm nodules of comparable size distributed throughout both lungs on cut surface examination. The tracheobronchial region demonstrated moderate mucosal thickening. No involvement of the pneumatized skeleton was grossly evident.

Same-day cytology of impression smears from an air sac nodule demonstrated numerous fungal hyphae with characteristic dichotomous branching at approximately 45-degree angles, septation, and parallel walls consistent with Aspergillus species; associated multinucleate giant cells and epithelioid macrophages with karyorrhectic neutrophil debris were present. The cytologic finding was diagnostic for pulmonary and air sac aspergillosis before histopathology was available. Fresh tissue was collected for aerobic fungal culture on Sabouraud dextrose agar, for polymerase chain reaction targeting Aspergillus-specific sequences with speciation, and for histopathology including special stains.

Cross-taxa reasoning at case interpretation drew on the extensive documented literature of avian aspergillosis. Aspergillus fumigatus is the dominant etiologic species in captive avian populations, with A. flavus, A. niger, and other species less commonly identified. Predisposing factors include environmental spore burden, stress, immunosuppression from concurrent disease, and species-specific susceptibility with African grey parrots documented at elevated susceptibility relative to other psittacine species. The gross pattern of multifocal firm pulmonary nodules with air sac plaque and nodule formation is the classical presentation, and the histopathologic recognition of fungal hyphae with granulomatous inflammation is transportable across avian species.

Histopathology confirmed pulmonary and air sac granulomatous inflammation with abundant septate fungal hyphae highlighted by Grocott-Gomori methenamine silver staining. The lesion architecture demonstrated epithelioid macrophage cuffs, multinucleate giant cells, central necrosis in mature lesions, and fungal hyphae radiating outward from lesion centers. Vascular invasion by fungal hyphae was present in several sections, indicating angioinvasive disease. Culture returned Aspergillus fumigatus within seven days; molecular speciation confirmed the identification. The final morphologic diagnosis was severe multifocal pulmonary and air sac granulomatous inflammation with fungal hyphae and angioinvasion. The etiologic diagnosis was aspergillosis with confirmed A. fumigatus species identification.

The institutional response addressed both the individual case and the collection-level implications. Environmental sampling of the collection was initiated to characterize Aspergillus spore burden, husbandry review addressed potential predisposing factors including exhibit ventilation and humidity, and additional psittacine individuals in the collection were placed on surveillance for compatible clinical signs. The case reinforced the recognition of aspergillosis as a leading cause of morbidity and mortality in captive psittacines and the utility of same-day cytology in directing appropriate ancillary workup before histopathology is available. The pattern of multifocal firm pulmonary nodules with air sac involvement is a Comparative Necropsy Pattern that repeats across the avian orders in the same recognizable form; cross-taxa recognition permits diagnostic direction regardless of individual pathologist experience with the specific species.

THE COMPARATIVE NECROPSY PATTERN SYSTEM — Pulmonary Mineralization Pattern in Captive Psittacines

The Pattern: Multifocal small firm mineralized foci distributed throughout the pulmonary parenchyma of a captive psittacine, often with concurrent renal or vascular mineralization.

Cross-Taxa Signature: Recognized principally in captive psittacines (particularly African grey parrots, Amazon parrots, and cockatoos) with chronic dietary imbalance producing hypervitaminosis D and hypercalcemia. Occasionally recognized in other captive avian species with similar dietary risk factors. The lesion is often accompanied by vascular mineralization and by renal tubular mineralization, indicating a systemic calcium-phosphate dysregulation.

Diagnostic Anchor: Gross recognition of multifocal firm parenchymal foci confirmed by histopathology with von Kossa staining. Serum biochemistry (calcium, phosphate) and dietary history contextualize the finding.

Trap Logic: The look-alike is granulomatous pneumonia with mineralized granulomas (mycobacterial disease, aspergillosis), which produces similar gross firm foci. Discrimination: granulomatous foci demonstrate epithelioid macrophage cuffs and multinucleate giant cells on histopathology; dystrophic mineralization does not. Special stains identify the etiologic agent in granulomatous disease.

Zoonotic/Reportable Flag: Not zoonotic. Institutionally reportable at collections managing psittacine populations for dietary reformulation.

Aspiration, Trauma, and Environmental Lung Injury

Aspiration Pneumonia Across Taxa

Aspiration pneumonia occurs when gastric contents, food material, water, or other extrinsic material is inhaled into the lower respiratory tract producing chemical and infectious pneumonia. In captive species, aspiration is recognized in the context of anesthetic recovery, disease-related regurgitation, hand-feeding technique errors in juvenile animals, and drowning or near-drowning events. The gross pattern includes cranioventral to diffuse consolidation with identifiable foreign material within airways and, on histopathology, multinucleate foreign body giant cells surrounding aspirated material. Aspiration pneumonia in marine mammals from seawater aspiration during stranding produces characteristic findings including foamy pulmonary edema and salt-water aspiration morphology.

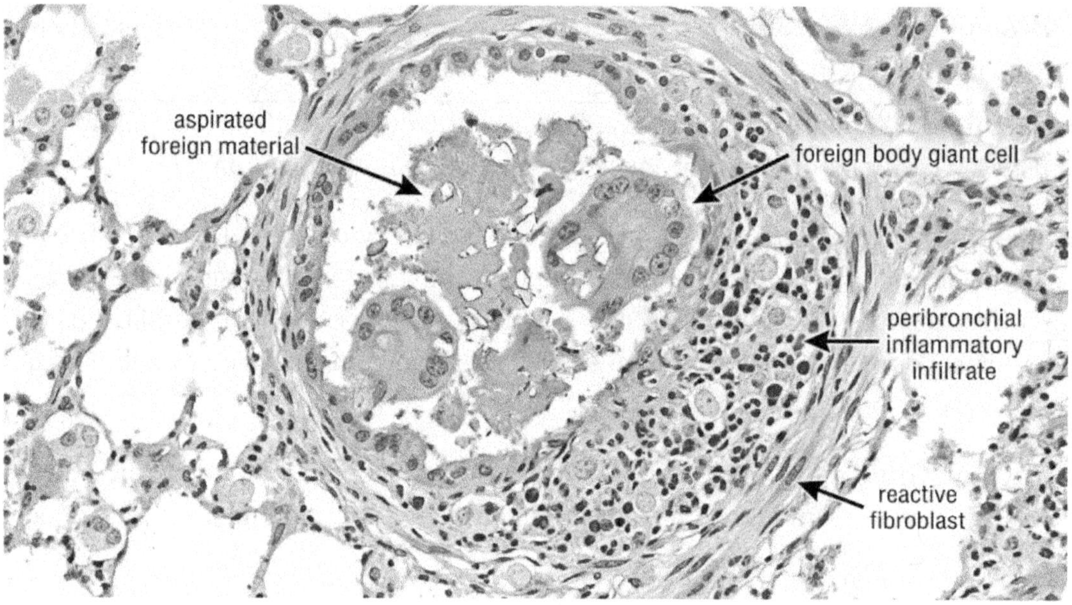

Pulmonary Trauma and Contusion

Pulmonary trauma produces contusion patterns that reflect the mechanism of injury. Vehicular collision produces broad pulmonary contusion with associated rib fracture and thoracic wall injury. Projectile injury produces pulmonary contusion along the projectile path with entrance and exit wounds. Falls and blunt trauma produce lobar contusion patterns. Barotrauma from rapid pressure changes (fish brought rapidly from depth, cetaceans with acoustic trauma) produces characteristic gas-associated lesions. Fat embolism secondary to long-bone fracture produces pulmonary microvascular occlusion with fat globules visible on histopathology with oil red O staining. Traumatic pneumothorax is recognized by lung collapse with pleural surface irregularities.

Environmental and Toxicologic Lung Injury

Environmental lung injury includes smoke inhalation from wildfire exposure with characteristic tracheal and bronchial epithelial necrosis, oxygen toxicity from prolonged high-concentration oxygen therapy in captive settings, and toxic gas exposure from ammonia, chlorine, or other reactive gases. Toxicologic lung injury includes paraquat toxicity with characteristic pulmonary fibrosis progression, anticoagulant rodenticide toxicosis with pulmonary hemorrhage, and mycotoxin-related respiratory disease. Marine mammal harmful algal bloom exposure produces respiratory lesions in populations exposed to aerosolized brevetoxin from red tide events.

Applied Case: Bacterial Bronchopneumonia in a Captive Reticulated Giraffe

A 7-year-old female reticulated giraffe (Giraffa reticulata) was found deceased in her exhibit on a cool autumn morning. Antemortem history included two days of reduced activity, nasal discharge, and reduced feed intake noted by keepers, with clinical evaluation planned for the day of death. The submission form recorded the antemortem observations and requested comprehensive necropsy with attention to respiratory disease. Necropsy was performed at the institutional pathology facility within four hours of discovery.

External examination demonstrated moderate body condition with mildly increased respiratory effort observed by keepers before death consistent with the postmortem finding of nasal mucopurulent discharge. Coelomic examination demonstrated no ascitic fluid. Thoracic examination demonstrated bilateral pulmonary consolidation involving the cranioventral aspects of both cranial and middle lung lobes with sparing of the caudal lung fields. Cut surface of the consolidated lung demonstrated purulent exudate within airways with expression of thick creamy material on pressure, and firm hepatization of the consolidated parenchyma. The pattern was classical bacterial bronchopneumonia with cranioventral distribution and prominent airway involvement. The tracheobronchial lymph nodes were moderately enlarged and edematous.

Same-day cytology of impression smears from cut lung surface demonstrated degenerate neutrophils with karyorrhectic nuclei, numerous extracellular bacterial rods and cocci, and reactive alveolar macrophages, consistent with acute bacterial bronchopneumonia. Cytology direction supported urgent aerobic and anaerobic culture of fresh lung tissue and of tracheobronchial lymph node. Sample collection followed the standard bacterial pneumonia workup including formalin-fixed pulmonary sections from multiple lobes, fresh-frozen tissue archive, aerobic culture in transport medium, and anaerobic culture in appropriate transport.

Cross-taxa reasoning at case interpretation drew on the extensive documented literature of bacterial bronchopneumonia in domestic ruminants and captive artiodactyls. The gross pattern of cranioventral consolidation with airway involvement is the classical morphology of ruminant bacterial bronchopneumonia, and the differential is dominated by Mannheimia haemolytica, Pasteurella multocida, Mycoplasma species, and, in some geographic contexts, Bibersteinia trehalosi. Species-specific considerations for captive giraffes include the recognized susceptibility of the species to respiratory stress under cold-weather conditions and the documented incidence of Mycoplasma species in giraffe respiratory disease.

Aerobic culture returned heavy growth of Mannheimia haemolytica from lung and lymph node within 48 hours; anaerobic culture demonstrated no anaerobic bacterial growth. Mycoplasma species-specific polymerase chain reaction was submitted in parallel and returned positive for Mycoplasma bovis-associated sequences, indicating a mixed infection with a bacterial-mycoplasmal component. Histopathology confirmed the gross impression of severe suppurative bronchopneumonia with airway-centered inflammation, and demonstrated the characteristic loss of ciliated epithelium with mucosal necrosis in bronchioles that has been associated with Mycoplasma infection in ruminants. The final morphologic diagnosis was severe cranioventral suppurative bronchopneumonia with bronchiolar epithelial necrosis; the etiologic diagnosis was Mannheimia haemolytica pneumonia with concurrent Mycoplasma infection.

The report was distributed to the collection veterinarian, the collection director, and the pathology archive. Antibiotic susceptibility of the Mannheimia isolate was assessed and reported. Institutional review of the case addressed environmental considerations (ambient temperature at exhibit, ventilation status, exhibit stress factors) as contributing components. The case reinforced the principle that infectious respiratory disease in captive artiodactyls follows the same pattern as domestic ruminant respiratory disease, that species-specific mycoplasma infections should be included in the differential, and that the comparative reasoning framework transports readily from domestic ruminant reference. Cross-taxa reasoning was the interpretive bridge that permitted rapid diagnostic conclusion in an unfamiliar-species case.

THE COMPARATIVE NECROPSY PATTERN SYSTEM — Aspiration Pattern Recognition Across Taxa

The Pattern: Cranioventral to diffuse pulmonary consolidation with identifiable foreign material within airways and, on histopathology, multinucleate foreign body giant cells surrounding aspirated material, indicating aspiration pneumonia.

Cross-Taxa Signature: Recognized across mammals, birds, and reptiles in specific contexts. In captive species, aspiration occurs during anesthetic recovery when protective airway reflexes are impaired, during disease-related regurgitation, during hand-feeding of juvenile animals when technique is inadequate, and during drowning or near-drowning events. In stranded marine mammals, seawater aspiration produces characteristic foamy pulmonary edema. In wildlife recovered from oil spill events, oil aspiration produces distinctive gross and histopathologic findings including oil droplets within airways.

Diagnostic Anchor: Identification of aspirated foreign material within airways on gross examination and multinucleate foreign body giant cells on histopathology surrounding aspirated material. Cranioventral distribution with airway involvement supports the diagnosis.

Trap Logic: The look-alike is primary bacterial bronchopneumonia with similar cranioventral distribution and airway involvement. Discrimination: aspiration demonstrates identifiable foreign material or foreign body giant cell reaction on histopathology; bacterial bronchopneumonia demonstrates neutrophil-rich exudate without foreign body reaction. Aspiration in an anesthetic recovery context may not demonstrate foreign material if aspirated liquid contents were absorbed rapidly.

Zoonotic/Reportable Flag: Aspiration itself is not zoonotic or reportable. Aspiration occurring during handling for regulatory purposes (capture, sampling, transport) requires documentation for institutional review. Oil-spill related aspiration in federally protected species requires coordination with regulatory partners including US Fish and Wildlife Service and NOAA Fisheries.

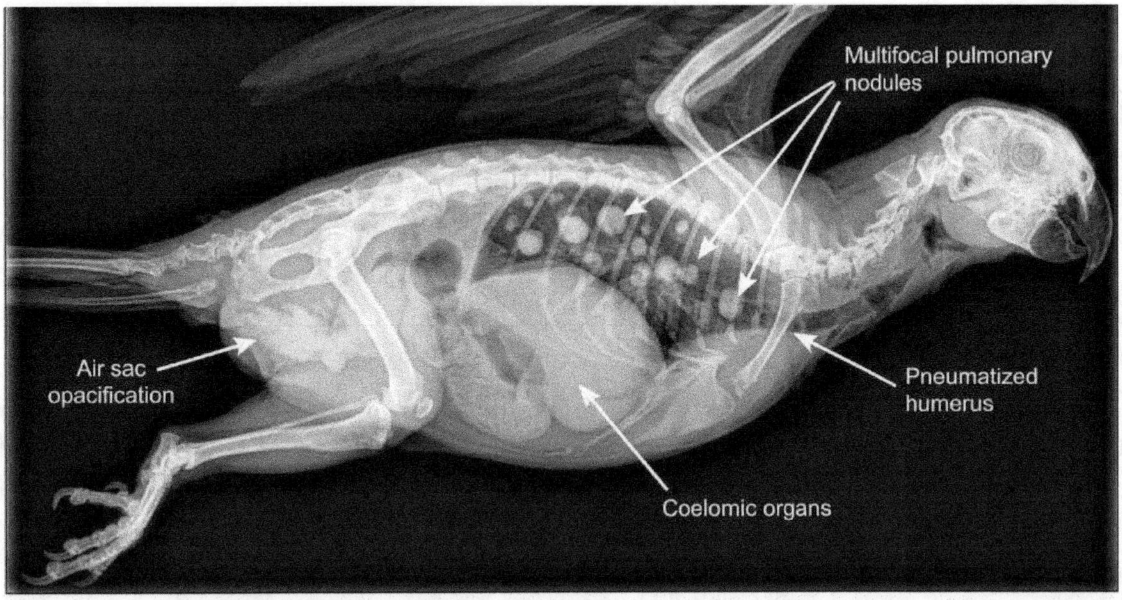

Figure 5.4: Post-Mortem Radiography of Multifocal Pulmonary Nodules in a Captive Psittacine with Aspergillosis.

Pneumonia Pattern	Gross Morphology	Histopathologic Hallmark	Common Etiology Across Taxa	Key Discriminator
Bacterial bronchopneumonia	Cranioventral consolidation with airway exudate	Suppurative inflammation with airway centered distribution	Mannheimia/Pasteurella in ungulates, Streptococcus in primates, E. coli in birds	Neutrophil-rich exudate without foreign material
Interstitial viral pneumonia	Diffuse parenchymal thickening without airway consolidation	Interstitial inflammation with syncytia (morbillivirus) or inclusions (herpesvirus, adenovirus)	Morbillivirus (cetaceans), influenza (mammals), herpesvirus (multiple), adenovirus (psittacines)	Diffuse interstitial distribution with viral inclusions or syncytia
Granulomatous pneumonia	Well-demarcated firm nodules, sometimes cavitary	Epithelioid granulomas with occasional multinucleate giant cells	Mycobacterium species, Aspergillus species, Cryptococcus	Granulomatous architecture with agent-specific stains
Aspiration pneumonia	Cranioventral to diffuse consolidation with foreign	Foreign body giant cells surrounding aspirated material	Anesthetic recovery aspiration, regurgitation,	Identifiable foreign material or foreign body giant cell reaction

	material in airways		drowning, oil-spill aspiration	
Pulmonary mineralization (dystrophic)	Multifocal small firm foci throughout parenchyma	Basophilic mineral deposition confirmed by von Kossa	Chronic dietary imbalance in captive psittacines	Mineral deposition without granulomatous or inflammatory reaction

CLINICAL PEARL: Air sacculitis is often the first sign of avian infectious respiratory disease and is identified during in-situ coelomic examination before organ displacement. Delayed identification after coelomic disruption compromises interpretation because environmental contamination reaches air sac surfaces. In-situ air sac examination is a standard step in every avian necropsy regardless of the anticipated differential.

EVIDENCE: Cetacean morbillivirus outbreaks have produced documented unusual mortality events in bottlenose dolphins across multiple regions, with characteristic multinucleate giant cell interstitial pneumonia as the diagnostic anchor at necropsy. Coordinated surveillance through the NOAA Fisheries Marine Mammal Health and Stranding Response Program has permitted population-level tracking of morbillivirus emergence.

CAUTION: Aspiration during anesthetic recovery may not demonstrate identifiable foreign material at necropsy if aspirated liquid contents were absorbed. The histopathologic finding of neutrophilic bronchopneumonia in an animal recently recovered from anesthesia should be interpreted with aspiration in the differential even without gross foreign material identification, and anesthetic technique review is warranted regardless of specific diagnostic confirmation.

THE COMPARATIVE NECROPSY PATTERN SYSTEM — Chapter 5 Respiratory Pattern Foundations

Faveolar Lung Consolidation Pattern in Reptiles Versus Alveolar Consolidation in Mammals: Firm mucoid consolidation filling faveolar spaces in reptiles versus alveolar hepatization in mammals. Anchor: species-appropriate architectural reference. Trap: normal faveolar architecture misread as consolidation. Flag: reptile mycobacterial and Salmonella pneumonias carry biosafety implications.

Cross-Taxa Bronchopneumonia Pattern Signaling Bacterial Pneumonia: Cranioventral airway-centered consolidation across ungulates, primates, birds, and marine mammals with species-specific etiologic profiles. Anchor: culture of fresh lung tissue with cranioventral distribution. Trap: aspiration pneumonia discriminated by foreign body giant cell reaction. Flag: some bacterial etiologies carry occupational health implications.

Pulmonary Mineralization Pattern in Captive Psittacines: Multifocal firm mineralized foci associated with chronic dietary imbalance and hypervitaminosis D. Anchor: histopathology with von Kossa confirmation. Trap: mineralized granulomas from mycobacterial or fungal disease discriminated by epithelioid architecture. Flag: institutionally reportable for dietary intervention.

Aspiration Pattern Recognition Across Taxa: Cranioventral consolidation with foreign material and foreign body giant cells across anesthetic recovery, regurgitation, drowning, and oil-spill contexts. Anchor: identifiable foreign material or foreign body reaction. Trap: primary bacterial bronchopneumonia discriminated by absent foreign material. Flag: oil-spill aspiration in federally protected species requires regulatory coordination.

Summary and Key Concepts

Comparative respiratory anatomy across taxa includes the avian air sac and parabronchial lung, the reptile faveolar lung, the marine mammal blowhole and diving-adapted lung, and the amphibian and fish respiratory systems; species-appropriate anatomic reference is prerequisite to pathologic interpretation.

Bacterial bronchopneumonia demonstrates a consistent cranioventral airway-centered pattern across taxa with species-specific etiologic profiles requiring appropriate culture and molecular workup.

Interstitial viral pneumonias including morbillivirus in cetaceans, influenza in mammalian spillover, and herpesvirus across multiple taxa demonstrate consistent histopathologic hallmarks including syncytia and viral inclusion bodies.

Granulomatous pneumonias including mycobacterial and fungal disease share gross morphology across taxa; histopathology and agent-specific stains discriminate etiologies.

Non-infectious respiratory disease includes primary and metastatic pulmonary neoplasia, pulmonary mineralization in captive psittacines, pulmonary fibrosis in aged captive species, and species-specific entities including air sac cystadenoma in psittacines.

Aspiration pneumonia, pulmonary trauma, and environmental and toxicologic lung injury each demonstrate characteristic patterns that must be distinguished from primary respiratory disease during interpretation.

CHAPTER 6: HEPATIC PATHOLOGY ACROSS TAXA

Learning Objectives

1. Recognize the major hepatic necrosis patterns across taxa and their species-specific etiologic profiles.
2. Distinguish dietary iron storage disease from hemolytic hemosiderosis, iatrogenic parenteral iron accumulation, and postmortem hemoglobin imbibition artifact.
3. Identify primary and metastatic hepatic neoplasia in non-domestic species with attention to species-specific tumor entities.
4. Interpret hepatobiliary parasitic and infectious disease across taxa with correlation to epidemiologic context.
5. Apply the Comparative Necropsy Pattern callout structure to hepatic lesion recognition across unfamiliar species.
6. Coordinate ancillary hepatic diagnostics including hepatic iron quantitation, hepatic biochemistry biomarkers, and molecular hepatic pathogen panels.

The liver occupies a privileged position in non-domestic species pathology because of its consistent involvement across a wide range of systemic disease processes and because of the interpretive information carried by hepatic lesion morphology alone. A pathologist can reason substantially about the underlying disease process from hepatic gross appearance and histopathologic findings even without antemortem history, and this reasoning is transportable across taxa with species-specific modifications. Multifocal hepatic necrosis in a mammal, in a bird, and in a reptile carries a similar differential list dominated by hematogenous infectious agents; the specific agents differ by taxonomic group, but the interpretive path is the same. Hepatic capsular fibrosis, hepatic congestion, and hepatic mass lesions each carry similar interpretive weight across vertebrate classes.

This chapter organizes hepatic pathology into four operational domains. Hepatic necrosis patterns across non-domestic species are considered by distribution (multifocal, centrilobular, midzonal, periportal, massive) and by associated cellular reaction. Iron storage disease and comparative hemosiderosis address the recurring interpretive challenge of iron-associated hepatic lesions in captive frugivorous primates, black rhinoceros, tapirs, and other predisposed species. Hepatic neoplasia in non-domestic species covers the range from primary hepatocellular and biliary tumors through metastatic disease. Hepatobiliary parasitic and infectious disease completes the chapter with attention to the specific parasitic and infectious differentials that dominate hepatobiliary disease in wildlife and zoo species.

Hepatic Necrosis Patterns Across Non-Domestic Species

Multifocal Random Hepatic Necrosis

Multifocal random hepatic necrosis is characterized by discrete foci of hepatocyte death distributed throughout the parenchyma without a lobular pattern. The distribution reflects hematogenous delivery of the injurious agent through the hepatic arterial and portal circulation. Across vertebrate taxa, the differential for multifocal random hepatic necrosis includes bacterial septicemia with hematogenous seeding, viral infection with hepatic tropism, protozoal infection with hepatic phase, hematogenous fungal infection, hematogenous embolic disease, and ingested hepatotoxin producing acute injury. The gross pattern is remarkably consistent: pale to red-tinged discrete foci ranging typically from 1 to 10 millimeters in diameter, sometimes with a central pale core and hyperemic margin. Histopathology confirms the discrete character with variable inflammatory response depending on the disease process.

The etiologic profile varies by taxonomic group. In carnivores, canine hepatozoonosis-like protozoal disease and infectious canine hepatitis (adenovirus) analogs produce multifocal random necrosis in captive wild carnivore populations. In birds, herpesvirus disease across multiple orders (psittacid herpesvirus 1, Pacheco disease; falconid herpesvirus; owl herpesvirus; falconid adenovirus) produces classical multifocal random necrosis. In reptiles, chelonian herpesvirus 1 and 3, snake herpesvirus, and ranavirus each produce multifocal random necrosis. In elephants, elephant endotheliotropic herpesvirus produces multifocal hepatic and other organ necrosis with prominent vascular involvement. In marine mammals, morbillivirus and herpesvirus disease produce multifocal necrosis as part of systemic disease presentation.

Centrilobular and Zonal Necrosis

Centrilobular necrosis (zone 3 necrosis in the Rappaport nomenclature) is characterized by hepatocyte death around the central vein with sparing of periportal hepatocytes. The pattern reflects the anatomic gradient of hepatic oxygenation and metabolic capacity; centrilobular hepatocytes have the highest cytochrome P450 activity and are consequently most vulnerable to toxicants requiring metabolic activation to a hepatotoxic intermediate. Across taxa, centrilobular necrosis carries a differential dominated by hepatotoxin exposure. Acetaminophen and related analgesic toxicity produce centrilobular necrosis in captive species with iatrogenic exposure. Pyrrolizidine alkaloid toxicity from consumed plants produces centrilobular necrosis with characteristic hepatocellular megalocytosis in exposed grazing species. Aflatoxin toxicity from mycotoxin-contaminated feed produces centrilobular necrosis with associated hepatic biliary hyperplasia and, in chronic exposure, hepatocellular carcinoma development. Chronic hypoxia from cardiovascular disease produces centrilobular necrosis of ischemic origin, distinguished from toxicologic centrilobular necrosis by absence of hepatocellular changes suggestive of metabolic activation and by concurrent cardiovascular disease.

Periportal and Massive Necrosis

Periportal necrosis (zone 1 necrosis) is less common than centrilobular necrosis and reflects toxicants that do not require metabolic activation or that preferentially affect zone 1 hepatocytes. Toxicants producing periportal necrosis include some heavy metals and some plant toxins. Massive necrosis involves the entire lobule with loss of the normal hepatic architecture, and reflects severe hepatocellular insult from any of several causes including acute viral hepatitis progression, toxic exposure with massive dose, and ischemic events with severe systemic compromise. Recognition of the pattern (periportal versus centrilobular versus massive) requires histopathology and provides substantial interpretive direction toward the underlying disease process.

Applied Case: Elephant Endotheliotropic Herpesvirus in a Captive Asian Elephant Calf

A 3-year-old male Asian elephant calf (Elephas maximus) housed in a Species Survival Plan managed collection was found deceased in the barn area during morning check with keepers reporting the calf had been in normal condition at the previous evening's feeding. Antemortem clinical signs had not been documented although the collection team maintained twice-weekly clinical monitoring of elephant calves consistent with published husbandry recommendations for the species. The submission form recorded sudden death without antemortem warning and requested comprehensive workup with attention to elephant endotheliotropic herpesvirus given the age and species predisposition. Elephant endotheliotropic herpesvirus is a documented cause of peracute mortality in captive Asian and African elephant calves, and the coordinated species-level surveillance response required documentation of confirmed and suspected cases through the Elephant Endotheliotropic Herpesvirus Advisory Group and Species Survival Plan structure.

External examination demonstrated appropriate body condition; no external trauma; and moderate volume of clear serous fluid at the trunk consistent with terminal event pulmonary edema. Necropsy was performed by adapted large-mammal technique with the calf positioned in lateral recumbency; systematic organ removal was modified for body size with standardized sampling from anatomically defined sites. Coelomic examination demonstrated moderate volume of serous fluid with fibrin flecks in the peritoneal cavity. Petechial and ecchymotic hemorrhages were prominent on the epicardium, on the serosal surface of the small intestine, and on the pleura. The heart demonstrated moderate volume of pericardial hemorrhage; the myocardium appeared unremarkable on gross examination.

The liver demonstrated the pattern that established the presumptive diagnosis at the necropsy table. Multiple discrete pale foci ranging from 3 to 15 millimeters in diameter were distributed randomly throughout both hepatic lobes; several foci had red-tinged hemorrhagic margins with central pallor consistent with the necrotic-hemorrhagic pattern characteristic of elephant endotheliotropic herpesvirus. Capsular petechiae were numerous. The gross appearance was highly compatible with published descriptions of elephant endotheliotropic herpesvirus hepatic disease and triggered immediate escalation of the diagnostic workup. The tongue, buccal mucosa, and cardiac endocardium demonstrated similar hemorrhagic lesions consistent with the vascular endothelial involvement characteristic of the disease.

Same-day cytology of impression smears from the hepatic necrotic foci demonstrated mixed inflammatory infiltrate with rare intranuclear inclusion bodies in hepatocytes at foci margins. The finding, combined with the gross pattern and species-age combination, was diagnostically compelling before histopathology was available. Fresh tissue was collected for elephant endotheliotropic herpesvirus polymerase chain reaction from liver, heart, tongue, spleen, and blood; for histopathology across a comprehensive panel of tissues; and for the standard elephant necropsy tissue archive maintained through the Species Survival Plan. Real-time polymerase chain reaction targeting the elephant endotheliotropic herpesvirus DNA polymerase gene was submitted to a reference laboratory with expedited turnaround given the case implications.

Histopathology confirmed multifocal random hepatic necrosis with Cowdry type A eosinophilic intranuclear inclusion bodies in hepatocytes and vascular endothelial cells at foci margins. Similar necrotic lesions with vascular endothelial inclusions were present in myocardium, tongue mucosa, and small intestinal serosa. Polymerase chain reaction returned positive for elephant endotheliotropic herpesvirus subtype 1A within 36 hours of submission, confirming the diagnosis and triggering the coordinated species-level response. The final morphologic diagnosis was severe multifocal necrotizing and hemorrhagic hepatitis with intranuclear viral inclusion bodies; systemic vascular endothelial infection with hemorrhage; and terminal event pulmonary edema. The etiologic diagnosis was elephant endotheliotropic herpesvirus subtype 1A.

The institutional response addressed several parallel channels. Individual case reporting to the collection veterinarian, curator, and director occurred within hours of the diagnostic result. Species-level reporting through the Elephant Endotheliotropic Herpesvirus Advisory Group followed the established protocol, contributing to the ongoing surveillance dataset. Herd biosecurity review at the affected collection addressed the exposure risk to other elephants in the herd, and clinical monitoring intensification was implemented for the remaining elephant calves. Necropsy reports were distributed to research collaborators contributing to elephant endotheliotropic herpesvirus vaccine development and to the molecular epidemiology characterization of the virus. The case illustrated the intersection between individual necropsy pathology and species-level conservation medicine that characterizes contemporary zoo pathology practice; the diagnostic finding was consequential not only for the individual case but for the coordinated species-level response to a documented threat to captive elephant populations.

THE COMPARATIVE NECROPSY PATTERN SYSTEM — Multifocal Random Hepatic Necrosis Signaling Systemic Infectious Disease Across Taxa

---

The Pattern: Discrete pale to red-tinged foci of hepatic necrosis distributed randomly throughout the parenchyma, indicating hematogenous delivery of an infectious agent or hematogenous embolic disease.

Cross-Taxa Signature: Recognized across mammals, birds, and reptiles with etiologic profiles varying by taxonomic group. In carnivores, protozoal and adenoviral disease dominates. In birds, herpesvirus disease across orders (psittacid, falconid, owl herpesvirus) and Chlamydia psittaci in psittacines produce classical multifocal necrosis. In reptiles, herpesvirus and ranavirus produce the pattern. In elephants, endotheliotropic herpesvirus produces multifocal necrosis with vascular endothelial involvement. In marine mammals, morbillivirus and herpesvirus produce multifocal necrosis as part of systemic disease. The gross morphology is transportable across taxa; the specific agent requires species-specific ancillary workup.

Diagnostic Anchor: Histopathologic characterization of the necrotic foci for inclusion bodies, agent-specific morphology, and inflammatory response, combined with polymerase chain reaction for taxon-appropriate agent panels. Cowdry type A intranuclear inclusion bodies in hepatocytes at foci margins support herpesvirus etiology; intracytoplasmic viral inclusion bodies support ranavirus etiology in ectothermic vertebrates.

Trap Logic: The look-alike is bacterial hepatic necrosis (particularly Yersinia species in psittacines and elephants, Clostridium piliforme across taxa, Salmonella species in reptiles and birds), which produces multifocal necrosis without viral inclusions but with neutrophil-rich exudate and gram-stainable bacterial organisms visible in tissue. Discrimination: bacterial necrosis demonstrates gram-stainable bacteria and neutrophil-rich response; viral necrosis demonstrates inclusion bodies with lymphocytic response.

Zoonotic/Reportable Flag: Herpes B in macaques with hepatic involvement is a hard-stop biosafety concern. Chlamydia psittaci in psittacines is zoonotic. Bacterial etiologies including Salmonella and Yersinia carry occupational health implications. Elephant endotheliotropic herpesvirus is institutionally reportable at Species Survival Plan facilities.

Figure 6.1: Multifocal Random Hepatic Necrosis in an African Elephant Calf: Herpesvirus-Associated Disease

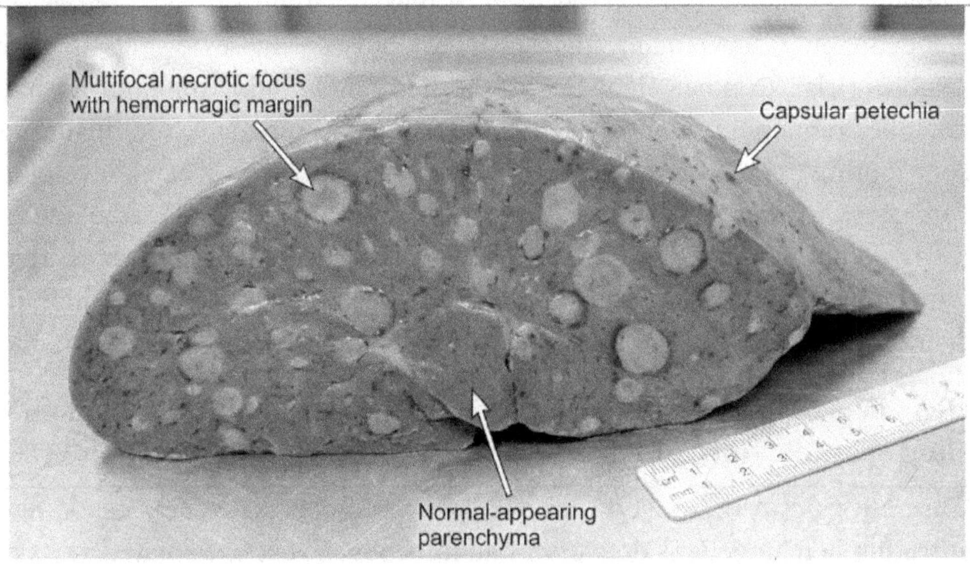

Iron Storage Disease and Comparative Hemosiderosis

Dietary Iron Storage Disease in Captive Populations

Dietary iron storage disease affects captive frugivorous primates (lemurs, marmosets, tamarins, some prosimians), black rhinoceros, tapirs, some frugivorous bats, and several passerine species. The unifying pathogenic feature is chronic dietary iron overload in species with intestinal absorptive machinery adapted to iron-poor natural diets, whose regulatory capacity to downregulate absorption is exceeded by captive diets. The natural diets of these species contain iron predominantly as non-heme iron in low absorbability form; captive diets containing pelleted feed with iron supplementation, iron-fortified fruit substitutes, or iron-supplemented insectivore diets deliver iron in higher absorbability form and at higher total quantity than the species evolved to handle. Chronic iron accumulation in hepatocytes proceeds over years and produces hemosiderin deposition prominently within hepatocyte cytoplasm and periportal Kupffer cells, with a periportal-to-midlobular gradient. Advanced cases demonstrate hepatocellular necrosis, periportal fibrosis, and, in some species, progression to hepatocellular carcinoma with iron association.

Hemolytic and Iatrogenic Hemosiderosis

Hemolytic hemosiderosis is characterized by iron accumulation within macrophages of the reticuloendothelial system with relative sparing of hepatocyte cytoplasm. The gross and histopathologic distribution is dominated by Kupffer cell prominence and by splenic macrophage hemosiderin. Underlying causes include recent hemolytic disease of any etiology (immune-mediated, infectious, mechanical) and recent blood transfusion. Iatrogenic parenteral iron accumulation produces Kupffer cell hemosiderin prominently with hepatocyte involvement only in late stages; the injection history distinguishes iatrogenic from dietary or hemolytic origin.

Hepatic Iron Quantitation and Species-Specific Thresholds

Hepatic iron quantitation provides objective interpretation of hepatic iron status in cases where the histopathologic distinction between physiologic accumulation and pathologic overload is ambiguous. Quantitative methods include atomic absorption spectroscopy and inductively coupled plasma mass spectrometry, both on dry-weight tissue basis. Species-specific reference thresholds are published for black rhinoceros and for a limited number of lemur species; for other species, comparative interpretation against the closest available published data is applied with explicit acknowledgment in the report. The distinction between physiologic iron accumulation (below species-appropriate threshold, without hepatocellular pathology) and pathologic iron overload (above threshold, with associated hepatocellular necrosis and fibrosis) has substantial implications for population-level dietary reformulation at Species Survival Plan facilities and drives management decisions across zoological institutions.

Species-Specific Predisposing Mechanisms and Management Implications

The species-specific predisposition to dietary iron storage disease reflects evolutionary adaptation to natural diets low in bioavailable iron. Frugivorous primates (lemurs, marmosets, tamarins) evolved in tropical habitats where their natural diets consist predominantly of fruits containing iron in low-absorbability non-heme form; the intestinal absorptive machinery of these species does not effectively downregulate iron absorption in the presence of iron surplus because the surplus condition is evolutionarily novel. Black rhinoceros, native to sub-Saharan African savanna and woodland habitats, evolved on browse containing tannins and other compounds that reduce dietary iron bioavailability; the substitution of captive diets lacking these compounds delivers iron in higher effective quantity. Frugivorous bats face similar constraints. In each case, the mechanistic pathway is chronic dietary iron delivery in bioavailable form exceeding the animal's regulatory capacity to downregulate absorption at the enterocyte level.

Population-level management follows from mechanistic understanding. At Species Survival Plan facilities managing affected species, dietary iron content is calculated for the full diet including all components, and iron content of pelleted feeds, fruits, and other diet components is verified through laboratory analysis rather than assumed from published feed composition data. Dietary tannin supplementation from grape pomace, tea powder, or other sources has been used in some captive black rhinoceros programs to reduce dietary iron bioavailability. Serum ferritin and transferrin saturation measurement in living animals permits antemortem monitoring of iron status; species-specific reference ranges are limited but longitudinal individual monitoring provides useful trend data. Reproductive management may consider iron status because reproductive iron demand may protect against tissue overload during periods of high demand. The linkage between necropsy findings, mechanistic understanding, and population-level management is a defining feature of contemporary zoo pathology practice.

THE COMPARATIVE NECROPSY PATTERN SYSTEM — Dietary Iron Storage Disease Pattern in Captive Frugivorous Primates and Perissodactyls

---

The Pattern: Periportal-to-midlobular hepatocyte cytoplasmic hemosiderin with periportal Kupffer cell involvement, in advanced cases accompanied by hepatocellular necrosis and periportal fibrosis, in a captive species with chronic dietary iron exposure.

Cross-Taxa Signature: Recognized in captive frugivorous primates (lemurs, marmosets, tamarins), black rhinoceros, tapirs, frugivorous bats, and some passerine species. The distribution and cellular localization are consistent across affected species; the etiologic profile is unified by chronic dietary iron exposure exceeding species-specific regulatory capacity.

Diagnostic Anchor: Prussian blue (Perls) staining confirms the pigment as ferric iron. Quantitative hepatic iron measurement against species-appropriate reference threshold provides objective distinction between physiologic and pathologic accumulation. Dietary history in the captive setting contextualizes the finding.

Trap Logic: The look-alike is hemolytic hemosiderosis, which produces Kupffer cell hemosiderin prominence with relative hepatocyte sparing. Discrimination: dietary iron storage demonstrates hepatocyte cytoplasmic dominance; hemolytic demonstrates macrophage dominance.

Zoonotic/Reportable Flag: Not zoonotic. Institutionally reportable at Species Survival Plan facilities managing black rhinoceros, lemurs, or other affected species because dietary reformulation is the population-level intervention required to prevent recurrence.

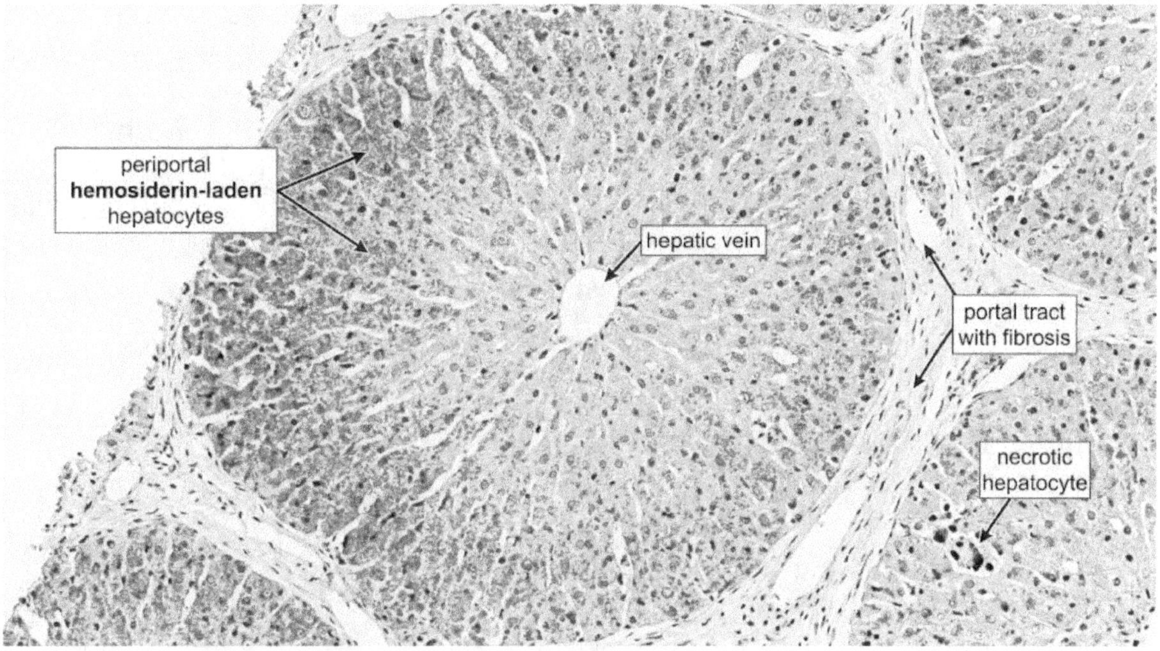

Hepatic Neoplasia in Non-Domestic Species

Primary Hepatocellular and Biliary Neoplasia

Primary hepatocellular carcinoma is documented in captive nonhuman primates, captive avian species (particularly aged psittacines), captive large mammals, and captive reptiles. The gross morphology of hepatocellular carcinoma is variable: solitary large mass, multifocal masses within the hepatic parenchyma, or diffuse infiltrative pattern. Histopathology demonstrates neoplastic hepatocytes with variable trabecular, acinar, or solid growth patterns. Immunohistochemistry with hepatocyte-specific markers (hepatocyte paraffin 1, arginase-1) supports the diagnosis when needed. Biliary tract neoplasms including cholangiocarcinoma and biliary cystadenoma are documented across taxa, with the biliary origin identified by cellular morphology and by immunohistochemistry for biliary markers (cytokeratin 7 in mammals with variable applicability across taxa).

Iron-Associated Hepatocellular Carcinoma

Iron-associated hepatocellular carcinoma has been documented in captive frugivorous primates and other species with chronic dietary iron storage disease. The mechanism involves chronic oxidative injury from iron overload producing cumulative DNA damage and hepatocellular transformation over years. Grossly, iron-associated hepatocellular carcinoma may present as one or more mass lesions in a background of iron storage disease with characteristic diffuse hepatocellular hemosiderin. Histopathologically, the neoplastic hepatocytes may retain iron accumulation, and Prussian blue staining of the tumor demonstrates ferric iron. Recognition of the association informs population-level management of species with dietary iron storage disease and reinforces the case for dietary reformulation.

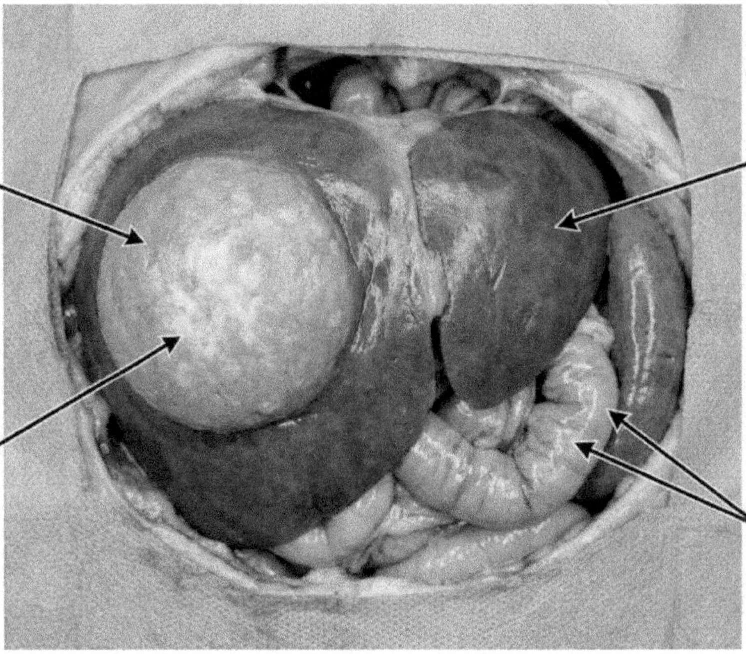

Metastatic Hepatic Disease

Metastatic hepatic disease is common in captive species with primary neoplasms elsewhere in the body. The hepatic distribution of metastatic disease reflects both the portal venous drainage pattern (metastases from gastrointestinal primary tumors) and the hepatic arterial delivery pattern (metastases from other sources). Gross pattern includes multifocal discrete masses of variable size, sometimes with umbilication (central depression) characteristic of some metastatic carcinomas. Histopathology of metastatic disease demonstrates the primary tumor cell type within the hepatic parenchyma; immunohistochemistry with tissue-of-origin markers supports the primary tumor identification when the primary site is not obvious.

Hepatobiliary Parasitic and Infectious Disease

Hepatic Trematode and Cestode Infections

Hepatic trematode infection is prominent across wildlife taxa. Fasciola hepatica and F. gigantica infect wild ruminants, wild suids, and occasionally other mammalian species. The gross pattern includes hepatic capsular thickening with adhesions, hemorrhagic tracts along migration paths in acute infection, and bile duct dilation with thickening in chronic infection. Adult flukes may be recovered from bile ducts. Cestode infection of the liver in wildlife includes hydatid disease (Echinococcus species) with characteristic cystic lesions containing daughter cysts and protoscolices, and, less commonly, other cestode species. Bile duct-associated cestodes and trematodes in wild carnivores include Opisthorchis species and related liver flukes.

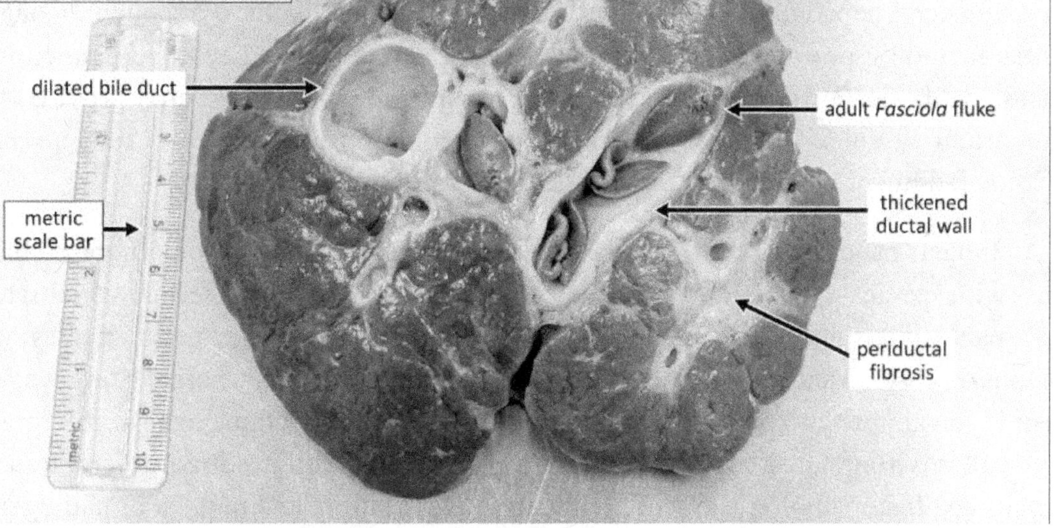

Figure 6.3: Bile Duct Fascioliasis in a Wild White-Tailed Deer: Cut Surface with Adult Flukes

Bacterial Hepatitis and Liver Abscess

Bacterial hepatitis in wildlife includes Yersinia pseudotuberculosis in psittacines, waterfowl, and some mammals producing multifocal necrosis with characteristic gram-negative bacterial rods on tissue Gram stain. Salmonella species produce hepatitis and hepatic granuloma formation in reptiles, birds, and mammals with associated systemic disease. Clostridium piliforme (Tyzzer disease) produces classical periportal hepatic necrosis with characteristic filamentous bacterial organisms within hepatocytes visualized by Warthin-Starry staining. Actinomyces and Fusobacterium species produce hepatic abscessation in some ungulate species.

Viral Hepatitis Across Taxa

Viral hepatitis across taxa includes herpesvirus disease as previously described, adenovirus infections in canid wildlife (canine adenovirus 1, infectious canine hepatitis) with characteristic hepatocellular intranuclear inclusions, and duck viral hepatitis in wild and captive anseriformes producing peracute mortality with characteristic hemorrhagic hepatitis. Reptile-specific hepatitis viruses including reptarenavirus in captive Boidae have been characterized more recently and produce chronic hepatic disease with associated inclusion body disease.

Ancillary Hepatic Diagnostics and Interpretive Integration

Ancillary hepatic diagnostics extend beyond histopathology to include serum or perimortem biochemistry, hepatic iron quantitation, hepatic mineral quantitation for heavy metal analysis, molecular pathogen panels, and hepatic tissue archives for downstream research and reference. Serum hepatic enzyme activities including alanine aminotransferase, aspartate aminotransferase, alkaline phosphatase, and gamma-glutamyltransferase provide functional information about hepatic status; species-specific reference ranges are limited for non-domestic species but longitudinal individual monitoring provides useful data. Serum bile acids provide sensitive information about hepatobiliary function and may reflect chronic hepatic disease that is not yet reflected in enzyme activities. Serum ammonia elevation may accompany advanced hepatic dysfunction with hepatic encephalopathy component. Coagulation profile abnormalities including prolonged prothrombin time reflect advanced hepatic dysfunction with reduced clotting factor synthesis. Perimortem or postmortem serum collection at necropsy provides these data even when antemortem samples were not obtained; species-appropriate reference ranges are applied with explicit acknowledgment of extrapolation.

Molecular pathogen panels for hepatic disease include organism-specific polymerase chain reaction for herpesvirus (with species-appropriate primer selection), ranavirus (in ectothermic vertebrates), Chlamydia species (in psittacines and other predisposed species), and mycobacterial species (in cases with granulomatous disease). Metagenomic sequencing approaches for cases where the target agent is unknown are increasingly available and permit unbiased identification of infectious agents; interpretation requires consideration of environmental contamination and of species-specific normal microbiota. Integration of gross morphology, histopathology, biochemistry, iron quantitation, and molecular pathogen identification into a coherent case narrative is the operative interpretive skill of hepatic pathology; the pathologist's obligation is to construct that narrative from the available data and to acknowledge the uncertainties that remain.

THE COMPARATIVE NECROPSY PATTERN SYSTEM — Bile Duct Trematode Pattern in Wild Ruminants and Wild Carnivores

---

The Pattern: Hepatic capsular thickening with adhesions and, on cut surface, dilated bile ducts with thickened walls containing adult flukes, indicating chronic bile duct trematode infection.

Cross-Taxa Signature: Recognized in wild ruminants and captive artiodactyls with Fasciola hepatica and F. gigantica infection, in wild carnivores with Opisthorchis and Clonorchis species infection, and in some avian species with bile duct-associated trematodes. The gross pattern is unified across species: dilated bile ducts, ductal wall thickening, and adult flukes recoverable from ducts. Hemorrhagic migration tracts in acute infection are recognized in ruminant fascioliasis.

Diagnostic Anchor: Recovery of adult flukes from bile ducts and identification to species based on morphology. Histopathology confirms ductal thickening with variable inflammatory infiltrate and, in chronic infection, biliary hyperplasia and periductal fibrosis.

Trap Logic: The look-alike is chronic biliary hyperplasia of non-parasitic etiology (chronic biliary obstruction, chronic cholangitis of other causes), which produces similar biliary thickening without recoverable parasites. Discrimination: parasitic biliary disease demonstrates recoverable parasites and characteristic parasite-associated inflammatory response; non-parasitic biliary disease demonstrates ductal changes without parasitic organisms.

Zoonotic/Reportable Flag: Fascioliasis has zoonotic potential from consumption of undercooked infected liver or contaminated aquatic vegetation. Opisthorchis and Clonorchis species infections in wild carnivores can indicate presence of the parasite in shared aquatic environments with human recreational or subsistence use.

Applied Case: Hepatic Disease in a Captive Black Rhinoceros

A 32-year-old female black rhinoceros (Diceros bicornis) housed in a Species Survival Plan managed collection had been in progressive decline for 18 months with weight loss, reduced feed intake, and evidence of chronic disease at annual physical examinations. Antemortem hepatic biochemistry demonstrated moderately elevated hepatic enzyme activities. Antemortem imaging was limited by species and body size. The animal was ultimately humanely euthanized for progressive quality of life decline. Necropsy focused on hepatic pathology given the antemortem findings and the well-recognized species predisposition to iron storage disease.

Coelomic necropsy demonstrated a moderately enlarged liver with markedly increased firmness on palpation. Cut surface demonstrated diffuse brown-orange discoloration of the parenchyma with prominent periportal fibrosis visible as pale linear patterns radiating from portal regions. Two discrete pale masses of 4 and 7 centimeters diameter were identified within the parenchyma with a hepatocellular appearance grossly. Regional lymph nodes were not enlarged. The remainder of the coelomic examination was consistent with age-related change without additional major findings.

Sample collection focused on the hepatic pathology. Multiple representative sections were formalin-fixed for histopathology; fresh-frozen samples were collected for hepatic iron quantitation and for molecular workup; the mass lesions were sampled for histopathology, cytology, and additional iron quantitation. Histopathology confirmed diffuse severe dietary iron storage disease with hepatocyte cytoplasmic hemosiderin, prominent periportal fibrosis extending to bridging fibrosis in some regions, hepatocellular necrosis, and biliary hyperplasia. The mass lesions demonstrated hepatocellular carcinoma with retained hepatocellular iron accumulation, consistent with iron-associated hepatocellular carcinoma. Hepatic iron quantitation by inductively coupled plasma mass spectrometry returned a value substantially above the published reference threshold for black rhinoceros, confirming pathologic overload.

Institutional response addressed the case at multiple levels. The individual case reinforced the established management principle that captive black rhinoceros dietary iron content requires ongoing management to prevent iron storage disease. The finding of iron-associated hepatocellular carcinoma in this individual added to the population-level surveillance data supporting the association. Dietary review at the institution was renewed with attention to iron content in the offered diet including all components, and cross-institutional coordination through the Species Survival Plan supported similar review at partner facilities. The case demonstrated how zoo pathology contributes to species-level conservation management: individual necropsy findings inform population-level dietary and health management, and coordinated surveillance across institutions permits detection of population-level trends that no single case can establish.

Multifocal Random Hepatic Necrosis Signaling Systemic Infectious Disease Across Taxa: Discrete random hepatic necrotic foci indicating hematogenous infectious agent across mammals, birds, and reptiles. Anchor: histopathologic characterization for inclusions and agent-specific morphology. Trap: bacterial necrosis discriminated by neutrophil-rich response and gram-stainable organisms. Flag: herpes B, elephant endotheliotropic herpesvirus, and Chlamydia psittaci carry zoonotic or institutional reporting implications.

Dietary Iron Storage Disease Pattern in Captive Frugivorous Primates and Perissodactyls: Periportal-to-midlobular hepatocyte hemosiderin with fibrosis in captive species with chronic dietary iron exposure. Anchor: Prussian blue confirmation with quantitative iron measurement against species-appropriate threshold. Trap: hemolytic hemosiderosis discriminated by Kupffer cell dominance. Flag: institutionally reportable at SSP facilities for dietary intervention.

Bile Duct Trematode Pattern in Wild Ruminants and Wild Carnivores: Bile duct dilation with wall thickening and recoverable adult flukes across ruminants, carnivores, and some birds. Anchor: parasite recovery with morphologic identification. Trap: non-parasitic biliary hyperplasia discriminated by absent parasites. Flag: fascioliasis has zoonotic potential from undercooked infected liver consumption.

Summary and Key Concepts

Hepatic necrosis patterns across taxa are interpreted by distribution (multifocal random, centrilobular, periportal, massive) with each distribution constraining the etiologic differential in transportable ways across taxonomic groups.

Multifocal random hepatic necrosis reflects hematogenous infectious agents with etiologic profiles varying by taxonomic group but a unified interpretive path from morphology to differential to ancillary workup.

Dietary iron storage disease affects captive frugivorous primates, black rhinoceros, tapirs, and other species with dietary regulatory capacity exceeded by captive diets; species-appropriate iron quantitation thresholds distinguish physiologic from pathologic accumulation.

Iron-associated hepatocellular carcinoma has been documented in captive species with chronic dietary iron storage disease, reinforcing the case for dietary reformulation and population-level management.

Hepatic neoplasia in non-domestic species includes primary hepatocellular carcinoma, biliary tract neoplasms, iron-associated hepatocellular carcinoma, and metastatic disease with recognition patterns transportable across taxa.

Hepatobiliary parasitic and infectious disease includes trematode and cestode infections.

CHAPTER 7: RENAL AND URINARY TRACT PATHOLOGY

Learning Objectives

1. Interpret comparative renal anatomic variation across taxa as it modifies pathologic interpretation.
2. Recognize the major nephropathy patterns in non-domestic species and their species-specific etiologic profiles.
3. Distinguish visceral gout, articular gout, renal urate tubular deposition, and postmortem urate artifact in uricotelic species.
4. Identify urinary tract neoplasia and traumatic urinary tract injury in non-domestic species.
5. Apply the Comparative Necropsy Pattern callout structure to renal and urinary tract lesion recognition across unfamiliar species.
6. Coordinate ancillary renal diagnostics including urinalysis at necropsy, renal biomarker analysis, and renal molecular pathogen panels.

Renal and urinary tract pathology in non-domestic species requires interpretive frames that vary substantially across taxonomic groups. The uricotelic strategy of birds and reptiles (excretion of nitrogen predominantly as insoluble urate) produces disease patterns absent from mammalian pathology: visceral gout, articular gout, and renal urate tubular deposition are recognizable across avian and reptile taxa but have no direct mammalian analog. The mammalian ureotelic strategy (nitrogen excretion as soluble urea) produces the familiar spectrum of glomerular, tubular, and interstitial disease. Fish osmoregulatory demands modify renal anatomy and disease patterns. The pathologist working across taxa must recognize the physiologic strategy before applying interpretive reasoning to renal lesions.

This chapter organizes renal and urinary tract pathology into four operational domains. Renal anatomy variation across taxa provides the interpretive frame; without species-appropriate anatomic reference, lesion interpretation fails. Nephropathies in non-domestic species address glomerular, tubular, and interstitial disease with attention to species-specific etiologies. Gout and uric acid deposition disease covers the uricotelic strategy diseases prominent in birds and reptiles. Urinary tract neoplasia and trauma complete the chapter with attention to the range of non-inflammatory lower urinary tract disease.

Renal Anatomy Variation Across Taxa

Mammalian Renal Anatomy and Species-Specific Variation

The mammalian kidney is characterized by a metanephric organization with cortical and medullary zones, glomeruli concentrated in the cortex, and a variable degree of medullary papillary development that determines urine concentration capacity. Species with strong urine concentration ability (desert-adapted rodents, some carnivores) demonstrate deep medullary papillae with substantial Henle loop length; species with lower concentration demand (fish-eating aquatic mammals) demonstrate shallower papillary development. Multi-lobar kidneys with distinct external lobation are characteristic of ursids, pinnipeds, cetaceans, and some other taxa; the reniculate kidney of cetaceans and pinnipeds consists of numerous small renal units (reniculi) each with its own cortex, medulla, and collecting system, creating an interpretive frame that differs substantially from unilobular mammalian kidneys. Recognition of reniculate architecture as normal is essential; interpretation of a reniculate cetacean kidney against a unilobular reference will produce systematic misinterpretation.

Avian Renal Anatomy

Avian kidneys are elongated structures embedded in the synsacrum with three lobes (cranial, middle, caudal) and a mixed nephron population combining reptile-type nephrons (short loops without Henle organization) and mammalian-type nephrons (longer loops with Henle organization). Urine concentration capacity in birds is generally lower than in mammals; the mammalian-type nephron population supports the concentration ability that exists. Urate excretion occurs through active tubular secretion in addition to glomerular filtration, and urate can precipitate within tubules under conditions of dehydration, obstruction, or hyperuricemia. Recognition of the avian nephron mixture is prerequisite to histopathologic interpretation of avian renal disease.

Reptile Renal Anatomy

Reptile kidneys are elongated paired structures typically located in the caudal coelom or associated with the pelvic canal in some species. The reptile nephron lacks the Henle loop organization of the mammalian nephron; urine concentration capacity is consequently limited, and reptiles rely on cloacal water reabsorption, bladder water storage (in species with bladders), and salt gland function (in species with salt glands) for osmoregulation. Uric acid excretion is the dominant nitrogen strategy and, similarly to birds, urate precipitation within tubules is a recurring finding in dehydrated or hyperuricemic animals. Sexual segments of the renal tubule (in males) produce secretions relevant to reproductive function; recognition of these normal structures as sexual dimorphism rather than as pathology is important.

Fish Renal Anatomy

Fish kidneys serve dual excretory and hematopoietic functions. The head kidney (pronephros in teleosts) is a lymphohematopoietic organ analogous to bone marrow and lymphoid tissue in higher vertebrates, without a significant excretory role in adult teleosts. The posterior kidney (mesonephros) performs the excretory function. Freshwater teleosts face constant water influx and produce copious dilute urine with active reabsorption of solutes; marine teleosts face constant water loss and produce small volumes of urine concentrated to isotonicity with plasma. Elasmobranchs employ urea retention as an osmoregulatory strategy, maintaining plasma urea at concentrations that would be pathologic in mammals. Recognition of these physiologic strategies is prerequisite to interpretation of fish renal biochemistry and pathology.

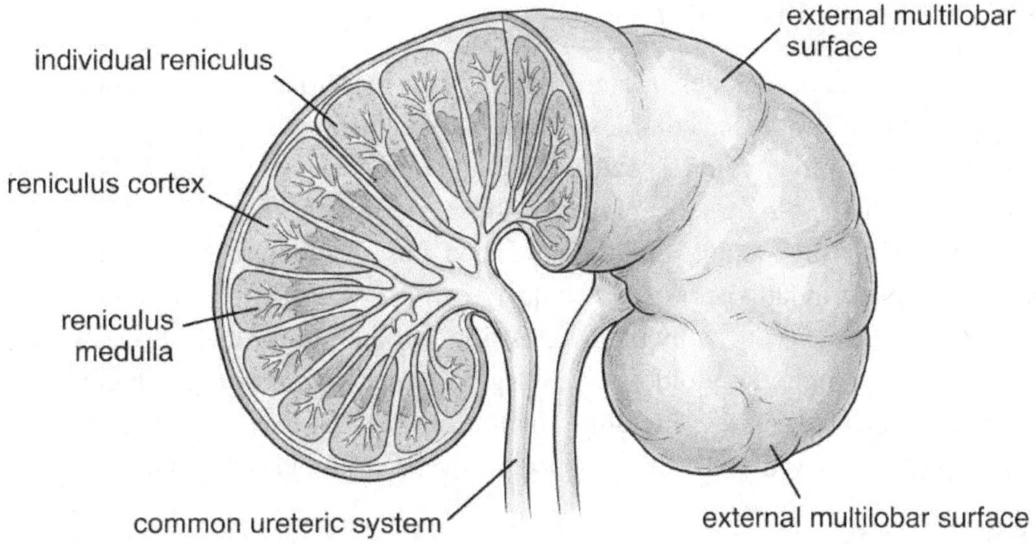

THE COMPARATIVE NECROPSY PATTERN SYSTEM — Reniculate Kidney Architecture Recognition in Marine Mammal Necropsy

---

The Pattern: The reniculate (multi-lobar) kidney architecture of cetaceans and pinnipeds, consisting of numerous small renal units (reniculi) each with independent cortex, medulla, and collecting system, recognized as normal anatomy before pathologic interpretation is applied.

Cross-Taxa Signature: Recognized in cetaceans (dolphins, whales, porpoises), pinnipeds (seals, sea lions, walruses), and, in modified form, in ursids. The number of reniculi varies by species and by body size; a single adult cetacean kidney may contain hundreds of individual reniculi. Each reniculus drains through a small collecting duct to the ureteric system. Disease processes that affect multiple reniculi produce lesions distributed across the renal parenchyma; processes affecting a single reniculus produce localized lesions that would be interpreted as multifocal in a unilobular kidney.

Diagnostic Anchor: Anatomic reference to reniculate architecture before applying pathologic interpretation. Systematic sampling from multiple reniculi during necropsy provides representative tissue for histopathologic characterization.

Trap Logic: The look-alike is generalized multifocal renal disease misinterpreted as a diffuse process, or single-reniculus disease misinterpreted as multifocal disease. Discrimination: recognition of the reniculate anatomy permits appropriate interpretation of lesion distribution as it relates to individual reniculi versus generalized process.

Zoonotic/Reportable Flag: Reniculate architecture is not itself infectious or reportable. Recognition matters because misinterpretation of the anatomy produces systematic error in marine mammal renal pathology reporting.

Nephropathies in Non-Domestic Species

Glomerular Disease Across Taxa

Glomerular disease across taxa includes immune complex glomerulonephritis, amyloidosis, and species-specific glomerulopathies. Immune complex glomerulonephritis has been documented in captive nonhuman primates, in captive avian species, and in some captive reptiles. The lesion pattern is comparable to mammalian glomerulonephritis with variable degrees of mesangial proliferation, glomerular capillary wall thickening, and, in advanced cases, glomerular sclerosis. Amyloidosis is prominent in some captive avian species (particularly captive waterfowl and some psittacines) and in captive nonhuman primates, with amyloid deposition producing glomerular basement membrane thickening and, in systemic amyloidosis, extraglomerular renal involvement. Species-specific glomerulopathies documented in the literature include some captive rodent glomerulopathies with distinctive morphology and some captive avian species-specific glomerular disease.

Tubulointerstitial Disease

Tubulointerstitial disease covers a range of processes affecting the tubular epithelium and interstitial tissue. Toxic nephropathy is prominent across captive and free-ranging species. Aminoglycoside toxicity, contrast media nephropathy, and heavy metal toxicity produce characteristic tubular epithelial necrosis with the specific tubular segment predominantly affected varying by the toxicant. Ethylene glycol toxicity produces characteristic calcium oxalate crystal deposition within tubules and is documented in accidental exposure cases in wildlife. Ochratoxin nephropathy from mycotoxin-contaminated feed produces distinctive tubular changes. Infectious nephropathy including leptospirosis in wildlife carnivores, tuberculosis with renal granuloma formation, and viral nephritis (adenovirus in reptiles, herpesvirus in some avian species) produces recognizable lesion patterns. Interstitial nephritis of unknown etiology is a recurring diagnosis in aged captive species.

Acute Kidney Injury and Chronic Kidney Disease

Acute kidney injury in non-domestic species reflects the same range of underlying processes as in domestic species: prerenal (volume depletion, hemodynamic compromise), intrinsic renal (toxic, ischemic, glomerular, tubulointerstitial), and postrenal (urinary tract obstruction). The histopathologic hallmarks of acute tubular injury including tubular epithelial swelling, tubular epithelial detachment, and intraluminal cellular debris are transportable across mammalian species with modifications for avian and reptile tubular architecture. Chronic kidney disease produces progressive tubulointerstitial fibrosis, glomerular sclerosis, and, in end-stage disease, the small firm shrunken kidney characteristic of end-stage renal disease across taxa. Species-specific chronic kidney disease predispositions include captive felid chronic kidney disease at high prevalence, aged captive nonhuman primate chronic kidney disease, and captive avian species chronic renal disease.

Applied Case: Amyloidosis in a Captive Cheetah With Chronic Kidney Disease

An 11-year-old female cheetah (Acinonyx jubatus) housed in a Species Survival Plan managed collection had been under veterinary care for six months for progressive weight loss, polyuria and polydipsia, and reduced appetite. Antemortem workup identified chronic kidney disease with elevated serum creatinine and blood urea nitrogen, moderate anemia consistent with chronic kidney disease, and moderate proteinuria on urinalysis. The proteinuria was a distinctive feature suggesting glomerular contribution to the renal disease process, and workup for amyloidosis was included in the differential given the well-documented predisposition of captive cheetahs to systemic AA amyloidosis. Renal biopsy under anesthesia was declined for animal welfare reasons; supportive management was maintained until humane euthanasia for progressive quality of life decline.

Coelomic necropsy demonstrated moderately enlarged, firm, waxy-appearing kidneys with a pale tan color and prominent lardaceous appearance on cut surface — the classical gross appearance of amyloidosis. The kidneys were surprisingly enlarged rather than the shrunken small firm kidneys of chronic tubulointerstitial nephritis, and the color change was characteristic. Concurrent findings included splenic enlargement with similar pale waxy appearance suggesting splenic amyloid deposition, mild hepatic capsular thickening with waxy appearance suggesting hepatic amyloid deposition, and adrenal enlargement with waxy appearance suggesting adrenal amyloid deposition. The pattern of multi-organ waxy enlargement was highly consistent with systemic AA amyloidosis, a well-recognized entity in captive cheetahs.

Cross-taxa reasoning at case interpretation drew on the extensive documented literature of captive cheetah amyloidosis. Systemic AA amyloidosis is documented in captive cheetahs at high prevalence and reflects chronic serum amyloid A protein elevation that has been associated with chronic inflammatory processes, potential horizontal transmission of amyloid fibrils, and species-specific predisposition. The disease has been the subject of extensive research including molecular characterization of the amyloid A protein sequence variants in cheetahs, epidemiological studies of the disease across captive populations, and intervention studies with anti-amyloid therapies. The finding in this individual added to the population-level surveillance dataset and reinforced the pattern well recognized in the species.

Histopathology confirmed the gross impression. Congo red staining of renal sections demonstrated apple-green birefringence under polarized light consistent with amyloid deposition, with amyloid predominantly localized to glomerular basement membranes and to the mesangium with extraglomerular medullary and interstitial deposition. Immunohistochemistry with anti-serum amyloid A antibody confirmed the AA (secondary or reactive) amyloid type. Similar amyloid deposition was demonstrated in spleen, liver, and adrenal. The final morphologic diagnosis was severe systemic AA amyloidosis with prominent renal, splenic, hepatic, and adrenal involvement, chronic kidney disease of secondary amyloidosis origin, and moderate anemia of chronic disease. The etiologic diagnosis was systemic AA amyloidosis characteristic of the well-documented captive cheetah disease phenotype.

Institutional response addressed the individual case and species-level implications. Distribution of the report followed the standard pathway with additional distribution to the Species Survival Plan coordinator and to the coordinated cheetah amyloidosis research programs. Fresh-frozen tissue was archived for potential downstream research use consistent with institutional protocols. The case reinforced the species-specific amyloidosis predisposition and contributed to the ongoing population-level surveillance for the disease. Comparative reasoning at case interpretation was again the interpretive bridge: the amyloidosis morphology was recognizable against the extensive human and domestic species amyloidosis literature; the Congo red apple-green birefringence and immunohistochemical characterization were transportable across species; the species-specific epidemiologic profile drove the clinical suspicion at antemortem workup and the interpretive weight granted at necropsy.

Ancillary Renal Diagnostics at Necropsy

Ancillary renal diagnostics at necropsy include urinalysis on bladder urine when available, renal biomarker analysis on perimortem serum, molecular renal pathogen panels where infectious etiology is suspected, and renal tissue archives for downstream research and reference. Postmortem urinalysis provides information about the urinary concentration, cellularity, protein content, and crystal presence at the time of death; abnormal findings including proteinuria, hematuria, and pathologic crystalluria support renal disease workup direction. Renal biomarker analysis on perimortem serum can include creatinine, blood urea nitrogen, symmetric dimethylarginine (an emerging marker of renal function), and serum ferritin or transferrin saturation when iron-associated renal disease is in the differential. Species-specific reference ranges for these biomarkers are limited in non-domestic species; comparative reference against the closest available species-specific data is applied with explicit acknowledgment of extrapolation.

THE COMPARATIVE NECROPSY PATTERN SYSTEM — Ethylene Glycol Toxicosis Pattern Across Wildlife Carnivores

The Pattern: Renal cortical and medullary tubular calcium oxalate crystal deposition with associated tubular epithelial necrosis in a wildlife carnivore, indicating ethylene glycol toxicosis from environmental exposure to antifreeze.

Cross-Taxa Signature: Recognized across wild carnivores with accidental antifreeze exposure. The gross pattern includes pale, mottled, sometimes edematous kidneys with variable degrees of hemorrhage; the histopathologic hallmark is the presence of refractile birefringent calcium oxalate crystals within tubular lumens, distributed throughout the cortex and medulla with concentration in the corticomedullary region. The crystal morphology (rosettes, sheaves, or fan-shaped clusters) is distinctive under polarized light. The pattern is documented in wild carnivores of many species with environmental exposure and is a recurring diagnosis in urban and suburban wildlife populations.

Diagnostic Anchor: Histopathologic identification of calcium oxalate crystals within renal tubules under polarized light. Ethylene glycol or ethylene glycol metabolite (glycolic acid, oxalic acid) quantitation in serum, urine, or fresh tissue confirms the toxicant.

Trap Logic: The look-alike is dietary oxalate nephropathy from consumed plant material (oxalate-containing plants), which produces similar crystal deposition without ethylene glycol exposure. Discrimination: environmental exposure history and toxicant quantitation distinguish the two; the dietary source may leave identifiable plant material in the gastrointestinal tract.

Zoonotic/Reportable Flag: Not zoonotic. Environmental exposure to antifreeze in wildlife may indicate improperly disposed or accessible antifreeze source; coordination with state wildlife authorities and, where relevant, environmental agencies supports source identification and mitigation.

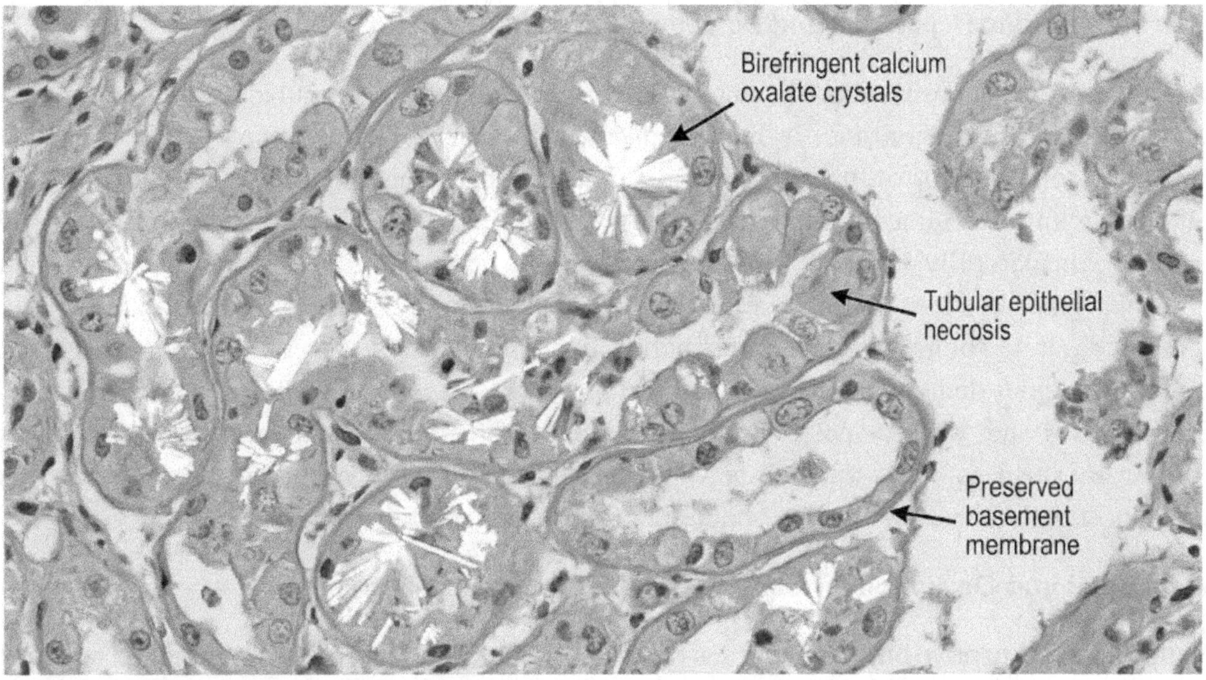

Gout and Uric Acid Deposition Disease

Visceral Gout in Birds and Reptiles

Visceral gout is characterized by deposition of urate crystals on the serosal surfaces of coelomic viscera, most prominently the pericardial surface, hepatic capsule, splenic capsule, and mesenteric surfaces. The condition reflects hyperuricemia sufficient to exceed the solubility limit of uric acid at physiologic conditions, driving crystal deposition on cool serosal surfaces where solubility is reduced. The gross pattern is highly recognizable: chalky white to yellow-white granular material adherent to serosal surfaces, sometimes coalescing to plaque-like deposits and, in advanced cases, producing serosal thickening and adhesions. Visceral gout in birds is documented across orders and reflects underlying renal disease, chronic dehydration, or dietary factors including chronic dietary protein excess. Visceral gout in reptiles is similarly documented across orders and reflects the same underlying processes.

Articular Gout and Tophi

Articular gout is characterized by deposition of urate crystals within joint spaces and periarticular tissues, producing swelling, pain, and reduced mobility antemortem. Grossly, articular gout demonstrates white to yellow-white chalky material within joint spaces and, in advanced cases, tophaceous nodules of urate accumulation in periarticular subcutaneous tissue. The condition is documented in birds and reptiles and reflects chronic hyperuricemia. Antemortem clinical presentation with progressive lameness in a captive avian or reptile species should prompt workup for articular gout among other differentials.

Renal Urate Tubular Deposition and Postmortem Urate Artifact

Renal urate tubular deposition is characterized by urate crystal accumulation within renal tubules, producing tubular obstruction and, in advanced cases, tubular epithelial necrosis. The condition may accompany visceral gout or occur independently. The histopathologic hallmark is the presence of urate crystals within tubular lumens, best appreciated on tissue fixed in non-aqueous fixative (alcohol, methanol) or on carefully handled formalin-fixed tissue because urate crystals dissolve in aqueous formalin over time. Postmortem urate artifact is the deposition of urate on serosal surfaces after death from continued urate solubility change; distinction from antemortem visceral gout requires recognition that antemortem gout demonstrates associated inflammatory response with foreign body giant cells and reactive fibrous tissue, whereas postmortem artifact does not. In cases with sudden death and coelomic urate on serosal surfaces, the distinction between antemortem visceral gout and postmortem artifact may not be diagnostically consequential but should be acknowledged in the report.

Environmental and Occupational Contributors to Uricotelic Disease

Uricotelic disease in captive birds and reptiles frequently reflects modifiable environmental and husbandry factors that produce chronic dehydration, chronic hyperuricemia, or both. Enclosure humidity, water availability, and thermal gradients each modify hydration status, and species-specific husbandry requirements must be met to prevent chronic subclinical dehydration that contributes to gout development. Dietary protein content, particularly in reptile diets containing high-protein invertebrate or vertebrate prey, may drive chronic hyperuricemia if intake exceeds the species' processing capacity. Vitamin A status modifies renal epithelial integrity, and vitamin A deficiency has been associated with renal disease and secondary hyperuricemia in some captive species. The pathologist reporting a case of visceral gout considers these environmental and dietary contributors and communicates the findings to the collection team for husbandry review; the individual necropsy finding often has population-level implications for other individuals of the species in the same collection.

Postmortem Recognition and Interpretive Limits

Postmortem recognition of urate deposition in birds and reptiles is straightforward when clear inflammatory response accompanies the deposition; without inflammatory response, distinction between antemortem visceral gout and postmortem urate artifact is more difficult. Postmortem urate deposition reflects the continued solubility change of urate after death, particularly on cool serosal surfaces. Freeze-thaw handling of carcasses may alter the appearance of both antemortem and postmortem urate. Formalin fixation dissolves urate over time, particularly with prolonged fixation in aqueous formalin; tissue destined for definitive characterization of urate deposition is fixed in non-aqueous fixative (alcohol) or is examined promptly after formalin fixation. Recognition of these interpretive limits is included in the necropsy report when the distinction between antemortem gout and postmortem artifact carries interpretive weight for the case.

Figure 7.3: Visceral Gout in a Captive Iguana: Serosal Urate Deposition at Coelomic Examination

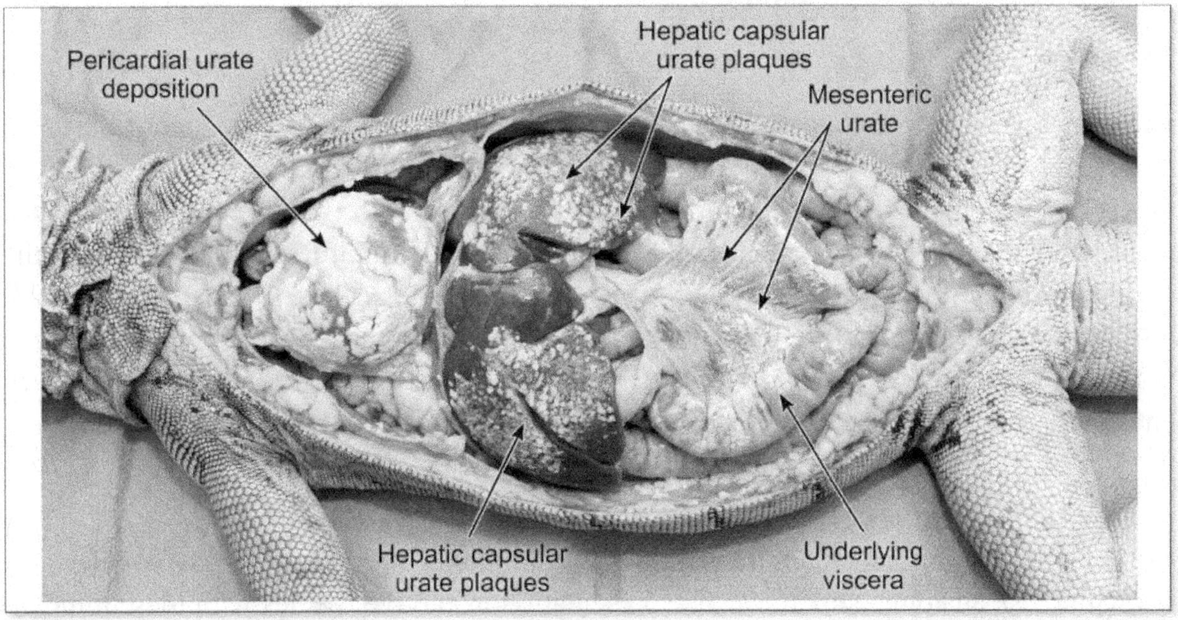

THE COMPARATIVE NECROPSY PATTERN SYSTEM — Visceral Gout Pattern in Captive Birds and Reptiles

---

The Pattern: Chalky white to yellow-white granular urate deposition on coelomic serosal surfaces (pericardial, hepatic, splenic capsules and mesentery) in captive birds or reptiles, indicating hyperuricemia with tissue urate deposition.

Cross-Taxa Signature: Recognized across avian orders (psittacines, waterfowl, gallinaceous birds, raptors, ratites) and across reptile orders (chelonians, squamates, crocodilians). The gross morphology is highly consistent across taxa; the etiologic profile includes chronic dehydration, primary renal disease, dietary protein excess in some captive settings, and vitamin A deficiency-associated renal disease. In each taxonomic group, the visceral gout reflects hyperuricemia that has been chronic or severe enough to exceed urate solubility at physiologic conditions.

Diagnostic Anchor: Gross recognition of chalky urate deposition on serosal surfaces confirmed by histopathology demonstrating urate crystals with associated inflammatory response including foreign body giant cells; polarized light demonstrates birefringent needle-shaped crystals characteristic of urate.

Trap Logic: The look-alike is postmortem urate artifact from urate solubility change after death without antemortem hyperuricemia. Discrimination: antemortem visceral gout demonstrates associated inflammatory response with foreign body giant cells and reactive fibrous tissue; postmortem artifact does not. The distinction may be difficult in cases with sudden death and minimal postmortem interval.

Zoonotic/Reportable Flag: Not zoonotic. Institutionally reportable at collections managing affected species for husbandry review addressing dehydration risk, dietary protein content, and vitamin A status.

Urinary Tract Neoplasia and Trauma

Renal Neoplasia

Primary renal neoplasia in non-domestic species includes renal cell carcinoma, transitional cell carcinoma of the renal pelvis, renal adenoma, and, in some captive species, embryonal renal neoplasms. Renal cell carcinoma is documented in captive nonhuman primates, captive large felids, captive avian species, and captive reptiles. The gross pattern includes solitary or occasionally multifocal mass lesions with variable degrees of hemorrhage, necrosis, and cystic change. Histopathology demonstrates neoplastic epithelial cells with variable growth patterns; immunohistochemistry with renal cell carcinoma-specific markers supports the diagnosis when needed. Metastatic renal disease from primary neoplasms elsewhere is documented across taxa with the renal distribution reflecting hematogenous delivery pattern.

Lower Urinary Tract Disease

Lower urinary tract neoplasia includes transitional cell carcinoma of the ureter, urinary bladder, or urethra in species with these anatomic structures. The presentation in captive species with these tumors includes hematuria, dysuria, and progressive obstructive uropathy. Non-neoplastic lower urinary tract disease includes urolithiasis with species-specific stone composition (struvite, urate, oxalate) and, in some species, chronic cystitis. Reptiles with bladders (some chelonian and some squamate species) may develop bladder pathology comparable to mammalian bladder disease with species-specific modifications. Cloacal pathology in birds and reptiles includes prolapse, neoplasia, and infectious disease as recurring recognitions.

Traumatic Urinary Tract Injury

Traumatic urinary tract injury reflects the mechanisms of trauma the animal has been exposed to. Vehicular collision may produce renal contusion, renal laceration, ureteral disruption, or bladder rupture. Projectile injury may produce renal or ureteric injury along the projectile path. Falls and blunt trauma produce renal contusion. Iatrogenic trauma from surgical or diagnostic procedures is recognized in captive settings. Traumatic urinary tract injury with disruption of urinary tract integrity produces peritoneal urine accumulation (uroperitoneum) with characteristic ascites and, in cases with delayed recognition, secondary chemical peritonitis. Recognition of the mechanism-appropriate injury pattern supports the necropsy interpretation.

Applied Case: Chronic Kidney Disease in an Aged Captive Amur Leopard

A 17-year-old female Amur leopard (Panthera pardus orientalis) housed in a Species Survival Plan managed collection had been under increasing veterinary care for approximately 18 months for progressive weight loss, polyuria, polydipsia, and reduced appetite. Antemortem workup had identified chronic kidney disease based on elevated serum creatinine and blood urea nitrogen, mild anemia, and hypertensive changes on retinal examination. Supportive management with dietary modification and medication had been implemented. The animal was ultimately humanely euthanized after progressive quality of life decline. Necropsy focused on characterization of the renal disease and identification of contributing or coincident conditions.

Coelomic necropsy demonstrated bilateral small, firm, irregular kidneys with reduced size compared to expected reference; the renal capsules were adherent to the underlying parenchyma; cut surface demonstrated loss of the normal corticomedullary distinction with pale patchy parenchymal changes throughout. Concurrent findings included moderate atherosclerotic change in coronary arteries and mild left ventricular hypertrophy consistent with hypertensive change; both findings supported the antemortem impression of hypertension secondary to chronic kidney disease. The remainder of the necropsy was consistent with age-related change without additional major primary disease.

Cross-taxa reasoning at case interpretation drew on the extensive documented literature of chronic kidney disease in aged domestic and non-domestic felids. Chronic kidney disease is a leading cause of morbidity and mortality in aged captive large felids and reflects the same range of underlying processes documented in aged domestic felids: chronic tubulointerstitial fibrosis of multifactorial origin, glomerulosclerosis, and end-stage kidney disease with the small firm irregular kidney characteristic of the process. Species-specific considerations for captive large felids include documented predisposition of certain lineages to chronic renal disease and the potential contribution of captive diet composition to progression.

Histopathology confirmed severe chronic tubulointerstitial nephritis with tubular loss, interstitial fibrosis, and residual tubular ectasia; glomerular sclerosis was prominent with globally sclerotic glomeruli intermixed with hypertrophic glomeruli in a pattern consistent with end-stage kidney disease. No infectious agents were identified. No neoplastic process was identified. The final morphologic diagnosis was severe bilateral chronic tubulointerstitial nephritis with glomerulosclerosis and end-stage kidney disease. Concurrent morphologic diagnoses included moderate coronary atherosclerosis and mild hypertensive left ventricular hypertrophy. The etiologic diagnosis was chronic kidney disease of multifactorial origin with hypertensive cardiovascular consequences.

The institutional response addressed both the individual case and population-level considerations. The report was distributed to the collection veterinarian and to the Species Survival Plan coordinator for Amur leopards. Cross-institutional coordination through the Species Survival Plan supports characterization of chronic kidney disease incidence and progression in the captive population; individual cases contribute to the surveillance dataset that informs management recommendations for the species. The case illustrated the contribution of aged individuals to population-level pathology surveillance and reinforced the recognition of chronic kidney disease as a leading cause of morbidity in aged captive large felids across taxa.

THE COMPARATIVE NECROPSY PATTERN SYSTEM — Chapter 7 Renal and Urinary Tract Pattern Foundations

---

Reniculate Kidney Architecture Recognition in Marine Mammal Necropsy: Multi-lobar reniculate architecture in cetaceans and pinnipeds recognized as normal anatomy before pathologic interpretation. Anchor: anatomic reference to reniculate structure. Trap: misinterpretation of anatomy as pathology or of lesion distribution as generalized when confined to reniculi. Flag: recognition matters because misinterpretation propagates through marine mammal renal pathology reports.

Ethylene Glycol Toxicosis Pattern Across Wildlife Carnivores: Renal tubular calcium oxalate crystal deposition in wildlife carnivores from environmental antifreeze exposure. Anchor: histopathologic identification of birefringent crystals with ethylene glycol quantitation. Trap: dietary oxalate nephropathy discriminated by exposure history and identifiable plant material. Flag: environmental antifreeze exposure indicates improperly disposed source warranting mitigation.

Visceral Gout Pattern in Captive Birds and Reptiles: Chalky urate deposition on coelomic serosal surfaces in uricotelic species indicating hyperuricemia. Anchor: gross recognition confirmed by histopathology with foreign body giant cell response. Trap: postmortem urate artifact discriminated by absent inflammatory response. Flag: institutionally reportable for husbandry review addressing dehydration, dietary protein, and vitamin A status.

Summary and Key Concepts

Renal anatomic variation across taxa includes the unilobular mammalian kidney, the reniculate marine mammal kidney, the mixed-nephron avian kidney, the loop-limited reptile kidney, and the dual-function fish kidney with head-kidney lymphohematopoietic role; species-appropriate anatomic reference is prerequisite to pathologic interpretation.

Nephropathies in non-domestic species include glomerular disease (immune complex, amyloidosis), tubulointerstitial disease (toxic, infectious, idiopathic), and species-specific patterns; acute kidney injury and chronic kidney disease reflect the same range of processes as in domestic species with taxonomic modifications.

Ethylene glycol toxicosis in wildlife carnivores produces characteristic tubular calcium oxalate deposition; environmental exposure to antifreeze warrants regulatory coordination for source mitigation.

Visceral gout, articular gout, and renal urate tubular deposition are recognizable across avian and reptile taxa and reflect hyperuricemia with tissue urate crystal deposition; postmortem urate artifact requires distinction from antemortem gout.

Urinary tract neoplasia in non-domestic species includes renal cell carcinoma and transitional cell carcinoma of the lower urinary tract; species-specific tumor entities and lower urinary tract disease occur across taxa.

Chronic kidney disease is a leading cause of morbidity and mortality in aged captive large felids and other captive species; individual necropsy findings contribute to population-level surveillance supporting species management through Species Survival Plans.

CHAPTER 8: GASTROINTESTINAL PATHOLOGY ACROSS TAXA

Learning Objectives

1. Interpret comparative gastrointestinal anatomic variation across mammalian, avian, reptile, amphibian, and fish taxa as it modifies pathologic interpretation.
2. Recognize the major enteric infectious disease patterns in non-domestic species with their species-specific etiologic profiles and zoonotic implications.
3. Identify foreign body obstruction, traumatic gastrointestinal injury, and iatrogenic gastrointestinal lesions across taxa.
4. Recognize primary and metastatic gastrointestinal neoplasia in non-domestic species with attention to species-specific tumor entities and predispositions.
5. Apply the Comparative Necropsy Pattern callout structure to gastrointestinal lesion recognition across unfamiliar species.
6. Coordinate ancillary gastrointestinal diagnostics including bacterial and molecular pathogen panels, parasitology, and toxicology on gastrointestinal contents.

The gastrointestinal tract in vertebrate diversity presents perhaps the widest anatomic variation of any organ system encountered in wildlife and zoo animal pathology. The compartmentalized ruminant forestomach, the crop and proventriculus and ventriculus of birds, the elongated single-chambered stomach of most carnivores, the gastric mill of some marine invertebrates, the hindgut-fermenting cecum of many herbivores, and the multi-compartmented stomach of cetaceans each represent distinct evolutionary adaptations to dietary strategy. Interpretation of gastrointestinal pathology requires the pathologist to hold the species-appropriate anatomic frame in mind before applying pathologic reasoning; without that frame, normal anatomy will be misread as pathology and true pathology will be missed. Comparative gastrointestinal knowledge is the interpretive foundation on which the remainder of this chapter is built.

This chapter organizes gastrointestinal pathology into four operational domains. Comparative gastrointestinal anatomy establishes the interpretive frames within which lesions are read. Enteric infectious disease across taxa considers bacterial, viral, protozoal, and parasitic infections with their species-specific etiologic profiles and their zoonotic implications. Foreign body, trauma, and iatrogenic gastrointestinal lesions cover the range of mechanical, thermal, and treatment-related injury to the gastrointestinal tract. Neoplasia of the non-domestic species gastrointestinal tract completes the chapter with attention to species-specific tumor entities and to the primary and metastatic disease patterns documented in captive and free-ranging populations.

Comparative Gastrointestinal Anatomy

Ruminant and Camelid Compartmentalized Stomach

The compartmentalized forestomach of ruminants (Bovidae, Cervidae, Giraffidae, Bovoidea) consists of the rumen, reticulum, omasum, and abomasum, each serving distinct fermentative and digestive functions. The rumen and reticulum together constitute the primary fermentation site where microbial digestion of cellulosic material occurs; the omasum performs absorption of water and short-chain fatty acids from the fermentation products; the abomasum is the true glandular stomach where enzymatic digestion begins. Recognition of the anatomy is prerequisite to interpretation of forestomach disease: parakeratosis of the rumen wall reflects chronic dietary acidosis and is distinguished from acute rumenitis; reticulopericarditis reflects foreign body penetration from the reticulum and is recognized by the anatomic relationship of reticulum to pericardium. Camelids (Camelidae including Old World and New World camels) demonstrate a three-compartmented forestomach with functional analogs to the ruminant compartments but distinct anatomic organization; the compartments are numbered C1, C2, and C3 and require species-specific reference for interpretation.

Avian Crop, Proventriculus, and Ventriculus

The avian upper gastrointestinal tract includes the crop (an outpouching of the esophagus serving as a food storage and softening organ), the proventriculus (the glandular stomach where enzymatic secretion occurs), and the ventriculus or gizzard (the muscular grinding organ that mechanically processes ingested material). Crop stasis with retention of ingesta reflects motility disorders or lower gastrointestinal obstruction and is a recurring clinical presentation in captive avian medicine. Proventricular lesions include gastric ulceration, proventricular dilation syndrome (associated with avian bornavirus in psittacines and passerines), and neoplasia. Ventricular impaction with foreign material or with excessive fibrous ingesta produces obstructive disease. Recognition of each of these compartments as anatomically distinct is prerequisite to lesion interpretation.

Reptile and Amphibian Gastrointestinal Anatomy

Reptile gastrointestinal anatomy varies by lineage. Snakes have an elongated single-chambered stomach followed by a variable small intestine and colon, with adaptations for infrequent large meal processing including the ability to rapidly upregulate gastric enzyme secretion and mucosal absorptive surface. Lizards have a stomach organization similar to mammals with a defined pyloric region. Chelonians have a stomach and intestinal organization adapted to their variable dietary strategies from strict herbivory to omnivory. Crocodilians have a two-chambered stomach with a glandular fundic region and a muscular gastric mill region containing gastroliths (swallowed stones) that assist mechanical digestion. Amphibian gastrointestinal anatomy is simpler with a single-chambered stomach and short intestine appropriate to the largely carnivorous diet of most adult amphibians.

Cetacean Multi-Chambered Stomach and Fish Gastrointestinal Anatomy

Cetacean gastrointestinal anatomy includes a multi-chambered stomach with three primary compartments in most species: the forestomach or fundic chamber (a large aglandular compartment), the main stomach (glandular chamber), and the pyloric chamber. Some cetacean species have additional connecting chambers. Interpretation of cetacean gastric disease requires species-specific anatomic reference. Fish gastrointestinal anatomy varies by species with substantial dietary adaptation: carnivorous teleosts have short intestines with strong gastric acid secretion, herbivorous teleosts have long intestines with modified fermentation adaptations, and some agastric species (cyprinids including carp and goldfish) lack a defined stomach entirely with continuous intestinal digestion. Elasmobranch gastrointestinal anatomy includes the distinctive spiral valve intestine which markedly increases mucosal absorptive surface within a compact body plan.

THE COMPARATIVE NECROPSY PATTERN SYSTEM — Compartmentalized Stomach Anatomy Recognition in Ruminants, Camelids, and Cetaceans

---

The Pattern: Recognition of the compartmentalized stomach anatomy specific to ruminants (four compartments), camelids (three compartments), and cetaceans (multi-chambered) as prerequisite to gastrointestinal pathologic interpretation.

Cross-Taxa Signature: Recognized across the taxa named. The compartmentalized stomach architectures represent convergent evolution toward multi-chambered digestive strategies from disparate evolutionary lineages, but each has species-specific anatomic organization. Ruminants demonstrate rumen, reticulum, omasum, and abomasum with characteristic mucosal architecture in each compartment. Camelids demonstrate three compartments (C1, C2, C3) with functional analogs but distinct anatomic organization. Cetaceans demonstrate two to four chambers depending on species with a large aglandular forestomach that has no ruminant or camelid analog.

Diagnostic Anchor: Anatomic reference to species-specific compartment identification before applying pathologic interpretation. Each compartment carries distinct disease susceptibilities and normal mucosal architecture; misidentification of compartments produces systematic error in gastric pathology reporting.

Trap Logic: The look-alike is misidentification of one compartment as another during necropsy, producing incorrect lesion attribution. Discrimination: systematic anatomic examination with reference to species-appropriate anatomic guides and, in unfamiliar species, consultation with published species-specific references.

Zoonotic/Reportable Flag: Not itself infectious or reportable. Recognition matters because misinterpretation of compartmentalized stomach anatomy produces error that propagates through case reports.

Figure 8.1: Comparative Compartmentalized Stomach Anatomy: Ruminant, Camelid, and Cetacean

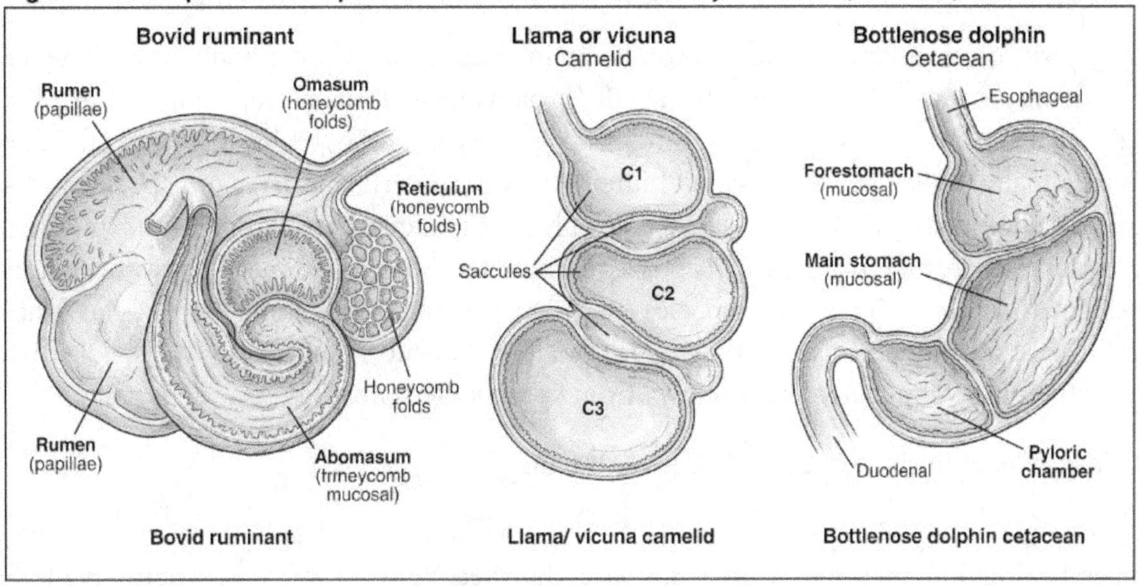

Enteric Infectious Disease Across Taxa

Bacterial Enteric Disease

Bacterial enteric disease across taxa includes Salmonella species infection in reptiles, birds, and mammals with variable clinical significance depending on host status. Salmonella species are commensal or near-commensal in many reptile species, and identification of Salmonella from a reptile carcass does not itself establish etiologic significance; clinical significance requires demonstration of enteric lesions with associated bacterial invasion. In captive avian and mammalian species, Salmonella species are typically pathogenic and produce enterocolitis with characteristic mucosal necrosis and, in systemic disease, hepatic and splenic granulomatous lesions. Escherichia coli enteric disease is documented across taxa with strain-specific virulence factors. Yersinia species produce enteric disease and, in cases with systemic spread, characteristic hepatic and splenic necrosis. Campylobacter species produce enteric disease in some captive species. Clostridial disease includes Clostridium perfringens-associated enteric disease, Clostridium difficile-associated enteric disease, and, in some captive species, Clostridium piliforme (Tyzzer disease) with characteristic hepatic involvement.

Viral Enteric Disease

Viral enteric disease across taxa includes parvovirus infection in captive carnivores with characteristic villus atrophy and cellular crypt necrosis, coronavirus infection in cetaceans and other captive species, rotavirus infection in juvenile captive mammals, and calicivirus infection in captive rabbits and hares producing severe hemorrhagic disease. Adenoviral enteric disease is documented in reptiles (particularly bearded dragons with adenovirus producing characteristic intranuclear inclusion bodies in enterocytes). Circovirus disease produces enteric involvement in some avian species. Ranavirus disease produces coelomic involvement including enteric mucosal necrosis in chelonians and anurans. Recognition of the viral etiologies requires histopathologic characterization and, in most cases, molecular confirmation.

Protozoal and Parasitic Enteric Disease

Protozoal enteric disease across taxa is prominent in wildlife and zoo populations. Cryptosporidium species infection produces characteristic intracellular parasites within enterocyte apical membranes with associated villus atrophy across mammals, birds, and reptiles. Giardia species infection produces mucosal disease across mammalian species. Coccidial infection with Eimeria and Isospora species is documented across taxa. Trichomonas gallinae in avian species produces characteristic upper gastrointestinal lesions. Entamoeba species are documented in captive reptiles and some mammals. Parasitic enteric disease includes nematode infection with species-specific parasites (ascarids, strongyles, hookworms, whipworms), cestode infection, and trematode infection. Parasite identification to species is important because population-level management follows from species identification.

Applied Case: Coccidiosis in a Captive Cheetah Cub

A 4-month-old male cheetah cub (Acinonyx jubatus), one of a litter of three born in a Species Survival Plan managed collection, presented with acute onset diarrhea, dehydration, and progressive lethargy over 48 hours. Clinical workup identified moderately elevated inflammatory markers and diarrheic fecal appearance with mucus and small volumes of frank blood. Supportive care with fluid therapy and empirical antibacterial treatment was initiated; the cub declined despite intervention and died approximately 72 hours after clinical presentation. Necropsy focused on characterization of the enteric disease and identification of the specific etiology given the population-level implications for the remaining littermates and the collection.

External examination demonstrated marked dehydration, thin body condition consistent with acute wasting, and no evidence of external trauma. Coelomic necropsy demonstrated marked serosal and mucosal congestion of the small intestine with moderate volume of hemorrhagic content within the small intestinal lumen. The colon demonstrated similar hemorrhagic content with mucosal congestion and multifocal small ulcerations. Mesenteric lymph nodes were moderately enlarged and edematous. The remainder of the coelomic examination demonstrated mild reactive changes secondary to the acute inflammatory process without additional primary disease. Same-day cytology of impression smears from small intestinal mucosa demonstrated numerous protozoal organisms consistent with coccidial oocysts and merozoites, and mixed inflammatory cell infiltrate with degenerate neutrophils and mononuclear cells.

Fresh fecal sample and intestinal content were submitted for parasitologic examination, and fresh intestinal tissue for histopathology and for molecular characterization of the parasitic agent. Aerobic and anaerobic bacterial culture were submitted in parallel to exclude concurrent bacterial disease. Histopathology confirmed severe multifocal coccidial enteritis with numerous protozoal life stages within enterocytes (schizonts, merozoites, and gametocytes) and associated villus atrophy, crypt cell necrosis, and mixed inflammatory cell infiltrate in the lamina propria. The coccidial organisms were identified as Cystoisospora species by morphology and confirmed by molecular sequencing as a Cystoisospora species previously documented in captive cheetah cubs. Aerobic culture was negative for significant bacterial growth.

Cross-taxa reasoning at case interpretation drew on the extensive documented literature of coccidial enteritis in captive carnivore cubs. Coccidiosis is a well-recognized cause of morbidity and mortality in captive cheetah cubs and in other captive carnivore neonates and juveniles; the species-specific predisposition reflects both host immunologic maturation and captive management factors. The pattern of severe coccidial enteritis with villus atrophy and associated inflammatory response is transportable across captive carnivore taxa; the specific coccidial species requires molecular or morphological characterization for definitive identification. Population-level intervention for the remaining littermates included prophylactic anticoccidial therapy and enhanced hygiene protocols; environmental sampling of the natal enclosure identified coccidial contamination that was addressed through enclosure sanitation and enclosure rotation practices.

The final morphologic diagnosis was severe multifocal coccidial enteritis with villus atrophy and crypt cell necrosis; the etiologic diagnosis was Cystoisospora species enteritis. Institutional response addressed the individual case and population-level implications for the collection's cheetah breeding program. The case reinforced the recognized coccidial disease susceptibility of captive cheetah cubs and contributed to the ongoing Species Survival Plan discussion of neonatal and juvenile disease management in the species. The interpretive pathway from clinical presentation through same-day cytology through histopathology through molecular characterization illustrated the integrated diagnostic workup applied to captive juvenile carnivore enteric disease.

THE COMPARATIVE NECROPSY PATTERN SYSTEM — Systemic Salmonellosis Pattern in Wild Ruminants and Captive Reptiles

The Pattern: Enterocolitis with fibrinonecrotic mucosal ulceration, mesenteric lymphadenopathy, and, in systemic disease, hepatic and splenic granulomatous lesions containing Salmonella organisms.

Cross-Taxa Signature: Recognized across wild ruminants (with clinical significance dominant), captive avian species (with clinical significance dominant), and captive reptiles (with commensal-to-pathogenic transition requiring histopathologic confirmation of enteric lesion). The gross enteric pattern is consistent across taxa; the interpretive weight granted to Salmonella isolation differs by taxonomic group and requires species-appropriate context.

Diagnostic Anchor: Aerobic bacterial culture of intestinal contents, mesenteric lymph node, or systemic tissue with identification of Salmonella species. Histopathologic demonstration of associated enteric mucosal lesions and, in systemic disease, of hepatic or splenic granulomatous lesions confirms clinical significance.

Trap Logic: The look-alike in reptiles is commensal Salmonella carriage without clinical significance, distinguished from clinically significant infection by absence of associated enteric lesions. In wild ruminants, the look-alike is other enteric bacterial disease including Yersinia species and Clostridium species, distinguished by culture and by histopathologic characterization.

Zoonotic/Reportable Flag: Salmonellosis is zoonotic across all taxonomic groups. Reptile salmonellosis carries particular public health significance because of the widespread reptile pet trade; educational and biosafety obligations apply. Human exposure through carcass handling requires occupational health awareness.

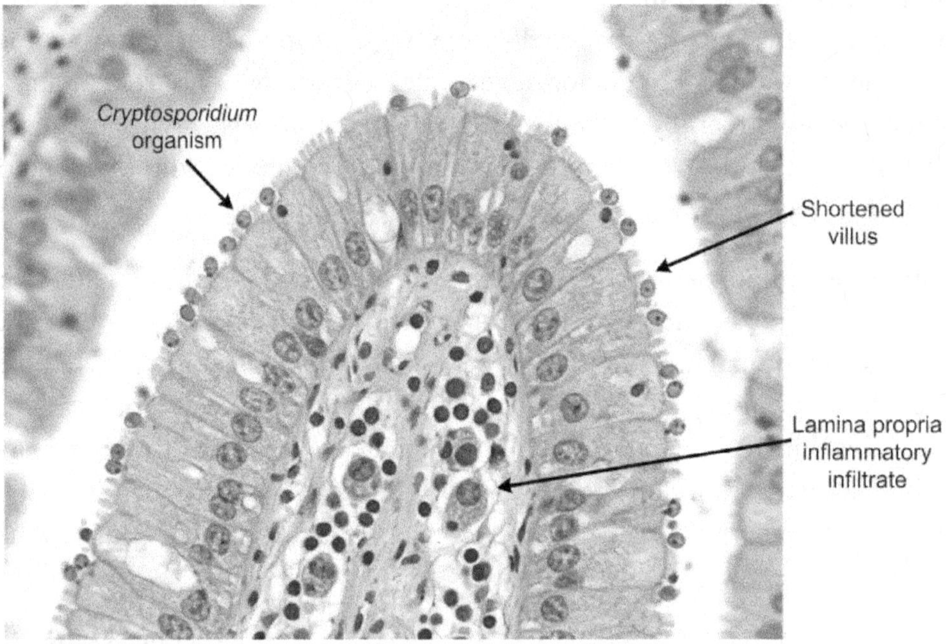

Applied Case: Foreign Body Obstruction in a Green Sea Turtle

A subadult female green sea turtle (Chelonia mydas) was recovered alive from a coastal stranding site with poor body condition, evidence of debilitation, and a history of buoyancy problems observed by beachgoers over several days before rescue. The animal was transported to a marine turtle rehabilitation facility where clinical examination and imaging identified probable gastrointestinal foreign body obstruction. Despite supportive care and attempted medical management, the animal declined over 72 hours and was euthanized for progressive quality of life decline. Necropsy focused on characterization of the gastrointestinal foreign body burden and identification of any concurrent disease processes.

External examination demonstrated the anticipated poor body condition, moderate carapace and plastron algal fouling consistent with reduced diving activity, and no evidence of external trauma. Necropsy proceeded by standard chelonian approach with plastron removal. Coelomic examination demonstrated marked distension of the stomach and small intestine with retained ingesta and non-food material. The stomach contained approximately 300 grams of mixed material including plastic fragments of various sizes, plastic bag fragments including a large intact fragment approximately 15 centimeters across, monofilament fishing line entangled through the gastric contents, and small quantities of natural prey remains suggesting the animal had continued to attempt feeding until obstruction became complete. The small intestine similarly contained plastic fragments and monofilament line with associated mucosal ulceration where the plastic edges had abraded the intestinal wall.

Coelomic examination further demonstrated multifocal serosal adhesions between intestinal loops and mesentery consistent with chronic peritonitis, and moderate volume of turbid coelomic fluid with fibrin flecks. The liver appeared moderately congested consistent with reduced perfusion secondary to chronic disease and dehydration. Additional systematic examination did not identify a primary infectious process, primary neoplasia, or evidence of vessel strike or projectile injury; the foreign body burden with associated mechanical and chemical gastrointestinal injury was the definitive cause of the debilitation and terminal event.

Cross-taxa reasoning at case interpretation drew on the extensive documented literature of marine debris ingestion in sea turtles and other marine wildlife. Ingestion of plastic material and fishing gear by marine turtles is documented at high prevalence across species and geographic regions; the impact on individual animals ranges from asymptomatic to severe with obstruction, gastrointestinal injury, and death. The pattern of mixed plastic and fishing gear ingestion with associated mucosal ulceration is well characterized in the marine turtle stranding pathology literature and reflects the marine environmental contamination that constitutes a substantial conservation threat to marine turtle populations. Sample collection followed the standard marine turtle stranding necropsy protocol including foreign body archival for material characterization, tissue archival for pathogen surveillance and biological reference, and photodocumentation appropriate for chain-of-custody purposes given the federal protection status of the species.

The final morphologic diagnosis was severe gastrointestinal foreign body impaction with plastic and fishing gear material, mucosal ulceration secondary to mechanical injury, and multifocal serosal adhesions and coelomitis consistent with chronic peritoneal inflammatory response. The etiologic diagnosis was marine debris ingestion. Institutional and regulatory reporting followed the marine turtle stranding pathway with distribution to the NOAA Fisheries Southeast Regional Stranding Coordinator, to the state marine turtle stranding program, and to the coordinated marine debris research community that uses stranding pathology data to inform environmental policy. The case reinforced the recognition of marine debris ingestion as a leading cause of morbidity and mortality in marine turtle populations and contributed to the population-level surveillance data supporting marine environmental protection advocacy.

Foreign Body, Trauma, and Iatrogenic GI Lesions

Foreign Body Ingestion and Obstruction

Foreign body ingestion producing gastrointestinal obstruction is documented across taxa. Captive nonhuman primates ingest enclosure furnishings, husbandry items, and cage substrate producing gastric or intestinal foreign body obstruction with characteristic radiographic and necropsy findings. Captive avian species with high foraging drive ingest small objects from enclosures. Captive reptiles ingest substrate material during feeding (particularly loose particulate substrates for insectivorous or carnivorous species) producing sand or gravel impaction. Marine wildlife including sea turtles, seabirds, and marine mammals ingest anthropogenic debris including plastic fragments, fishing gear, and balloon material producing gastrointestinal obstruction and, in some cases, translocation of ingested material through the gastrointestinal wall with peritoneal involvement. Foreign body ingestion in wild ruminants includes metallic hardware ingestion with reticular penetration and reticulopericarditis, historically a leading cause of morbidity in ruminants and remaining relevant in captive collections.

Traumatic Gastrointestinal Injury

Traumatic gastrointestinal injury reflects the mechanism of trauma sustained. Vehicular collision produces gastric or intestinal rupture with peritonitis. Projectile injury produces perforation along the projectile path with associated mesenteric hemorrhage and peritoneal contamination. Falls and blunt trauma produce mesenteric hemorrhage, gastric or intestinal contusion, and, in severe cases, rupture. Iatrogenic gastrointestinal injury includes injection site injury from parenteral medications, endoscopic biopsy site injury, and surgical anastomosis site complications. Recognition of the mechanism-appropriate pattern supports the necropsy interpretation and, in cases with legal implications, the chain-of-custody documentation and reporting.

Iatrogenic Gastrointestinal Lesions

Iatrogenic gastrointestinal lesions in captive populations reflect the range of clinical interventions applied. Nonsteroidal anti-inflammatory drug (NSAID) toxicity produces characteristic gastric ulceration with associated hemorrhage; the toxicity is species-variable with some species particularly susceptible (nonhuman primates, some carnivores, and, notably, vultures with catastrophic species-level population impact from diclofenac exposure in the Indian subcontinent). Corticosteroid-associated gastric ulceration is documented in captive species receiving therapeutic corticosteroids. Antibiotic-associated colitis is documented in some captive species. Anesthetic-related aspiration during recovery may produce upper gastrointestinal effects. Recognition of the iatrogenic origin requires correlation with clinical history and consideration of the specific therapeutic interventions applied.

THE COMPARATIVE NECROPSY PATTERN SYSTEM — Marine Debris Ingestion Pattern in Marine Turtles and Marine Birds

---

The Pattern: Retained ingested plastic material, fishing gear, or other anthropogenic debris within the gastrointestinal tract of marine turtles or marine birds, with associated mucosal ulceration, obstruction, or perforation.

Cross-Taxa Signature: Recognized across marine turtle species (green, loggerhead, hawksbill, olive ridley, Kemp's ridley, leatherback), marine bird species (albatrosses, petrels, gulls, terns, penguins), and, less commonly, other marine wildlife. The pattern reflects marine environmental contamination and is documented at high prevalence in some populations. The specific material profile varies with the animal's foraging strategy: leatherbacks specifically ingest plastic bags mistaken for jellyfish prey, filter-feeding marine birds ingest microplastic and mesoplastic material, and predatory marine species ingest fishing gear during interaction with human fisheries.

Diagnostic Anchor: Gross identification of retained anthropogenic debris within the gastrointestinal tract with associated mucosal injury or obstruction. Debris archival for material characterization supports downstream research and environmental policy applications.

Trap Logic: The look-alike is incidental postmortem ingestion or transit of debris in a carcass with debris present in the gastrointestinal tract but without associated mucosal injury or antemortem clinical significance. Discrimination: clinically significant debris ingestion demonstrates associated mucosal injury, chronic gastrointestinal inflammatory response, or acute obstruction; incidental transit does not.

Zoonotic/Reportable Flag: Not zoonotic. Federally protected species (marine turtles, marine mammals, migratory birds) with debris-associated mortality require reporting through the appropriate federal stranding coordinator and support the marine debris research and policy advocacy community.

Neoplasia of the Non-Domestic Species Gastrointestinal Tract

Primary Gastrointestinal Neoplasia

Primary gastrointestinal neoplasia in non-domestic species includes gastric adenocarcinoma in captive nonhuman primates (particularly aged individuals of some species), intestinal adenocarcinoma across taxa, colonic adenocarcinoma in some species, gastrointestinal stromal tumors, and lymphoma with intestinal or gastric primary involvement. Gastric adenocarcinoma in aged captive lemurs, aged captive great apes, and aged captive some other species is a recurring necropsy finding with variable antemortem clinical presentation. Intestinal adenocarcinoma is documented in captive carnivores, captive nonhuman primates, and other captive species with predisposition varying by lineage. Neuroendocrine tumors of the gastrointestinal tract including gastrinomas and other functional and non-functional neuroendocrine neoplasms are documented in some captive species.

Gastrointestinal Lymphoma

Gastrointestinal lymphoma is documented across taxa and may present as a diffuse infiltrative process with mucosal or transmural involvement, as one or more discrete mass lesions with obstructive potential, or as a component of systemic lymphoma with gastrointestinal involvement. Histopathologic characterization with immunohistochemistry to determine T-cell or B-cell origin supports the diagnosis and, in some species with published prognostic data, has implications for antemortem management decisions when the disease is identified before death. Species-specific lymphoma predispositions are documented in captive ferrets, some captive nonhuman primates, and other captive species.

Metastatic Gastrointestinal Disease

Metastatic gastrointestinal disease from distant primary neoplasms is documented across taxa with the pattern reflecting hematogenous delivery of tumor cells or serosal seeding from adjacent primary tumors. Ovarian carcinoma with omental and intestinal serosal metastases is documented in captive nonhuman primates. Hemangiosarcoma with intestinal metastases is documented in captive carnivores. Recognition of metastatic disease is by gross morphology with characteristic multifocal serosal or transmural masses and by histopathologic characterization identifying the primary tumor cell type. Immunohistochemistry with tissue-of-origin markers supports identification of the primary site when it is not clinically obvious.

Applied Case: Gastric Adenocarcinoma in an Aged Captive Ring-Tailed Lemur

A 22-year-old male ring-tailed lemur (Lemur catta) housed in a Species Survival Plan managed collection had been in clinical decline for several months with progressive weight loss, reduced appetite, and intermittent vomiting. Antemortem workup had identified evidence of chronic upper gastrointestinal disease including modestly elevated hepatic enzymes and evidence of gastric wall thickening on ultrasonographic imaging. Endoscopic biopsy under anesthesia had returned a diagnosis of gastric adenocarcinoma with modestly differentiated glandular pattern; clinical staging had suggested advanced local disease with regional lymph node involvement. Palliative supportive management was elected in consultation with the collection team; the animal was humanely euthanized after progressive decline and demonstration of intractable clinical signs. Necropsy focused on characterization of the gastric neoplasia and identification of metastatic disease.

Coelomic necropsy demonstrated a large gastric mass occupying approximately 60 percent of the gastric wall with prominent transmural involvement and serosal involvement. The mass demonstrated ulcerated mucosal surface with associated adherent fibrin and necrotic debris and firm to hard consistency on palpation. Regional gastric lymph nodes were markedly enlarged, firm, and pale on cut surface consistent with metastatic involvement. Small multifocal peritoneal implants were identified on the mesentery and on the omentum consistent with peritoneal carcinomatosis. Hepatic surface demonstrated several small firm pale nodules consistent with hepatic metastases. Body condition was thin consistent with the chronic disease. The remainder of the necropsy was consistent with age-related change without additional major primary disease.

Histopathology confirmed moderately differentiated gastric adenocarcinoma with transmural gastric wall involvement, lymphatic invasion, and metastatic disease in gastric regional lymph nodes, peritoneal implants, and hepatic parenchyma. Immunohistochemistry with cytokeratin markers supported the epithelial origin. The final morphologic diagnosis was moderately differentiated gastric adenocarcinoma with widespread metastatic disease including regional lymph nodes, peritoneal carcinomatosis, and hepatic metastases. Cross-taxa reasoning at case interpretation drew on the documented literature of gastric adenocarcinoma in aged captive lemurs; the disease is documented as a recurring cause of morbidity and mortality in the species, and the individual case contributed to the Species Survival Plan population-level surveillance data. The report distribution followed the standard SSP pathway.

The case illustrated the interpretive integration required in geriatric zoo pathology: antemortem clinical workup identified the disease process, endoscopic biopsy provided histopathologic diagnosis before death, palliative decision-making was informed by staging, and postmortem confirmation and characterization added to the population-level surveillance data. The interpretive pathway drew heavily on cross-taxa reasoning against the extensive human and domestic species gastric adenocarcinoma literature; species-specific considerations for captive lemurs included the documented predisposition and the SSP surveillance context. The pattern of gastric adenocarcinoma with metastatic disease in an aged captive nonhuman primate is a recognizable Comparative Necropsy Pattern that repeats across primate lineages with predisposition varying by species.

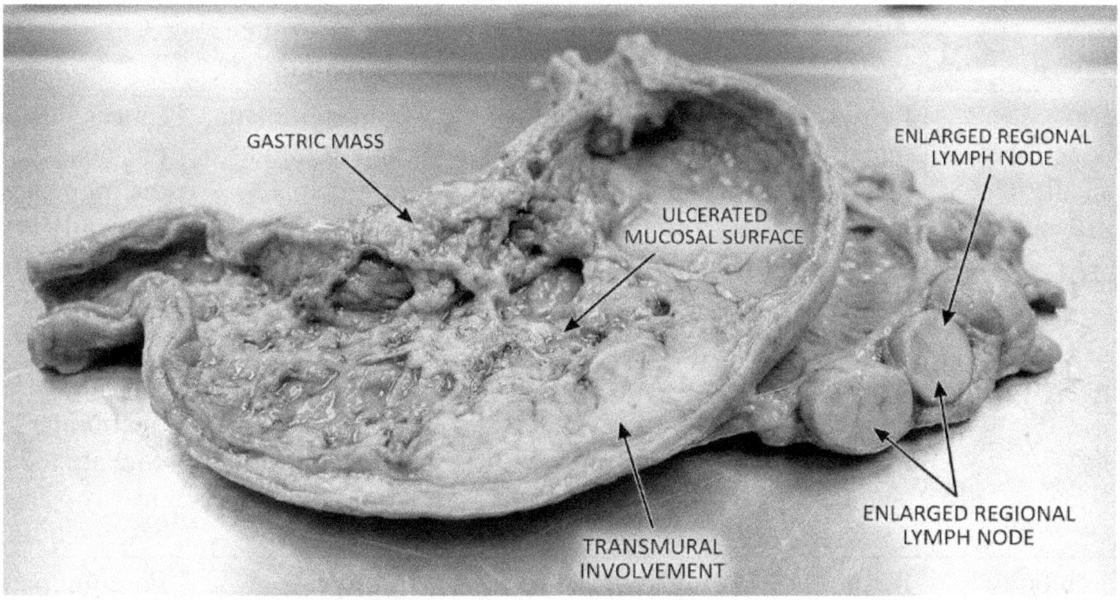

THE COMPARATIVE NECROPSY PATTERN SYSTEM — Gastric Adenocarcinoma Pattern in Aged Captive Nonhuman Primates

The Pattern: Gastric mass with mucosal ulceration, transmural involvement, regional lymph node metastasis, and, in advanced cases, peritoneal carcinomatosis and hepatic metastases in an aged captive nonhuman primate.

Cross-Taxa Signature: Recognized in aged captive lemurs, captive great apes, and other captive nonhuman primate species with species-specific predisposition varying by lineage. The gross and histopathologic patterns are transportable across primate taxa; the epidemiologic profile requires species-specific reference.

Diagnostic Anchor: Gross recognition of gastric mass with characteristic morphology confirmed by histopathology of the primary mass and of metastatic sites. Immunohistochemistry with epithelial markers supports the diagnosis when needed.

Trap Logic: The look-alike is chronic gastric ulceration of non-neoplastic origin (NSAID-associated, stress-associated, infectious), which produces mucosal disease without the transmural mass component or metastatic pattern. Discrimination: histopathology of the mass demonstrates neoplastic epithelium with characteristic architectural patterns; non-neoplastic ulceration demonstrates inflammatory and reparative response without neoplastic component.

Zoonotic/Reportable Flag: Not zoonotic or regulatorily reportable. Institutionally reportable at Species Survival Plan facilities for lineage documentation and population-level surveillance.

GI Disease Pattern	Gross Morphology	Histopathologic Hallmark	Species Predisposed	Key Discriminator
Enteric salmonellosis (clinically significant)	Fibrinonecrotic mucosal ulceration with mesenteric lymphadenopathy	Suppurative enterocolitis with bacterial invasion; systemic granulomatous lesions	Wild ruminants, captive birds (dominant); reptiles (requires lesion confirmation)	Enteric lesion presence distinguishes clinically significant from commensal carriage
Cryptosporidiosis	Intestinal thickening and mild mucosal changes	Apical enterocyte parasites with villus atrophy	Juvenile mammals, birds, and reptiles across taxa	Apical membrane parasite location on histopathology
Foreign body obstruction	Retained material with mucosal injury and possible perforation	Mucosal ulceration with mechanical injury pattern	Captive primates, marine turtles, marine birds, ratites	Foreign material identification with associated antemortem injury
Marine debris ingestion	Retained plastic or fishing gear with mucosal injury	Mechanical ulceration with foreign body inflammatory response	Marine turtles (all species), marine birds	Anthropogenic material with antemortem obstruction or chronic ingestion pattern
Gastric adenocarcinoma	Gastric mass with transmural involvement and metastasis	Neoplastic glandular epithelium with characteristic architectural patterns	Aged captive lemurs, aged captive great apes, other aged primates	Transmural mass with metastatic disease distinguishes from non-neoplastic ulceration
Reticulopericarditis (traumatic)	Reticular foreign body with pericardial involvement	Fibrinopurulent pericarditis with reticular perforation	Wild ruminants, captive artiodactyls with metallic foreign body exposure	Anatomic relationship of reticulum to pericardium with penetrating foreign body

CLINICAL PEARL: The commensal-to-pathogenic transition of Salmonella species in reptiles is one of the more interpretively challenging patterns in wildlife pathology. Isolation of Salmonella from a reptile carcass does not itself establish etiologic significance; clinically significant infection requires demonstration of associated enteric lesions with bacterial invasion. Report interpretation must reflect this distinction, and the zoonotic implications apply regardless of the individual case's disease significance.

EVIDENCE: Diclofenac exposure in vultures through consumption of livestock carcasses treated with the NSAID produced catastrophic population-level decline in Asian vulture species during the 1990s and early 2000s, with more than 95 percent population loss in some species. The recognition of the vulture-specific NSAID vulnerability and subsequent regulatory action illustrates how wildlife pathology findings inform species-level conservation policy at the highest stakes.

CAUTION: Reptile Salmonella carriage is nearly ubiquitous in some species and does not itself indicate clinical disease; however, the zoonotic significance of reptile Salmonella carriage is independent of the individual reptile's disease status. Human exposure through carcass handling requires appropriate personal protective equipment and hand hygiene regardless of the individual case's clinical relevance.

KEY POINT: The compartmentalized ruminant stomach carries the anatomic relationship between reticulum and pericardium that produces traumatic reticulopericarditis when metallic foreign bodies penetrate the reticular wall. In captive artiodactyls, exhibit hardware, wire fencing, and other metallic objects remain relevant sources of foreign body exposure; recognition of reticulopericarditis at necropsy prompts investigation of the exhibit environment for source identification and mitigation.

THE COMPARATIVE NECROPSY PATTERN SYSTEM — Chapter 8 Gastrointestinal Pattern Foundations

---

Compartmentalized Stomach Anatomy Recognition in Ruminants, Camelids, and Cetaceans: Species-specific compartment identification prerequisite to gastric pathologic interpretation. Anchor: anatomic reference before interpretation. Trap: compartment misidentification producing incorrect lesion attribution. Flag: recognition matters for accurate reporting.

Systemic Salmonellosis Pattern in Wild Ruminants and Captive Reptiles: Enterocolitis with systemic granulomatous lesions across taxa with species-specific clinical significance. Anchor: culture with histopathologic confirmation of lesions. Trap: commensal reptile carriage discriminated by absent enteric lesion. Flag: zoonotic across all taxa with public health obligations.

Marine Debris Ingestion Pattern in Marine Turtles and Marine Birds: Retained anthropogenic material with mucosal injury and obstructive potential. Anchor: gross material identification with antemortem injury correlation. Trap: incidental postmortem debris discriminated by absent mucosal injury. Flag: federally protected species require regulatory coordination.

Gastric Adenocarcinoma Pattern in Aged Captive Nonhuman Primates: Gastric mass with transmural involvement, regional lymph node metastasis, and peritoneal or hepatic metastatic disease in aged primates. Anchor: histopathologic characterization of primary and metastatic sites. Trap: non-neoplastic gastric ulceration discriminated by absent mass component. Flag: institutionally reportable at SSP facilities for lineage surveillance.

Summary and Key Concepts

Comparative gastrointestinal anatomy across taxa includes the compartmentalized ruminant and camelid forestomachs, the crop-proventriculus-ventriculus of birds, the elongated single-chambered stomach of most carnivores, the multi-chambered cetacean stomach, and the diverse reptile, amphibian, and fish gastrointestinal arrangements; species-appropriate anatomic reference is prerequisite to pathologic interpretation.

Bacterial enteric disease across taxa includes Salmonella (with reptile commensal-to-pathogenic transition requiring interpretive care), Escherichia coli, Yersinia, Campylobacter, and clostridial disease with species-specific etiologic profiles.

Viral enteric disease includes parvovirus, coronavirus, rotavirus, calicivirus, adenovirus, circovirus, and ranavirus with species-specific patterns and histopathologic characteristics.

Foreign body obstruction is documented across taxa with recurring recognition of substrate ingestion in captive reptiles, enclosure furnishing ingestion in captive primates, and marine debris ingestion in marine turtles and seabirds as leading causes of morbidity and mortality.

Traumatic and iatrogenic gastrointestinal injury including NSAID-associated ulceration, reticulopericarditis, and species-specific drug toxicities (diclofenac in vultures) contribute to the differential across captive and free-ranging populations.

Gastrointestinal neoplasia in non-domestic species includes primary gastric adenocarcinoma (aged captive nonhuman primates), intestinal adenocarcinoma, gastrointestinal lymphoma, and metastatic disease with recognition patterns transportable across taxa.

CHAPTER 9: NERVOUS SYSTEM PATHOLOGY

Learning Objectives

1. Interpret comparative neuroanatomic variation across vertebrate taxa as it modifies pathologic interpretation.
2. Recognize the transmissible spongiform encephalopathies in wildlife and their regulatory reporting requirements.
3. Identify viral, bacterial, parasitic, and fungal encephalitides in non-domestic species with their species-specific etiologic profiles.
4. Distinguish non-infectious neurologic disease including neoplasia, degenerative disease, and traumatic and toxic injury.
5. Apply the Comparative Necropsy Pattern callout structure to nervous system lesion recognition across unfamiliar species.
6. Coordinate ancillary neurologic diagnostics including cerebrospinal fluid analysis, molecular pathogen panels, and prion diagnostic submission.

Nervous system pathology in wildlife and zoo species carries interpretive weight disproportionate to the anatomic space the nervous system occupies. Neurologic disease often produces terminal event mortality with characteristic antemortem clinical signs; the necropsy diagnosis carries substantial implications for regulatory reporting when a transmissible spongiform encephalopathy is confirmed, for biosafety when a zoonotic viral encephalitis is confirmed, and for population-level surveillance when an emerging neurotropic pathogen is identified. The chapter addresses the interpretive frames required to work through neurologic cases across taxonomic groups and the recognition patterns that recur across disparate diseases affecting the central and peripheral nervous system.

The chapter organizes nervous system pathology into four operational domains. Comparative neuroanatomy provides the interpretive frame within which lesions are read. Transmissible spongiform encephalopathies in wildlife address the prion diseases including chronic wasting disease and their regulatory reporting pathways. Viral, bacterial, and parasitic encephalitides cover the range of infectious neurologic disease across taxa. Non-infectious neurologic disease completes the chapter with neoplasia, degenerative disease, traumatic injury, and toxic neurologic injury.

Comparative Neuroanatomy Relevant to Pathology

Mammalian Central Nervous System Organization

The mammalian central nervous system organization provides the interpretive baseline for most non-domestic species neurology. The cerebrum with characteristic cortical gyri and sulci, the cerebellum with its distinctive foliation, the brainstem with cranial nerve origins, and the spinal cord with segmental organization together constitute the anatomic frame. Species-specific variation includes brain-to-body-mass ratio (varying substantially across mammalian orders), cerebral cortical folding complexity (increased in cetaceans, most carnivores, and primates; reduced in some smaller mammals), cerebellar prominence (increased in species with complex motor demands including cetaceans and some birds despite the mammalian anatomic frame), and species-specific brainstem organization. Interpretation of gross brain lesions requires species-appropriate anatomic reference; a cerebellar mass in a cetacean is interpreted against the cetacean cerebellar anatomy, not against generic mammalian cerebellar reference.

Avian Central Nervous System Organization

The avian central nervous system organization differs from mammalian organization in specific and important ways. The avian telencephalon is organized as pallial nuclear clusters rather than as the columnar cortical arrangement of mammals, producing a smooth external brain surface without prominent gyri and sulci. Nucleus-specific pathology is more characteristic of avian neurologic disease than the diffuse cortical patterns of mammalian pathology. The avian cerebellum is prominent with characteristic foliation. The optic tectum is highly developed reflecting the visual acuity that dominates avian sensory processing. Cranial nerve organization varies from mammalian organization in several respects. Recognition of the avian anatomic frame is prerequisite to interpretation of avian neurologic pathology.

Reptile, Amphibian, and Fish Central Nervous System

Reptile central nervous system anatomy is intermediate between the avian and mammalian arrangements with a smooth cortical surface, prominent optic tectum, and defined cerebellar architecture. Amphibian central nervous system anatomy is smaller and less complex with anatomic organization reflecting the aquatic-to-terrestrial transition. Fish central nervous system anatomy includes distinct forebrain, midbrain, hindbrain, and cerebellar organization with substantial species-specific variation reflecting the ecological diversity of the taxonomic group. Elasmobranch central nervous systems demonstrate relatively large brains for the body mass compared to teleosts. Species-specific reference is required for interpretation of central nervous system pathology in these lower vertebrate classes.

Meninges, Ventricles, and Peripheral Nervous System

The meningeal covering of the central nervous system varies subtly across taxa but retains the interpretive weight of meningeal inflammatory changes as diagnostic findings. Ventricular anatomy varies across taxa with characteristic patterns in each vertebrate class. The peripheral nervous system including cranial nerves, spinal nerves, and autonomic ganglia demonstrates species-specific organization but retains the interpretive utility of peripheral nerve pathology recognition. Recognition of the peripheral nervous system anatomy supports identification of peripheral neuropathy patterns, cranial nerve involvement, and autonomic ganglion pathology.

Figure 9.1: Comparative Vertebrate Brain Organization: Mammalian, Avian, and Reptile

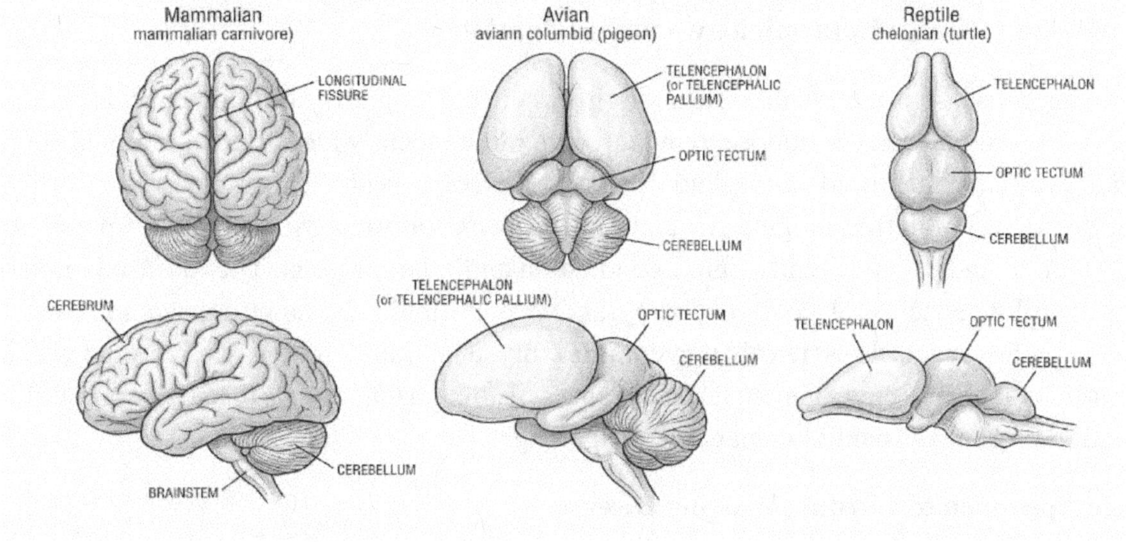

THE COMPARATIVE NECROPSY PATTERN SYSTEM — Meningoencephalitis Pattern Recognition Across Mammalian and Avian Taxa

The Pattern: Grossly recognized meningeal congestion or opacification and, on histopathology, inflammatory infiltrate involving meninges and underlying brain parenchyma indicating meningoencephalitis of infectious or immune-mediated origin.

Cross-Taxa Signature: Recognized across mammals, birds, and reptiles with variable etiologic profiles. In mammals, viral meningoencephalitis (rabies, morbillivirus, herpesvirus, arbovirus, and others), bacterial meningitis (Streptococcus, Listeria, and other bacteria), protozoal encephalitis (Toxoplasma, Sarcocystis, and others), and fungal encephalitis (Cryptococcus, Aspergillus with CNS extension) are documented. In birds, viral encephalitis (West Nile virus, eastern equine encephalitis virus, and others), bacterial disease, and protozoal disease produce comparable gross and histopathologic patterns.

Diagnostic Anchor: Systematic histopathologic examination of brain sections with attention to meningeal infiltrate, perivascular cuffing, gliosis, and inflammatory cell type composition. Molecular pathogen panels appropriate to the species and epidemiologic context identify specific agents. Cerebrospinal fluid analysis when antemortem samples are available complements the postmortem workup.

Trap Logic: The look-alike is agonal meningeal congestion in a carcass with terminal event circulatory changes, distinguished by absent inflammatory cell infiltrate on histopathology. Another look-alike is postmortem meningeal contamination during necropsy handling, distinguished by absence of vital response and by contamination pattern.

Zoonotic/Reportable Flag: Rabies in a carnivore or bat, West Nile virus in birds or mammals, and several arboviral encephalitides carry zoonotic and public health reporting obligations. Biosafety escalation to appropriate PPE and, in rabies suspects, notification of public health authorities and occupational health precede continued dissection of central nervous system tissue.

Transmissible Spongiform Encephalopathies in Wildlife

Chronic Wasting Disease Epidemiology and Distribution

Chronic wasting disease is a transmissible spongiform encephalopathy affecting cervid species including mule deer, white-tailed deer, elk, moose, reindeer, and, more recently identified, additional cervid species. The disease was first identified in the late 1960s in captive cervids at a research facility in Colorado; subsequent recognition in free-ranging populations has been followed by geographic spread across much of North America and, more recently, into Scandinavia and other regions. The disease is invariably fatal following a prolonged clinical course of progressive neurologic dysfunction, weight loss, behavioral changes, and, in advanced cases, terminal event mortality. The transmissibility of chronic wasting disease among cervids and the environmental persistence of the prion agent through soil and vegetation contamination present substantial management challenges.

Diagnostic Approach to Chronic Wasting Disease

Diagnostic approach to chronic wasting disease at necropsy centers on collection of specific tissues for prion testing. The obex region of the brainstem and the retropharyngeal lymph nodes are the primary tissues submitted for the standard testing algorithm using immunohistochemistry and enzyme-linked immunosorbent assay methods. Additional lymphoid tissues including tonsils may be sampled for research or for surveillance purposes. Standard biosafety practices during collection include personal protective equipment appropriate to prion handling and disposable instruments where feasible; reusable instruments require specific decontamination protocols that exceed standard biological decontamination. Confirmed positive results trigger the state-specific regulatory response coordinated through the state wildlife agency and USDA APHIS.

Other Transmissible Spongiform Encephalopathies and Regulatory Response

Other transmissible spongiform encephalopathies relevant to wildlife pathology include scrapie in wild ovid populations (rare but documented), bovine spongiform encephalopathy in captive artiodactyls (with historical outbreak in captive ungulates at zoological institutions during the 1990s bovine spongiform encephalopathy epidemic), and feline spongiform encephalopathy in captive felids from the same historical period. Regulatory response to any suspected transmissible spongiform encephalopathy is coordinated through state animal health authority and USDA APHIS with rapid confirmation testing at the National Veterinary Services Laboratories. Chain of custody documentation and specific tissue archival requirements apply.

THE COMPARATIVE NECROPSY PATTERN SYSTEM — Chronic Wasting Disease Pattern in Free-Ranging Cervids

The Pattern: Cervid carcass with poor body condition, characteristic clinical history of progressive neurologic dysfunction and weight loss, and diagnostic tissue submission for prion testing.

Cross-Taxa Signature: Recognized in cervid species including mule deer, white-tailed deer, elk, moose, and reindeer with expanding taxonomic and geographic distribution documented since the disease's first identification. Species-specific susceptibility varies with reindeer historically thought less susceptible until recent Scandinavian identification demonstrated significant vulnerability. The clinical and pathologic patterns are broadly consistent across affected species with the characteristic progressive neurologic decline preceding terminal event.

Diagnostic Anchor: Immunohistochemistry or enzyme-linked immunosorbent assay demonstration of pathologic prion protein accumulation in obex or retropharyngeal lymph node from the affected animal. Confirmation testing at reference laboratories for regulatory submission.

Trap Logic: The look-alike is any other cause of progressive weight loss and neurologic decline in cervids, distinguished by prion testing. Other look-alikes include chronic mycobacterial disease and chronic parasitism which may produce similar body condition changes without the neurologic component.

Zoonotic/Reportable Flag: Chronic wasting disease is a reportable disease in the United States with state-specific and federal reporting pathways. While zoonotic potential to humans has not been established, precautionary handling guidance for hunters and consumers has been issued by public health authorities. All suspected cases require appropriate tissue submission through the coordinated surveillance network.

Viral, Bacterial, and Parasitic Encephalitides

Viral Encephalitides

Viral encephalitides across taxa include rabies with its characteristic Negri bodies in Purkinje cells and cerebral cortical neurons, arboviral encephalitides including West Nile virus with prominent involvement of the brainstem and thalamus and eastern equine encephalitis virus with similar distribution, herpesvirus encephalitides with characteristic intranuclear inclusion bodies, morbillivirus encephalitides with multinucleate giant cells in cetaceans and other affected species, and, more recently identified, several emerging neurotropic viruses. Species-specific viral encephalitides include Borna disease virus in some captive avian species (avian bornavirus complex) producing proventricular dilation syndrome with neurologic component, and species-specific herpesvirus encephalitides in various captive collections. Recognition of viral encephalitis requires histopathologic characterization with attention to inclusion body morphology, inflammatory cell type composition, and vascular involvement, complemented by molecular pathogen identification.

Bacterial Encephalitides and Meningitis

Bacterial encephalitides and meningitis across taxa include Streptococcus species meningitis in captive nonhuman primates and other captive mammals, Listeria monocytogenes encephalitis in captive ruminants and other species with characteristic brainstem localization, and species-specific bacterial encephalitides in various taxa. Fungal encephalitis with central nervous system extension of systemic mycoses including cryptococcosis is documented in captive mammals and some avian species. Bacterial and fungal encephalitides require culture-based identification and, in some cases, specific stains on histopathology (Gram stain for bacteria, Grocott-Gomori methenamine silver for fungi).

Parasitic and Protozoal Encephalitides

Parasitic and protozoal encephalitides across taxa include Sarcocystis species meningoencephalomyelitis in wild birds and mammals with characteristic protozoal cyst formation in neural tissue, Toxoplasma gondii encephalitis in immunocompromised captive marsupials and some other species, cerebrospinal parelaphostrongylosis in cervids with aberrant migration of Parelaphostrongylus tenuis larvae producing characteristic neurologic disease, and other parasitic neurologic diseases with species-specific presentations. Recognition of parasitic neurologic disease requires histopathologic identification of the specific parasitic form and, in some cases, molecular confirmation.

Applied Case: Rabies Diagnosis in a Wild Striped Skunk

A wild striped skunk (Mephitis mephitis) was found alive but severely abnormal in a residential neighborhood, exhibiting daytime activity, apparent disorientation, and lack of fear of human observers. Animal control services humanely euthanized the animal in accordance with local protocols for rabies-suspect wildlife and submitted the carcass to the state diagnostic laboratory for rabies testing. The submission form recorded the abnormal behavioral observations and the potential human exposure concern related to a neighborhood resident who had contact with the animal before animal control response. Necropsy was performed under strict biosafety protocols with attention to rabies suspect handling requirements including enhanced personal protective equipment, disposable instruments where feasible, and containment of tissue during processing.

Necropsy focused on brain removal and appropriate tissue submission for rabies testing following standard protocols. External examination demonstrated appropriate body condition for the species, no evidence of external trauma, and no other significant abnormalities. Coelomic examination was performed briefly with attention to any additional differential considerations but was not the primary focus. Brain removal proceeded by standard technique with the entire brain submitted for direct fluorescent antibody testing at the state diagnostic laboratory. Portions of brainstem were also archived for potential downstream molecular characterization. Standard biosafety practices during brain removal included appropriate personal protective equipment, containment of tissue, and appropriate instrument handling for the rabies suspect designation.

Cross-taxa reasoning at case interpretation drew on the extensive documented literature of terrestrial rabies in North American wildlife. Skunks are an important reservoir species for terrestrial rabies with regional variant strains circulating across different geographic regions of North America; the north-central skunk variant, south-central skunk variant, and other regional variants each demonstrate characteristic epidemiology and, in some cases, distinctive molecular characteristics. Behavioral abnormalities in a wild skunk during daytime activity are highly suspicious for rabies and require the standard diagnostic and public health response regardless of any additional clinical features. The species is an important sentinel for terrestrial rabies presence in an area.

The direct fluorescent antibody test returned positive for rabies virus antigen in brain tissue, confirming the diagnosis. Molecular characterization identified the north-central skunk variant strain, consistent with the geographic region of the case. Public health response was immediate and coordinated. The neighborhood resident who had contact with the animal was notified through the state health department and evaluated for potential rabies exposure with post-exposure prophylaxis initiated in accordance with standard public health protocols. Local animal control was notified with recommendations regarding potential enhanced surveillance in the affected area. The state wildlife health veterinarian was notified as part of the ongoing state rabies surveillance program. The case reinforced the recognition of wildlife rabies as an ongoing public health concern requiring coordinated response between wildlife pathology, veterinary diagnostic services, and public health authorities.

Applied Case: Cerebrospinal Parelaphostrongylosis in a Captive Moose

A 6-year-old male moose (Alces alces) housed in a northern facility with mixed hoofstock collection developed progressive neurologic clinical signs over several weeks including hind limb ataxia, weakness, and, in the terminal stages, inability to stand. Antemortem clinical assessment identified progressive neurologic disease of undetermined etiology despite empirical antiparasitic treatment; the animal was humanely euthanized for progressive quality of life decline. The facility was located in a geographic region with sympatric white-tailed deer populations. Necropsy focused on characterization of the neurologic disease with attention to cerebrospinal parelaphostrongylosis given the geographic context and species predisposition.

External examination confirmed poor body condition with reduced muscle mass consistent with chronic disease and disuse. Systematic necropsy demonstrated no significant abnormalities in most organ systems. Central nervous system examination demonstrated mild meningeal congestion without gross parenchymal lesions. Cerebellum and spinal cord were examined with attention to potential parasitic tract lesions. Fresh tissue was collected for standard histopathologic examination and for potential parasite recovery.

Cross-taxa reasoning at case interpretation drew on the documented pathology of cerebrospinal parelaphostrongylosis in captive and wild moose. Parelaphostrongylus tenuis is a metastrongylid nematode that uses white-tailed deer as its normal definitive host without producing significant clinical disease; the larvae migrate through the central nervous system of the deer host as a normal component of the life cycle without producing pathology. In aberrant hosts including moose, elk, caribou, and captive artiodactyls of many species, the larval migration produces significant parenchymal damage in the central nervous system and clinical neurologic disease that is often progressive and fatal. The pattern is well documented and represents a substantial threat to captive artiodactyl collections in geographic regions with sympatric white-tailed deer populations.

Histopathology confirmed multifocal meningeal and parenchymal inflammatory tract lesions in cerebrum and spinal cord consistent with parasitic tract migration; occasional larval sections were identified in tissue confirming Parelaphostrongylus species. The final morphologic diagnosis was multifocal meningoencephalomyelitis with parasitic tract lesions and identifiable larval nematode sections consistent with cerebrospinal parelaphostrongylosis. Institutional response addressed the collection-level considerations including recognition of the ongoing risk to other susceptible species in the collection given the geographic context, coordination with state wildlife health authorities regarding regional white-tailed deer population dynamics, and consideration of preventive antiparasitic management for other susceptible species in the collection.

Ancillary Neurologic Diagnostics at Necropsy

Ancillary neurologic diagnostics at necropsy include cerebrospinal fluid analysis when antemortem or immediate postmortem samples are available, molecular pathogen panels for the anticipated infectious differential, immunohistochemistry for viral antigen identification, prion testing following specific protocols for transmissible spongiform encephalopathy suspects, and toxicology panels for suspected toxic exposures. Cerebrospinal fluid analysis in postmortem samples provides information about protein content, cellularity, and specific pathogen presence; the interpretive limitations of postmortem samples include the effects of red blood cell contamination and of postmortem cellular changes but do not preclude diagnostic use. Molecular pathogen panels should be selected based on the anticipated differential and the species-specific pathogen profile; comprehensive syndromic panels may be appropriate when the differential is broad. Immunohistochemistry with virus-specific antibodies provides definitive characterization when the differential is narrower and when appropriate species-specific antibodies are available. Prion testing follows the specific protocols established for the taxonomic group and requires appropriate tissue selection at collection.

THE COMPARATIVE NECROPSY PATTERN SYSTEM — West Nile Virus Encephalitis Pattern in Corvids and Raptors

The Pattern: Nonsuppurative meningoencephalitis with prominent brainstem, thalamic, and cerebellar involvement, associated cardiac and renal changes, and clinical history of neurologic dysfunction preceding death in a corvid or raptor received during warm season.

Cross-Taxa Signature: Recognized across corvid species (crows, ravens, jays, magpies) with catastrophic population impact in some species, raptor species (particularly Cooper's hawk, red-tailed hawk, great horned owl), and other avian species with variable susceptibility. In mammals, West Nile virus produces neurologic disease in captive nonhuman primates, in some captive equids and cervids, and, less commonly, in other captive mammals. The pattern in birds includes prominent central nervous system involvement with characteristic distribution.

Diagnostic Anchor: Polymerase chain reaction targeting West Nile virus RNA from brain or other affected tissue confirms the etiology. Histopathologic hallmark is nonsuppurative meningoencephalitis with lymphocytic infiltrate. Immunohistochemistry with West Nile virus antibody demonstrates viral antigen in affected neurons.

Trap Logic: The look-alike is eastern equine encephalitis virus disease with similar distribution and histopathologic pattern, distinguished by molecular characterization. Another look-alike is bacterial or fungal encephalitis producing similar gross meningeal changes but with different inflammatory cell composition and characterized by culture.

Zoonotic/Reportable Flag: West Nile virus is a zoonotic pathogen with mosquito vector transmission and endemic circulation across much of North America. Case detection contributes to public health surveillance systems coordinated through state departments of health. Biosafety awareness during necropsy and appropriate PPE for suspected cases are standard.

Figure 9.2 West Nile Virus Encephalitis in a Wild American Crow: Nonsuppurative Meningoencephalitis at 20× Magnification

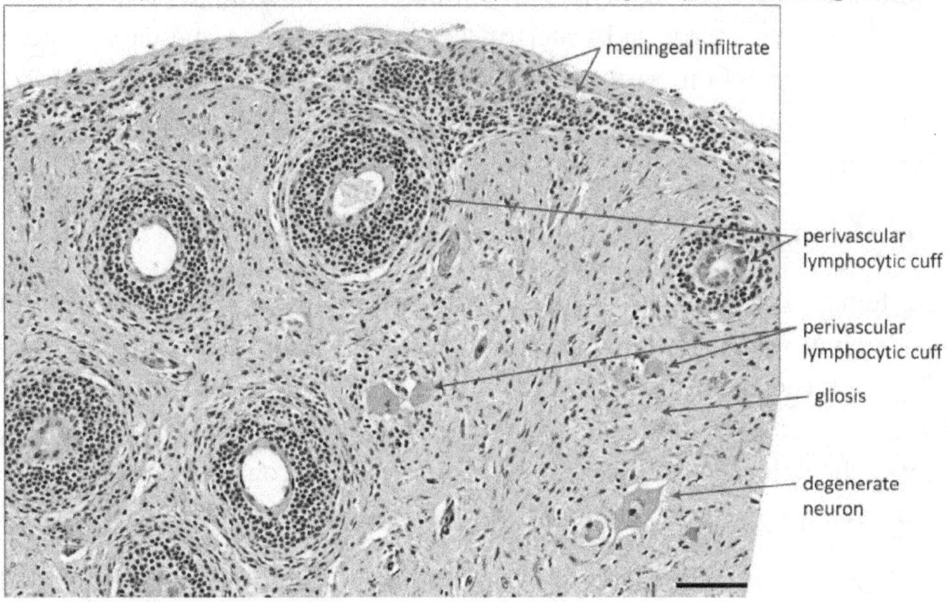

Non-Infectious Neurologic Disease

Central Nervous System Neoplasia

Central nervous system neoplasia in non-domestic species includes primary tumors (meningioma, glioma, ependymoma, choroid plexus tumors, primary CNS lymphoma) and metastatic disease. Meningioma in aged captive nonhuman primates and captive marine mammals is documented at recognizable frequency. Glial tumors including astrocytoma and oligodendroglioma are documented in captive mammals. Choroid plexus tumors are documented in some captive species. Metastatic CNS disease from primary neoplasms elsewhere is documented across taxa with the CNS distribution reflecting hematogenous delivery.

Recognition of CNS neoplasia requires antemortem imaging when available and definitive histopathologic characterization at necropsy.

Neurodegenerative Disease

Neurodegenerative disease in aged captive species includes cognitive dysfunction analogs comparable to canine cognitive dysfunction with characteristic amyloid plaque formation in some captive species, Parkinsonian-like disease with substantia nigra pathology documented in some individual cases, and species-specific age-related neurologic changes. Recognition of neurodegenerative disease is by antemortem clinical assessment complemented by postmortem histopathologic characterization with attention to characteristic pathologic protein deposition (amyloid, tau, alpha-synuclein) using appropriate immunohistochemistry.

Traumatic and Toxic Neurologic Injury

Traumatic neurologic injury reflects the mechanisms of trauma including vehicular collision, projectile injury, and blunt trauma with characteristic contusion patterns and, in severe cases, intracranial hemorrhage or contrecoup injury. Iatrogenic neurologic injury includes injection-site injury and, in captive settings, complications of neurosurgical intervention. Toxic neurologic injury includes lead toxicosis with characteristic sequelae in raptors and waterfowl, organophosphate and carbamate pesticide toxicity with acetylcholinesterase depression, harmful algal bloom neurotoxin exposure in marine wildlife (particularly domoic acid causing seizures and hippocampal lesions in California sea lions), and species-specific neurotoxic exposures.

Applied Case: Meningioma in an Aged Captive Grizzly Bear

A 24-year-old female grizzly bear (Ursus arctos horribilis) housed in a Species Survival Plan managed collection had been in progressive decline for approximately eight months with subtle neurologic clinical signs including reduced coordination, occasional stumbling, and, in the terminal weeks before death, apparent visual dysfunction affecting the right side. Antemortem workup was limited by species and body size constraints. The animal was humanely euthanized after progressive quality of life decline. Necropsy focused on comprehensive characterization with attention to the antemortem neurologic clinical signs.

External examination demonstrated appropriate body condition for the aged animal. Coelomic necropsy demonstrated no significant primary abnormalities in most organ systems with modest age-related changes throughout. Brain removal by standard technique demonstrated a large discrete mass approximately 4 centimeters in maximum diameter attached to the meninges over the left cerebral cortex in the region of the parietal and occipital lobes. The mass appeared firm, well-demarcated from adjacent tissue, and produced local compression of the underlying cortex with associated distortion of adjacent structures. Histopathology confirmed meningioma with characteristic whorled cellular architecture, occasional psammoma bodies, and immunohistochemical positivity for meningeal markers. The final morphologic diagnosis was left cerebral cortical meningioma with associated cortical compression.

Cross-taxa reasoning at case interpretation drew on the documented literature of meningioma in aged captive nonhuman primates, aged captive carnivores, and aged captive marine mammals. Meningioma is a recognized age-related tumor across mammalian taxa with recognizable gross morphology and histopathologic characteristics that are transportable across species. The clinical presentation of unilateral neurologic dysfunction in an aged captive animal should include meningioma among the differentials, and the postmortem finding provides the definitive diagnosis when antemortem imaging is limited. Institutional response addressed the individual case and contributed to the population-level surveillance data through the Species Survival Plan reporting pathway.

TSE Regulatory Framework and Sample Handling Standards

The regulatory framework for transmissible spongiform encephalopathies requires specific handling of sample tissues, chain of custody documentation, and coordinated response with state and federal animal health authorities. Chronic wasting disease in cervids is managed through state-specific surveillance programs with USDA APHIS coordination; specific tissue sampling requirements including obex and retropharyngeal lymph node are standardized across surveillance programs. Bovine spongiform encephalopathy testing in captive artiodactyls follows the historical protocols established during the bovine spongiform encephalopathy epidemic; while active testing volume has decreased since the epidemic period, protocols remain in place for suspect cases. Feline spongiform encephalopathy testing in captive felids follows similar protocols. Confirmed prion disease detection in any species triggers specific institutional response including tissue archival for reference, appropriate biosafety practices during any subsequent handling of tissue, and coordination with public health authorities regarding potential zoonotic implications where relevant.

Applied Case: Domoic Acid Toxicosis in a California Sea Lion

An adult female California sea lion (Zalophus californianus) was recovered alive from a stranding site during a period of documented harmful algal bloom activity along the central California coast. Antemortem clinical presentation included seizures, disorientation, head-weaving, and characteristic behavioral changes consistent with domoic acid toxicosis. Marine mammal stranding rehabilitation was attempted with anticonvulsant therapy and supportive care; the animal declined despite intervention and died approximately 96 hours after stranding. Necropsy focused on characterization of the neurologic disease and confirmation of the presumptive domoic acid diagnosis.

External examination demonstrated appropriate body condition consistent with recent good health before the acute illness, and no evidence of external trauma. Systematic marine mammal necropsy by adapted terrestrial mammal approach demonstrated no significant abnormalities in most organ systems. Brain examination demonstrated bilateral hippocampal atrophy with characteristic gross appearance of pallor and shrinkage in the hippocampal formation region; this finding is the pathognomonic gross lesion of chronic domoic acid toxicosis and is recognized on gross examination when present. Sample collection included fresh-frozen brain tissue for domoic acid quantitation and standard histopathologic sampling.

Cross-taxa reasoning at case interpretation drew on the extensive documented literature of domoic acid toxicosis in California sea lions and other marine wildlife during Pseudo-nitzschia harmful algal bloom events along the Pacific coast. Domoic acid is a glutamate receptor agonist neurotoxin produced by certain Pseudo-nitzschia diatom species that accumulates in filter-feeding organisms and ascends the marine food web through anchovy and sardine intermediate hosts. Marine mammals exposed through prey consumption develop acute neurologic disease and, with chronic exposure, characteristic hippocampal atrophy. The pattern is well documented and has become a leading cause of morbidity and mortality in California sea lions during bloom events.

Histopathology confirmed severe bilateral hippocampal atrophy with characteristic loss of pyramidal neurons in the CA1, CA3, and CA4 hippocampal regions, associated gliosis with reactive astrocytes and microglia, and preserved dentate gyrus consistent with the well-characterized pattern of domoic acid-induced hippocampal injury. Domoic acid quantitation on fresh-frozen brain returned a value consistent with recent significant exposure. The final morphologic diagnosis was severe bilateral hippocampal atrophy consistent with domoic acid toxicosis, and terminal event neurologic dysfunction consistent with the same. Institutional reporting followed the marine mammal stranding pathway with distribution to the NOAA Fisheries regional coordinator and to the coordinated harmful algal bloom research community.

THE COMPARATIVE NECROPSY PATTERN SYSTEM — Chapter 9 Nervous System Pattern Foundations

Meningoencephalitis Pattern Recognition Across Mammalian and Avian Taxa: Meningeal congestion with parenchymal inflammatory infiltrate across taxa indicating infectious or immune-mediated CNS disease. Anchor: histopathologic characterization with molecular pathogen panels. Trap: agonal meningeal congestion discriminated by absent inflammatory infiltrate. Flag: rabies, arboviral encephalitides, and several other zoonotic agents carry public health obligations.

Chronic Wasting Disease Pattern in Free-Ranging Cervids: Cervid carcass with progressive neurologic decline requiring prion testing on obex and retropharyngeal lymph node. Anchor: immunohistochemistry or ELISA for pathologic prion protein. Trap: other chronic weight loss diseases in cervids discriminated by prion testing. Flag: reportable disease with coordinated state and federal surveillance.

West Nile Virus Encephalitis Pattern in Corvids and Raptors: Nonsuppurative meningoencephalitis with brainstem and thalamic involvement across corvids, raptors, and other affected species. Anchor: PCR for West Nile virus with immunohistochemistry demonstrating viral antigen. Trap: EEE virus discriminated by molecular characterization. Flag: zoonotic pathogen contributing to public health surveillance.

Summary and Key Concepts

Comparative neuroanatomic knowledge is prerequisite to nervous system pathology interpretation across taxa; species-appropriate anatomic reference must be established before pathologic interpretation is applied.

Meningoencephalitis pattern recognition supports the interpretive path from gross observation through histopathology through molecular pathogen identification across a wide range of etiologies.

Chronic wasting disease in cervids is a reportable transmissible spongiform encephalopathy with expanding geographic and taxonomic distribution requiring coordinated surveillance response.

Viral encephalitides across taxa include rabies, arboviral encephalitides including West Nile virus, herpesvirus, morbillivirus, and emerging pathogens each with characteristic patterns and specific reporting obligations.

Bacterial encephalitides and meningitis, fungal encephalitis with CNS extension, and parasitic and protozoal encephalitides each contribute to the CNS disease differential with species-appropriate ancillary workup.

Non-infectious neurologic disease including central nervous system neoplasia, neurodegenerative disease, traumatic injury, and toxic injury (with domoic acid toxicosis in marine mammals as a leading exemplar) each carry recognizable patterns transportable across taxa.

CHAPTER 10: MUSCULOSKELETAL, INTEGUMENTARY, AND OCULAR PATHOLOGY

Learning Objectives

1. Recognize metabolic bone disease patterns in managed captive populations across mammalian, avian, and reptile taxa.
2. Identify major skin disease patterns in non-domestic species including infectious, parasitic, and non-infectious disease.
3. Interpret ocular pathology in non-domestic species with attention to species-specific ocular anatomy and disease patterns.
4. Distinguish traumatic and developmental musculoskeletal disease from primary bone disease.
5. Apply the Comparative Necropsy Pattern callout structure to musculoskeletal, integumentary, and ocular lesion recognition across unfamiliar species.
6. Coordinate ancillary diagnostics for musculoskeletal, integumentary, and ocular disease including bone histomorphometry, dermatopathology stains, and ocular histopathology.

The musculoskeletal, integumentary, and ocular systems together carry a substantial proportion of the recognizable disease burden in captive and free-ranging wildlife. Metabolic bone disease affects juvenile animals of many captive species and remains a leading cause of morbidity in poorly managed collections. Skin disease is often the earliest recognized clinical presentation of infectious or systemic disease and provides antemortem accessibility that internal organ disease does not. Ocular pathology carries interpretive weight for both individual health and for population-level surveillance because ocular disease may reflect systemic conditions or specific infectious processes. This chapter organizes these three organ systems together not because they are anatomically related but because they are frequently accessible for antemortem clinical assessment and because the pathology of each carries distinctive interpretive frameworks that support diagnostic reasoning.

The chapter organizes musculoskeletal, integumentary, and ocular pathology into four operational domains. Metabolic bone disease addresses the calcium, phosphorus, and vitamin D-related bone disease patterns that dominate captive juvenile animal pathology. Skin disease across taxa covers infectious, parasitic, and non-infectious skin disease. Ocular pathology in non-domestic species addresses the recurring ocular disease patterns including species-specific ocular disease entities. Traumatic and developmental musculoskeletal disease completes the chapter with attention to the range of non-primary bone disease that produces musculoskeletal clinical presentation.

Metabolic Bone Disease in Managed Populations

Nutritional Secondary Hyperparathyroidism

Nutritional secondary hyperparathyroidism is the most common metabolic bone disease pattern in captive populations and reflects dietary calcium-to-phosphorus imbalance producing chronic parathyroid hormone elevation with characteristic skeletal consequences. In captive reptiles, the disease is particularly prominent in growing individuals fed invertebrate-heavy diets without appropriate calcium supplementation; the gross pattern includes rubber jaw with palpably softened mandibles, curvature of long bones with characteristic bowing, pathologic fractures at sites of skeletal weakness, and, in advanced cases, generalized skeletal deformity. Histopathology demonstrates fibrous osteodystrophy with peritrabecular fibrosis, thinned cortical bone, and reactive periosteal changes. In captive juvenile mammals and juvenile avian species, similar patterns are recognized with species-appropriate modifications. Recognition of the pattern at necropsy prompts institutional review of the affected animal's diet history and consideration of other individuals at similar risk in the collection.

Hypovitaminosis D and Rickets

Hypovitaminosis D produces rickets in growing captive animals and osteomalacia in adult animals. The disease reflects inadequate ultraviolet B exposure required for endogenous vitamin D synthesis in captive housing without appropriate lighting, inadequate dietary vitamin D content, or both. In captive reptiles maintained without appropriate ultraviolet B lighting, rickets is a recurring disease with characteristic skeletal deformities. In captive avian species similar patterns are documented. In captive juvenile mammals, dietary vitamin D content is typically the primary consideration because most mammalian species do not require ultraviolet B exposure for adequate vitamin D synthesis under normal conditions. The gross and histopathologic patterns include growth plate widening with disorganized cartilage architecture, defective mineralization of osteoid, and characteristic radiographic and gross changes at long bone metaphyses.

Hypervitaminosis D and Metastatic Mineralization

Hypervitaminosis D from excessive dietary vitamin D supplementation produces the opposite pattern: hypercalcemia with metastatic mineralization of soft tissues including kidneys, blood vessels, gastrointestinal tract, and lung. The condition is documented in captive psittacines with chronic dietary vitamin D excess and, less commonly, in other captive species with iatrogenic vitamin D toxicity. The gross pattern includes multifocal firm gritty deposits within affected soft tissues, and the histopathologic pattern includes basophilic mineral deposition confirmed by von Kossa staining. Recognition of the pattern prompts institutional dietary review addressing supplementation practices and vitamin D content of offered diets.

THE COMPARATIVE NECROPSY PATTERN SYSTEM — Nutritional Secondary Hyperparathyroidism Pattern in Captive Juvenile Reptiles and Birds

The Pattern: Juvenile captive reptile or bird with softened mandible (rubber jaw), long bone bowing and pathologic fractures, and generalized skeletal deformity indicating nutritional secondary hyperparathyroidism from dietary calcium-phosphorus imbalance.

Cross-Taxa Signature: Recognized across captive juvenile reptile species (particularly herbivorous species fed diets without appropriate calcium supplementation, and insectivorous species fed unsupplemented invertebrate diets), captive juvenile avian species (particularly gallinaceous and psittacine species), and, less commonly, captive juvenile mammalian species with similar dietary risk factors. The gross patterns are broadly consistent across affected taxa with species-appropriate modifications.

Diagnostic Anchor: Radiographic and gross recognition of characteristic skeletal changes confirmed by histopathology demonstrating fibrous osteodystrophy. Serum calcium, phosphorus, and parathyroid hormone measurement supports the diagnosis when antemortem samples are available.

Trap Logic: The look-alike is rickets from hypovitaminosis D with similar skeletal patterns but distinguished by growth plate architecture on histopathology. Discrimination: nutritional secondary hyperparathyroidism demonstrates fibrous osteodystrophy predominantly; rickets demonstrates growth plate widening with disorganized cartilage predominantly.

Zoonotic/Reportable Flag: Not zoonotic or regulatorily reportable. Institutionally reportable for dietary and husbandry review to prevent additional cases in the collection.

Figure 10.1: Nutritional Secondary Hyperparathyroidism in a Juvenile Captive Bearded Dragon: Radiographic and Gross Appearance.

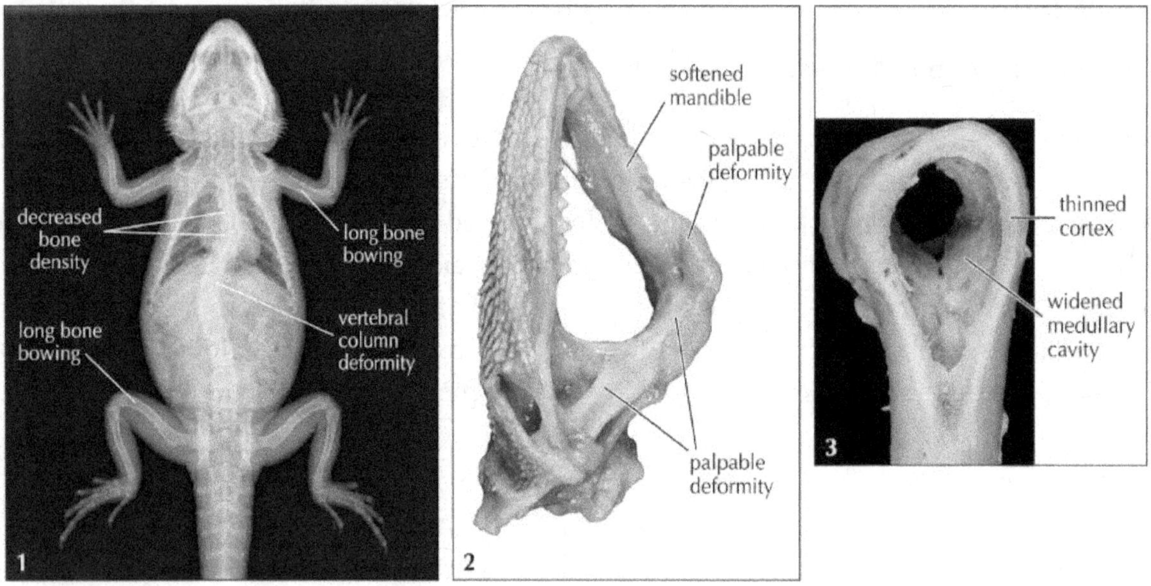

Skin Disease Across Taxa

Bacterial and Fungal Skin Disease

Bacterial skin disease across taxa includes Dermatophilus congolensis infection in wild ruminants producing characteristic exudative dermatitis with crust formation, Staphylococcus and Streptococcus species pyoderma in captive species, and species-specific bacterial dermatitis. Fungal skin disease includes dermatophytosis with Microsporum and Trichophyton species infection in captive mammals, Malassezia species yeast dermatitis in some captive species, and chromoblastomycosis and phaeohyphomycosis in captive reptiles and amphibians. Chytridiomycosis in amphibians is caused by Batrachochytrium dendrobatidis and B. salamandrivorans and produces characteristic epidermal thickening with fungal thalli visible on histopathology; the disease is a leading conservation threat to amphibian populations worldwide. Snake fungal disease caused by Ophidiomyces ophiodiicola produces characteristic dermatologic lesions in captive and free-ranging snakes with expanding geographic distribution.

Parasitic Skin Disease

Parasitic skin disease across taxa includes sarcoptic and demodectic mange in wild carnivores with characteristic scaling and alopecia and, in severe cases, systemic debilitation from chronic disease; Notoedres cati and related mite infections in captive felids; louse infestation across taxa with species-specific louse-host associations; and tick infestation with associated tick-borne disease transmission. Ectoparasitism in wildlife carries interpretive weight beyond the individual disease because ectoparasite species identification informs regional vector-borne disease surveillance and provides baseline data on wildlife-vector interactions.

Non-Infectious and Neoplastic Skin Disease

Non-infectious skin disease includes autoimmune disease, allergic dermatitis, and species-specific skin conditions. Neoplastic skin disease across taxa includes squamous cell carcinoma with predisposition in captive white-haired felids and captive avian species with reduced pigmentation, mast cell tumors in captive mammals, melanoma in captive species with pigmented skin, and species-specific tumor entities. Iridovirus disease in captive gilthead seabream and other fish species produces characteristic dermatologic changes. Poxvirus disease in captive avian species produces characteristic proliferative dermatologic lesions with intracytoplasmic viral inclusion bodies on histopathology.

Applied Case: Sarcoptic Mange in a Wild Coyote

A wild coyote (Canis latrans) was recovered dead from a suburban area with a submission history noting extensive alopecia, poor body condition, and evidence of chronic disease before death. Similar cases had been submitted from the same geographic region over the preceding 18 months, suggesting an ongoing outbreak of ectoparasitism in the local coyote population. Necropsy focused on characterization of the skin disease and confirmation of the ectoparasite species.

External examination demonstrated extensive alopecia affecting greater than 60 percent of the body surface with characteristic distribution over the flanks, hindquarters, and dorsum sparing the head. The affected skin was markedly thickened, hyperkeratotic, and covered with dry crusts and scaling. Body condition was poor with prominent skeletal features. Systematic necropsy demonstrated the anticipated poor body condition, hepatic congestion consistent with terminal event, and no significant primary organ disease. Skin scrapings from affected areas demonstrated numerous sarcoptic mites and multiple mite eggs on wet-mount microscopy, confirming Sarcoptes scabiei var. canis infestation.

Cross-taxa reasoning at case interpretation drew on the documented epidemiology of sarcoptic mange in wild carnivore populations. Sarcoptic mange in wild canids is documented at variable prevalence across geographic regions and can produce catastrophic population-level impacts during outbreak periods. The disease produces the individual-level pathology of chronic skin disease with associated debilitation while also serving as an important indicator of population health and environmental stress. Case surveillance provides data on outbreak dynamics and, in some cases, informs regulatory or management responses. Institutional response included submission of case data to the state wildlife health veterinarian for regional surveillance and coordination with the state wildlife agency for consideration of broader population monitoring.

Applied Case: Uveal Melanoma in an Aged Captive Snow Leopard

An aged captive snow leopard (Panthera uncia) had been diagnosed clinically with a progressive ocular mass affecting the left eye. Antemortem clinical assessment identified the mass as an intraocular tumor with prominent uveal involvement; enucleation was elected after progressive tumor growth. The animal was subsequently maintained in the collection for approximately two years after enucleation without evidence of tumor recurrence or metastatic disease before dying of unrelated causes. Necropsy focused on comprehensive assessment with attention to potential late metastatic disease.

Necropsy examination demonstrated no evidence of metastatic disease at any site examined. The previously enucleated orbit demonstrated appropriate surgical healing without local recurrence. The final assessment concluded that the enucleation had achieved definitive local control of the primary tumor without subsequent metastatic disease during the observation period. Histopathologic re-examination of the original enucleation specimen (retained in the institutional archive) confirmed the diagnosis of uveal melanoma with cellular features supporting a favorable local prognosis. The case illustrated the utility of definitive local treatment for uveal melanoma in captive felids and reinforced the value of retained tissue archives for retrospective analysis when subsequent case outcomes provide interpretive context.

Species-Specific Ocular Conditions and Population Surveillance

Species-specific ocular conditions across captive collections include documented cataract clusters in some captive fish species related to dietary nucleotide content, riboflavin deficiency-associated cataracts in some captive avian species with historic dietary formulation problems, and species-specific ocular disease patterns in captive aged animals of many species. Population-level ocular surveillance at Species Survival Plan facilities contributes to species management by identifying environmental, nutritional, or genetic contributors to disease clusters. Individual necropsy findings inform population-level management decisions when interpreted in the context of collection-level surveillance data. The pathologist's obligation extends to appropriate reporting of ocular findings to the collection team and to the coordinated species management structure.

THE COMPARATIVE NECROPSY PATTERN SYSTEM — Chytridiomycosis Pattern in Free-Ranging and Captive Amphibians

The Pattern: Amphibian carcass with characteristic epidermal thickening, hyperkeratosis of skin covering the digits and body, and, on histopathology, fungal thalli within the epidermal keratin layer indicating chytridiomycosis.

Cross-Taxa Signature: Recognized across amphibian species with variable susceptibility; anuran species have been most severely affected with catastrophic population declines documented in some Neotropical and Australian species. Batrachochytrium dendrobatidis produces the classical presentation; Batrachochytrium salamandrivorans produces similar lesions with predilection for caudate amphibians (salamanders and newts) and has emerged as a distinct threat to European caudate populations with active surveillance to prevent North American introduction.

Diagnostic Anchor: Histopathologic demonstration of fungal thalli within the epidermal keratin layer with characteristic morphology. Molecular confirmation by polymerase chain reaction targeting Batrachochytrium-specific sequences confirms the diagnosis and permits species-level identification.

Trap Logic: The look-alike is normal epidermal thickening in some amphibian species during specific physiologic states (breeding season in some species), distinguished by absence of fungal thalli. Another look-alike is other fungal skin disease in amphibians distinguished by the specific chytrid morphology.

Zoonotic/Reportable Flag: Chytridiomycosis is a World Organisation for Animal Health-notifiable disease requiring reporting through state and federal wildlife health authorities. Not zoonotic. Detection triggers biosecurity review of the affected population or collection, source investigation, and coordinated conservation response.

Ocular Pathology in Non-Domestic Species

Comparative Ocular Anatomy

Comparative ocular anatomy varies substantially across vertebrate taxa in ways that modify pathologic interpretation. Avian eyes are relatively large for the body size with a distinctive pecten oculi projecting into the vitreous, an intraocular vascular structure with no mammalian analog; disease of the pecten is a recognized entity in avian ocular pathology. Reptile eyes include species-specific features such as spectacles (fused eyelids covering the eye in snakes and some geckos) that modify examination approach. Fish eyes include species-specific features and, in deep-water species, adaptations for low-light vision. Marine mammal eyes include species-specific adaptations for underwater vision. Mammalian eye anatomy demonstrates species-specific variation in tapetum lucidum, pupil shape, and other features that modify interpretation.

Infectious and Inflammatory Ocular Disease

Infectious and inflammatory ocular disease across taxa includes bacterial conjunctivitis and keratitis, viral ocular disease including herpesvirus involvement of ocular tissues, fungal ocular disease particularly in captive avian species, and parasitic ocular disease including onchocercid nematode infections in wildlife and Thelazia species eye worms. Chlamydial conjunctivitis produces characteristic findings in captive avian species and in some captive reptiles. Mycobacterial ocular disease is documented in captive species with systemic mycobacteriosis.

Non-Infectious Ocular Disease and Neoplasia

Non-infectious ocular disease includes cataract formation with recognized associations to species, age, and diet in some captive populations; glaucoma with primary and secondary presentations; retinal degeneration with variable etiologies; and traumatic ocular injury. Ocular neoplasia includes uveal melanoma in captive mammals, squamous cell carcinoma of the eyelid and periocular tissue, retrobulbar tumors with associated exophthalmos, and species-specific ocular tumor entities. Ocular pathology in wildlife often provides early clinical recognition of systemic disease because ocular examination is accessible during clinical assessment.

Applied Case: Snake Fungal Disease in a Wild Timber Rattlesnake

A wild adult timber rattlesnake (Crotalus horridus) was submitted for necropsy after being found dead by a herpetological monitoring program in a documented population under active conservation assessment. Antemortem observation had identified evidence of dermatologic disease with characteristic gross appearance including facial swelling, crusting lesions, and dysecdysis affecting multiple body regions. The individual had been observed with progressive clinical signs for several weeks before death. Timber rattlesnake populations in the eastern United States have been subject to substantial declines from habitat loss, illegal collection, and, more recently, from snake fungal disease caused by Ophidiomyces ophiodiicola.

External examination confirmed severe dermatologic disease with facial swelling, ulcerated and crusted lesions distributed asymmetrically across the head and rostrum, and evidence of chronic dysecdysis with retained shed material adherent to multiple body regions. Body condition was thin consistent with chronic disease affecting normal feeding and activity. Systematic necropsy demonstrated no significant abnormalities in most internal organ systems; the disease was predominantly dermatologic with secondary systemic effects. Fresh tissue samples of affected skin were collected for histopathology and for molecular characterization; environmental swabs from the recovery area were coordinated with the ongoing surveillance program.

Cross-taxa reasoning at case interpretation drew on the extensive documented literature of snake fungal disease. Ophidiomyces ophiodiicola produces characteristic dermatologic disease across snake species with well-documented outbreaks in wild North American populations. The pattern includes facial and rostral involvement, ulcerated and crusted skin lesions, and dysecdysis; histopathology demonstrates fungal thalli within affected skin layers with associated granulomatous inflammatory response. Molecular characterization confirmed Ophidiomyces ophiodiicola in this individual. The final morphologic diagnosis was severe fungal dermatitis with associated granulomatous inflammatory response and secondary poor body condition; the etiologic diagnosis was snake fungal disease caused by Ophidiomyces ophiodiicola. Case data were coordinated with the state wildlife health veterinarian, the herpetological conservation research community, and the surveillance program that supports snake population health assessment.

Bone Histomorphometry and Ancillary Musculoskeletal Diagnostics

Bone histomorphometry provides quantitative assessment of bone mass, structure, and remodeling activity through analysis of undecalcified bone sections. In metabolic bone disease cases where quantitative characterization supports clinical decision-making or contributes to population-level surveillance, bone histomorphometry provides interpretive detail beyond routine histopathology. Serum biomarkers of bone metabolism including alkaline phosphatase (particularly the bone isoenzyme), calcium, phosphorus, and, when species-appropriate assays are available, parathyroid hormone and vitamin D metabolites support the diagnosis and management of metabolic bone disease. Radiographic assessment of skeletal density and structure, when antemortem imaging is available or when postmortem imaging is performed, provides additional characterization. Species-appropriate reference ranges for these biomarkers are limited across non-domestic species; comparative interpretation against the closest available species-specific data supports interpretation.

Dermatopathology Special Stains and Molecular Techniques

Dermatopathology special stains support the identification of specific etiologic agents in skin disease cases. Periodic acid-Schiff and Grocott-Gomori methenamine silver stains highlight fungal organisms in cases of dermatophytosis, chytridiomycosis, chromoblastomycosis, and other fungal skin disease. Gram stain identifies bacterial organisms in cases of bacterial dermatitis. Ziehl-Neelsen acid-fast staining identifies mycobacterial organisms in cases of cutaneous mycobacteriosis. Immunohistochemistry supports the identification of viral antigens in cases of viral dermatologic disease including poxvirus and herpesvirus infections. Molecular techniques including polymerase chain reaction for chytrid fungi, snake fungal disease, and other emerging pathogens support the definitive characterization of dermatologic disease in captive and free-ranging populations. Standard collection of fresh skin samples for potential molecular analysis complements the routine formalin-fixed sampling for histopathology.

THE COMPARATIVE NECROPSY PATTERN SYSTEM — Cataract Pattern Across Aged Captive Species

The Pattern: Lens opacification with characteristic gross and histopathologic changes across aged captive species indicating cataract formation of primary or secondary origin.

Cross-Taxa Signature: Recognized across mammalian, avian, and reptile taxa in aged captive animals. Species-specific predispositions include documented cataract associations in captive fish species (some cataracts related to dietary factors), captive nonhuman primates (age-related predisposition varying by species), and captive marine mammals. Diabetic cataract has been documented in captive species with diabetes mellitus. Congenital cataract is documented in some captive species with genetic predisposition.

Diagnostic Anchor: Gross recognition of lens opacification confirmed by histopathologic characterization of lens fiber changes. Underlying etiology assessment includes evaluation for diabetes, chronic uveitis, or other associations.

Trap Logic: The look-alike is postmortem lens changes in a carcass with prolonged postmortem interval, distinguished by lens architecture on histopathology. Another look-alike is nuclear sclerosis in aged animals which does not progress to true cataract.

Zoonotic/Reportable Flag: Not zoonotic. Institutionally documented for species and individual clinical records; population-level cataract clustering may indicate dietary or environmental factors warranting collection-level review.

Traumatic and Developmental Musculoskeletal Disease

Traumatic Fracture Patterns

Traumatic fracture patterns in non-domestic species reflect the mechanism of injury sustained. Vehicular collision produces long bone fractures with characteristic distribution reflecting the impact vector, associated soft tissue injury, and radiographic changes recognizable at necropsy. Projectile injury produces fractures along the projectile path with associated tissue disruption. Falls produce distinctive fracture patterns at anatomic sites of impact. Intraspecific and interspecific trauma produces characteristic patterns reflecting the specific interaction. Fracture healing patterns provide interpretive information about the timing of injury; callus formation at various stages of maturation indicates injury timing and permits reasoning about the case history.

Developmental Musculoskeletal Disease

Developmental musculoskeletal disease in captive species includes osteochondrosis and osteochondritis dissecans in captive large ungulates, angular limb deformities in captive juveniles, congenital vertebral malformations documented in various captive species, and species-specific developmental patterns. Osteochondrosis is documented in captive rhinoceros, captive giraffe, and some other large captive ungulates and reflects combined genetic and nutritional factors during development. Recognition of the developmental pattern requires evaluation of both individual case features and, at Species Survival Plan facilities, consideration of population-level breeding management implications.

Applied Case: Osteochondrosis in a Juvenile Captive Giraffe

A 2-year-old female reticulated giraffe (Giraffa reticulata) was euthanized after a fall in her exhibit produced a comminuted long bone fracture with a poor prognosis for return to function. Antemortem history included documented lameness of the affected limb over several weeks prior to the fall; the fall itself was likely secondary to the pre-existing lameness. Antemortem workup had identified the lameness as musculoskeletal in origin without complete characterization due to species-related imaging constraints. Necropsy focused on characterization of both the acute fracture and the underlying musculoskeletal disease process.

Systematic examination of the affected limb demonstrated the acute comminuted fracture with associated soft tissue injury. Additional evaluation of joint surfaces demonstrated multifocal osteochondrotic lesions affecting several joints including the affected fracture site, several other joints in the affected limb, and the contralateral limb. The osteochondrotic lesions demonstrated the characteristic gross appearance of joint surface irregularity, occasional cartilage flap formation, and subchondral bone changes. Histopathology confirmed osteochondrosis with characteristic changes including disruption of the growth plate architecture, subchondral bone cyst formation, and reactive changes.

Cross-taxa reasoning at case interpretation drew on the documented literature of osteochondrosis in captive large ungulates. Osteochondrosis is documented in captive giraffe, captive rhinoceros, and other captive large ungulates and reflects combined genetic predisposition and nutritional factors during rapid growth phases. The pattern in this individual was consistent with published descriptions and contributed to the ongoing Species Survival Plan discussion of osteochondrosis management in the species. Institutional response addressed the individual case and considered implications for other juvenile giraffes in the collection with attention to growth rate management, nutritional supplementation, and exercise programming.

THE COMPARATIVE NECROPSY PATTERN SYSTEM — Chapter 10 Musculoskeletal, Integumentary, and Ocular Pattern Foundations

---

Nutritional Secondary Hyperparathyroidism Pattern in Captive Juvenile Reptiles and Birds: Rubber jaw and skeletal deformity from dietary calcium-phosphorus imbalance in captive juveniles. Anchor: histopathology demonstrating fibrous osteodystrophy. Trap: rickets discriminated by growth plate architecture. Flag: institutionally reportable for dietary review.

Chytridiomycosis Pattern in Free-Ranging and Captive Amphibians: Amphibian epidermal thickening with fungal thalli indicating Batrachochytrium infection. Anchor: histopathologic and molecular characterization. Trap: normal breeding-season epidermal changes discriminated by absent fungal thalli. Flag: WOAH-notifiable amphibian disease with conservation implications.

Cataract Pattern Across Aged Captive Species: Lens opacification across aged mammals, birds, and reptiles with variable etiologic profiles. Anchor: histopathologic lens fiber characterization. Trap: postmortem lens changes discriminated by architectural assessment. Flag: population-level clustering may indicate dietary or environmental factors.

Summary and Key Concepts

Metabolic bone disease in managed captive populations includes nutritional secondary hyperparathyroidism (most common), rickets from hypovitaminosis D, and hypervitaminosis D with metastatic mineralization; recognition prompts institutional dietary and husbandry review.

Skin disease across taxa includes bacterial and fungal disease with amphibian chytridiomycosis and snake fungal disease as leading conservation-relevant entities, parasitic disease with ectoparasitism carrying vector-borne surveillance implications, and non-infectious and neoplastic conditions.

Ocular pathology in non-domestic species requires comparative ocular anatomic knowledge; infectious, non-infectious, and neoplastic ocular disease patterns are documented across taxa with species-specific presentations.

Traumatic musculoskeletal disease patterns reflect injury mechanism; fracture healing timing supports case history reconstruction.

Developmental musculoskeletal disease including osteochondrosis in captive large ungulates and angular limb deformities in captive juveniles reflects combined genetic and nutritional factors during development.

Musculoskeletal, integumentary, and ocular pathology recognition at necropsy carries substantial implications for population-level management at Species Survival Plan facilities and for conservation-relevant disease surveillance.

CHAPTER 11: ENDOCRINE, REPRODUCTIVE, AND HEMATOLYMPHATIC PATHOLOGY

Learning Objectives

1. Recognize endocrinopathy patterns in non-domestic species including thyroid, adrenal, pancreatic, and pituitary disease.
2. Identify reproductive pathology in captive and free-ranging populations including infertility patterns, dystocia complications, and reproductive tract neoplasia.
3. Interpret splenic and lymph node pathology across taxa with attention to reactive, infectious, and neoplastic changes.
4. Recognize hematopoietic neoplasia including lymphoma and leukemia patterns across taxa.
5. Apply the Comparative Necropsy Pattern callout structure to endocrine, reproductive, and hematolymphatic lesion recognition across unfamiliar species.
6. Coordinate ancillary endocrine, reproductive, and hematolymphatic diagnostics including hormone assays, reproductive tract histopathology, and flow cytometry for hematopoietic neoplasia characterization.

The endocrine, reproductive, and hematolymphatic organ systems together carry substantial interpretive weight in wildlife and zoo animal pathology. Endocrinopathies in captive species reflect the interpretive challenge of maintaining physiologic hormone regulation in animals whose evolutionary context differs from their captive conditions; the disease patterns recognized in domestic animals recur in non-domestic species with species-specific modifications. Reproductive pathology carries dual significance because reproductive success drives population-level conservation management at Species Survival Plan facilities and because reproductive tract disease produces recognizable pathology at necropsy. Splenic and lymph node pathology serves as a sentinel indicator of systemic disease processes because these organs participate in immunologic response to nearly every infectious and neoplastic disease affecting the host. Hematopoietic neoplasia including lymphoma and leukemia is recognized across taxa with species-specific predispositions that inform population-level management.

This chapter organizes the three combined organ systems into four operational domains. Endocrinopathies in non-domestic species address the thyroid, adrenal, pancreatic, and pituitary disease patterns documented across captive and free-ranging populations. Reproductive pathology covers the range of reproductive tract disease affecting captive breeding programs and free-ranging population health. Splenic and lymph node pathology across taxa considers reactive, infectious, and neoplastic changes as diagnostic anchors for systemic disease. Hematopoietic neoplasia completes the chapter with attention to lymphoma, leukemia, and related hematopoietic neoplastic entities documented across taxa.

Endocrinopathies in Non-Domestic Species

Thyroid Disease Across Taxa

Thyroid disease in non-domestic species includes both hyperthyroidism and hypothyroidism with species-specific presentations and recognitions. Hyperthyroidism in captive felids follows the well-documented domestic feline pattern with thyroid adenoma or adenomatous hyperplasia producing chronic thyroid hormone excess; the disease has been documented in captive large felids at recognizable prevalence and follows a clinical course comparable to domestic felid hyperthyroidism with progressive weight loss despite adequate intake, cardiovascular consequences, and eventual terminal event mortality without appropriate management. Hypothyroidism is documented in captive canids and in some captive avian species with characteristic clinical and gross pathologic changes including alopecia in mammalian cases and reproductive dysfunction across affected species. Thyroid neoplasia including thyroid carcinoma is documented across taxa in aged captive individuals. Iodine deficiency-associated goiter has been documented historically in captive collections with inadequate iodine supplementation and remains relevant in some geographic regions with iodine-poor water and food sources. Recognition of thyroid disease at necropsy requires attention to thyroid gland size, texture, and cut surface appearance with comparison against species-appropriate reference where available.

Adrenal Disease Patterns

Adrenal disease in non-domestic species includes hyperadrenocorticism in captive ferrets (a species-specific pattern with adrenal tumor formation producing hormonally active neoplasia with characteristic clinical presentation), hyperadrenocorticism in captive nonhuman primates with pituitary or adrenal origins, adrenal cortical neoplasia in aged captive species across taxa, and pheochromocytoma with catecholamine-producing tumor formation. The hyperadrenocorticism of captive ferrets warrants specific mention because the disease is one of the most common endocrine diseases in captive ferret populations and reflects both genetic predisposition and management factors including early gonadectomy affecting subsequent adrenal steroidogenesis. Recognition of adrenal disease at necropsy requires systematic bilateral adrenal examination with attention to gland size (both absolute and relative to body size), texture, cut surface appearance, and any evidence of mass lesions.

Pancreatic Endocrine Disease and Diabetes Mellitus

Pancreatic endocrine disease across taxa includes diabetes mellitus with characteristic hyperglycemia and metabolic consequences. Diabetes mellitus is documented in captive nonhuman primates (with recognized dietary and genetic contributions in some captive populations), captive great apes with substantial documented case series in some collections, captive avian species (particularly captive psittacines), captive dolphins, and other captive species. Type 1 diabetes with pancreatic beta cell destruction and type 2 diabetes with insulin resistance are both documented across taxa. Recognition of chronic diabetes mellitus at necropsy includes assessment of pancreatic islet architecture on histopathology with immunohistochemistry for insulin, glucagon, and somatostatin supporting characterization of the specific beta cell versus alpha cell versus mixed patterns. Diabetes complications including nephropathy, retinopathy, and neuropathy analogs are documented in captive species with chronic disease. Pancreatic islet neoplasia including insulinoma and glucagonoma is documented in aged captive species across taxa.

Pituitary and Reproductive Endocrine Disease

Pituitary disease in non-domestic species includes pituitary adenoma with characteristic gross and histopathologic features, pituitary macroadenoma producing local mass effect with compression of adjacent structures, and pituitary carcinoma (less common than adenoma). Pituitary disease with cortisol excess (Cushing analog) or with growth hormone excess (acromegaly analog) is documented in captive species. Reproductive endocrine disease including chronic anovulation, chronic reproductive hormone dysregulation, and reproductive senescence patterns is documented across captive species with implications for breeding program management at Species Survival Plan facilities.

THE COMPARATIVE NECROPSY PATTERN SYSTEM — Diabetes Mellitus Pattern in Captive Nonhuman Primates and Captive Psittacines

The Pattern: Chronic hyperglycemia with associated metabolic consequences including glycosuria, cataract formation, and, in advanced cases, diabetic nephropathy and neuropathy analogs in captive nonhuman primates, captive psittacines, and other affected captive species.

Cross-Taxa Signature: Recognized across captive nonhuman primates (particularly great apes and some cercopithecine species with documented dietary and genetic contributions), captive psittacines (with well-documented species predisposition in some species), captive dolphins (with documented cases in aged managed care populations), and other captive species. The clinical and pathologic patterns are broadly comparable across taxa with species-specific modifications reflecting metabolic and dietary differences.

Diagnostic Anchor: Histopathologic assessment of pancreatic islet architecture with immunohistochemistry for beta cells (insulin), alpha cells (glucagon), and delta cells (somatostatin) supporting characterization of the specific islet pattern. Serum biochemistry with elevated glucose, glycated hemoglobin measurement when species-appropriate assays are available, and urinalysis with documented glycosuria support the antemortem or perimortem diagnosis.

Trap Logic: The look-alike is stress hyperglycemia with transient elevation of glucose in the terminal event context, distinguished by absence of chronic metabolic consequences and by histopathologic characterization of pancreatic islets. Another look-alike is postmortem glucose changes distinguished by fresh vitreous humor glucose measurement or by other tissue chemistry.

Zoonotic/Reportable Flag: Not zoonotic or regulatorily reportable. Institutionally documented for individual and population-level dietary and husbandry review, particularly at collections with recognized species predispositions.

Figure 11.1: Pancreatic Islet Amyloidosis (Congo Red, 20×)

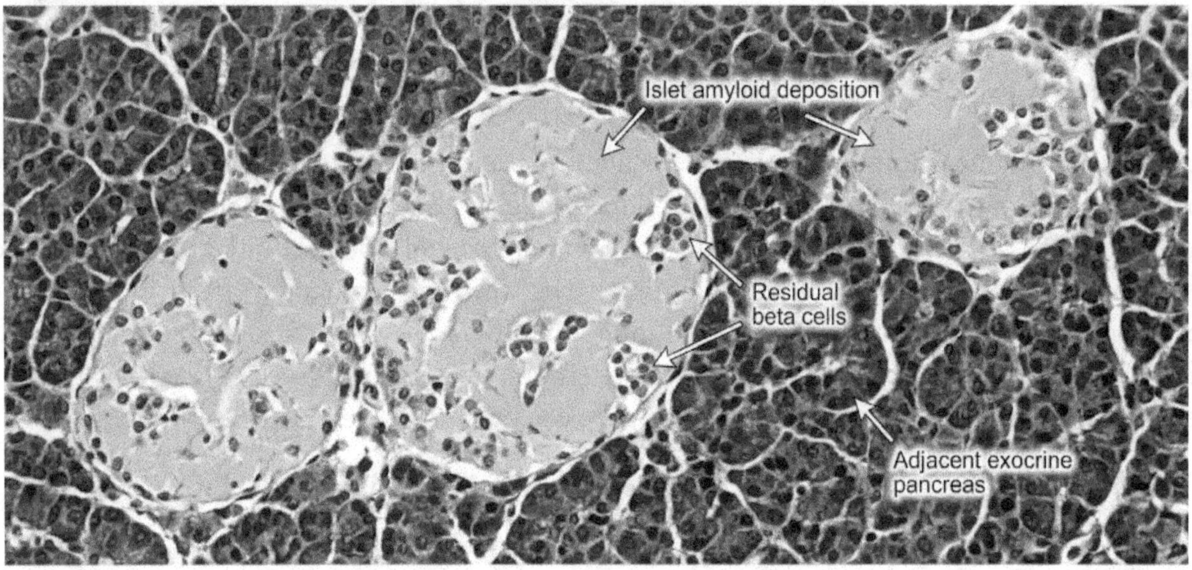

Histopathological photomicrograph of pancreatic tissue from a captive olive baboon with type 2 diabetes mellitus — Congo red stain at 20× magnification showing pancreatic islets containing prominent salmon-pink amyloid deposition throughout the islet architecture; adjacent exocrine pancreas appears normal; the amyloid deposition displaces beta cells and disrupts normal islet organization.

Reproductive Pathology in Zoo and Wildlife Populations

Female Reproductive Tract Disease

Female reproductive tract disease in non-domestic species includes ovarian disease with the range of primary neoplasia (granulosa cell tumor, ovarian cystadenoma, ovarian teratoma, ovarian carcinoma), ovarian cystic disease, and ovarian hemorrhage; uterine disease with endometrial hyperplasia, endometritis, pyometra, uterine neoplasia including leiomyoma and leiomyosarcoma, and adenocarcinoma of the uterus; cervical and vaginal disease with characteristic patterns; and mammary disease with primary neoplasia and mastitis. Endometrial hyperplasia and pyometra in captive nonhuman primates and other captive species reflects chronic reproductive cyclicity without pregnancy in captive management; the pattern is well documented and reflects a management-related pathology contrast with wild populations. Uterine leiomyoma is documented in aged captive great apes at recognizable prevalence. Mammary neoplasia in captive species includes both benign and malignant patterns with species-specific predispositions.

Male Reproductive Tract Disease

Male reproductive tract disease in non-domestic species includes testicular neoplasia (Sertoli cell tumor, seminoma, interstitial cell tumor), testicular degeneration in aged individuals, orchitis of infectious or immune-mediated origin, and prostatic disease in species with prostates. Prostatic hyperplasia in aged captive males of susceptible species has been documented across mammalian taxa. Testicular neoplasia including bilateral testicular tumors is documented in captive species with genetic predispositions in some lineages. Cryptorchidism with associated increased testicular neoplasia risk is documented across species.

Reproductive Disease and Population-Level Management

Reproductive disease in captive populations carries direct population-level management implications at Species Survival Plan facilities because reproductive success is a central component of species conservation strategy. Individual necropsy findings of reproductive tract disease contribute to Species Survival Plan population data supporting management decisions including breeding recommendations, medical intervention protocols, and, in some cases, contraceptive management for genetic diversity purposes. Neonatal and juvenile mortality from congenital disease, infectious disease, or dystocia complications is systematically tracked at Species Survival Plan facilities with necropsy findings informing prevention strategies. Dystocia at parturition with characteristic maternal and fetal pathology is documented across species with implications for individual case management and for institutional protocols governing parturition monitoring and intervention.

Applied Case: Hyperadrenocorticism in a Captive Domestic Ferret

A 5-year-old male neutered domestic ferret (Mustela putorius furo) had been under veterinary care for progressive symmetric alopecia over the trunk, progressive lethargy, and, over the preceding month, evidence of urinary tract obstruction related to prostatic disease. Antemortem clinical workup identified hyperadrenocorticism with adrenal-origin disease based on adrenal ultrasonographic imaging demonstrating enlargement of the left adrenal gland and appropriate hormonal profile. Adrenalectomy was performed with initial clinical improvement; the animal died approximately 8 months later from unrelated cardiovascular disease. Necropsy focused on comprehensive assessment with retrospective correlation to the adrenalectomy specimen and evaluation for any residual or contralateral adrenal disease.

Systematic necropsy demonstrated appropriate healing at the adrenalectomy site with no evidence of residual neoplastic tissue. The contralateral right adrenal gland demonstrated modest enlargement with characteristic cortical changes on cut surface; histopathology confirmed cortical hyperplasia with occasional small nodules consistent with early adrenal-origin hyperadrenocorticism developing in the contralateral gland. Retrospective review of the adrenalectomy specimen histopathology confirmed the original diagnosis of adrenal cortical carcinoma with characteristic cellular features. The final assessment concluded that the initial adrenalectomy had achieved appropriate local control of the primary disease with subsequent development of contralateral adrenal disease consistent with the well-documented pattern of bilateral or sequential adrenal disease in ferret hyperadrenocorticism.

Cross-taxa reasoning at case interpretation drew on the extensive documented literature of ferret hyperadrenocorticism. The disease is one of the most common endocrine disorders in captive ferret populations with well-recognized clinical presentations, hormonal profiles, imaging findings, and histopathologic patterns. Species-specific predisposition has been characterized including the recognized association with early gonadectomy and its effect on adrenal steroidogenesis through pituitary-adrenal axis modification. The species-specific presentation differs from the pattern of hyperadrenocorticism in other species (canine hyperadrenocorticism, feline hyperadrenocorticism, human Cushing disease) but shares the underlying pattern of adrenal hormone excess with characteristic clinical consequences. Cross-taxa reasoning permits rapid diagnostic direction while species-specific reference guides interpretation of the specific clinical and pathologic patterns.

Reproductive Neoplasia Case Series in Aged Captive Great Apes

Reproductive tract neoplasia in aged captive great apes has been documented at recognizable prevalence across Species Survival Plan facilities including uterine leiomyoma and, less commonly, leiomyosarcoma in aged female great apes; ovarian neoplasia including cystadenoma and, in some cases, granulosa cell tumor; endometrial adenocarcinoma with characteristic gross and histopathologic features; and mammary neoplasia including mammary adenocarcinoma in aged female great apes. Recognition of reproductive neoplasia patterns contributes to Species Survival Plan population-level surveillance for the species and informs medical management protocols for individual cases identified antemortem. Postmortem confirmation of reproductive neoplasia in cases with antemortem clinical suspicion supports the clinical diagnostic pathway and provides interpretive weight for future case interpretation.

Ancillary Reproductive Diagnostics

Ancillary reproductive diagnostics at necropsy include reproductive hormone assays on perimortem or postmortem serum when species-appropriate assays are available, reproductive tract histopathology with attention to endometrial cycle stage assessment when this information is relevant to case interpretation, immunohistochemistry for reproductive-associated markers (estrogen and progesterone receptor when species-appropriate antibodies are available), and molecular characterization of reproductive tract neoplasms with attention to specific tumor markers. Antemortem reproductive hormone monitoring at Species Survival Plan facilities provides longitudinal data supporting individual and population-level reproductive management; postmortem correlation of reproductive tract pathology with the longitudinal hormonal data supports interpretive integration of individual case findings within the population-level context.

THE COMPARATIVE NECROPSY PATTERN SYSTEM — Endometrial Hyperplasia and Pyometra Pattern in Captive Nonhuman Primates

The Pattern: Endometrial hyperplasia with cystic dilation and, in advanced cases, purulent uterine content indicating pyometra in captive nonhuman primate females with chronic reproductive cyclicity without pregnancy.

Cross-Taxa Signature: Recognized across captive nonhuman primate species including great apes, cercopithecine species, and callitrichid species. The pattern reflects chronic reproductive cyclicity without pregnancy that occurs in captive management differing from wild reproductive patterns where regular pregnancy interrupts continuous cyclicity. The pathology varies from mild endometrial changes to severe pyometra with associated systemic sepsis potential.

Diagnostic Anchor: Gross recognition of uterine enlargement with cystic endometrial changes confirmed by histopathologic characterization of endometrial hyperplasia and, in pyometra cases, of purulent content with bacterial culture identifying the etiologic organism.

Trap Logic: The look-alike is normal luteal phase endometrial changes in a reproductively cycling individual, distinguished by degree of endometrial change and by the presence or absence of cystic dilation and inflammatory response. Another look-alike is postmortem uterine autolysis distinguished by architectural preservation and by inflammatory cell characterization.

Zoonotic/Reportable Flag: Not zoonotic. Institutionally reportable at Species Survival Plan facilities for reproductive management program review and for consideration of hormonal or surgical intervention protocols.

Splenic and Lymph Node Pathology Across Taxa

Reactive Splenic and Lymph Node Changes

Reactive splenic and lymph node changes across taxa reflect immunologic response to systemic disease processes and provide diagnostic anchors for characterization of underlying disease. Splenomegaly with follicular hyperplasia reflects antigenic stimulation; splenic congestion reflects circulatory and hemodynamic factors; splenic infarction reflects vascular events. Lymph node hyperplasia with follicular expansion reflects immunologic activation; sinus histiocytosis reflects reactive macrophage activation; granulomatous lymphadenitis reflects specific infectious or inflammatory processes. Recognition of these reactive changes supports the diagnostic workup by directing attention to the underlying disease process rather than serving as a primary diagnosis.

Infectious Splenic and Lymph Node Disease

Infectious splenic and lymph node disease across taxa includes bacterial disease with characteristic gross and histopathologic changes; viral disease with specific viral inclusion body patterns and characteristic inflammatory response; and mycobacterial disease with granulomatous lymphadenitis. Mycobacterial disease produces characteristic gross and histopathologic patterns including well-demarcated granulomas with central caseation, epithelioid macrophage cuffs, multinucleate giant cells, and, in advanced disease, cavitation. Special stains identify acid-fast bacilli. Systemic salmonellosis, brucellosis, and yersiniosis each produce recognizable patterns. Fungal disease with granulomatous inflammatory response is documented across taxa.

Splenic and Lymph Node Neoplasia

Splenic and lymph node neoplasia across taxa includes lymphoma with characteristic architectural effacement and neoplastic lymphocyte populations, hemangiosarcoma with characteristic vascular architecture and, in some captive species, aggressive metastatic behavior, mast cell tumors particularly in captive small mammals, and metastatic neoplasia from distant primary tumors. Splenic neoplasia may present as a discrete mass with variable degrees of hemorrhage and necrosis or as a diffuse infiltrative pattern. Recognition of splenic neoplasia requires histopathologic characterization with immunohistochemistry for specific lineage markers when needed.

Applied Case: Mycobacterial Lymphadenitis in a Captive Asian Elephant

A 42-year-old female Asian elephant (Elephas maximus) housed in a Species Survival Plan managed collection had been under long-term surveillance for tuberculosis given the well-documented species susceptibility and the extensive management protocols developed for captive elephant tuberculosis surveillance. Antemortem screening including trunk wash and serologic testing had returned occasional weakly reactive results over the preceding five years without confirmed disease. The animal died acutely of unrelated cardiovascular disease; comprehensive necropsy was performed with attention to tuberculosis assessment given the surveillance context.

Systematic necropsy identified multiple enlarged tracheobronchial and mesenteric lymph nodes with characteristic granulomatous appearance on cut surface including central caseation and, in some nodes, mineralization. The pulmonary parenchyma demonstrated small multifocal firm nodules with similar granulomatous features. Sample collection followed standard elephant tuberculosis protocols including fresh tissue for mycobacterial culture, formalin-fixed tissue for histopathology with acid-fast staining, and fresh-frozen tissue archive for molecular characterization. Culture returned Mycobacterium tuberculosis complex growth within 6 weeks with subsequent identification as Mycobacterium tuberculosis; molecular strain characterization identified a strain type documented in the elephant tuberculosis surveillance program. Regulatory reporting followed the coordinated elephant tuberculosis response pathway including institutional biosafety review, occupational health assessment for personnel with elephant contact history, and state animal health authority notification. The case reinforced the ongoing tuberculosis surveillance requirements at facilities managing captive elephants and contributed to the coordinated species-level surveillance data.

Species-Specific Hematopoietic Anatomic Considerations

Species-specific hematopoietic anatomic considerations modify the interpretation of splenic and lymph node pathology across non-domestic taxa. The avian spleen differs from mammalian anatomy in several respects including the absence of a discrete white pulp and red pulp organization and the presence of ellipsoid-associated cells with immunologic function. The reptile spleen demonstrates variable organization with species-specific patterns. The fish head kidney serves the hematopoietic function that mammalian bone marrow serves and interpretation of fish hematologic disease requires recognition of this anatomic distinction. Cetacean and pinniped spleens demonstrate species-specific size relationships and organizational patterns. Recognition of these species-specific anatomic considerations is prerequisite to accurate interpretation of hematopoietic pathology in non-domestic species.

Applied Case: Adrenal Cortical Adenoma in an Aged Captive Rhesus Macaque

An aged captive rhesus macaque (Macaca mulatta) housed in a research collection had been under long-term care with routine health monitoring. The animal died acutely of unrelated cardiac disease in the terminal event; comprehensive necropsy was performed with attention to age-related pathology assessment. Systematic necropsy identified a discrete adrenal cortical mass approximately 2 centimeters in maximum diameter affecting the left adrenal gland. The mass demonstrated characteristic gross appearance of a well-demarcated cortical nodule with yellow-orange color on cut surface consistent with lipid-rich cortical origin. Histopathology confirmed adrenal cortical adenoma with characteristic cellular features and no evidence of vascular invasion or metastasis. The finding was an incidental postmortem discovery without documented antemortem clinical significance. The case contributed to the ongoing surveillance of age-related endocrine findings in captive nonhuman primate populations and reinforced the recognition of adrenal cortical adenoma as a common incidental finding in aged captive individuals of the species.

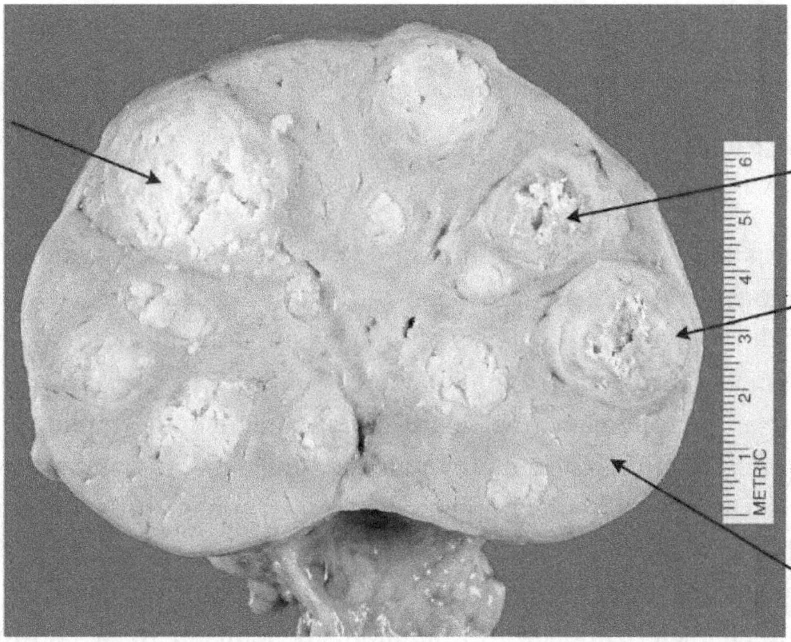

THE COMPARATIVE NECROPSY PATTERN SYSTEM — Granulomatous Lymphadenitis Pattern Signaling Mycobacterial Disease Across Taxa

The Pattern: Enlarged lymph nodes with well-demarcated granulomatous foci demonstrating central caseation, epithelioid macrophage cuffs, occasional multinucleate giant cells, and, in advanced disease, mineralization or cavitation indicating mycobacterial disease.

Cross-Taxa Signature: Recognized across mammalian taxa including captive elephants (Mycobacterium tuberculosis), captive artiodactyls (Mycobacterium bovis), captive nonhuman primates (Mycobacterium tuberculosis and Mycobacterium bovis), captive avian species (Mycobacterium avium complex), captive reptiles (non-tuberculous mycobacteria), and other captive species with mycobacterial exposure or predisposition. The gross morphology of the granulomatous pattern is highly consistent across affected taxa; the specific mycobacterial species requires species-specific culture and molecular characterization.

Diagnostic Anchor: Histopathologic recognition of granulomatous architecture confirmed by acid-fast staining demonstrating acid-fast bacilli. Culture and molecular species identification confirms the specific mycobacterial etiology. Comprehensive tissue sampling with attention to lymph nodes, spleen, liver, and lungs identifies the disease distribution.

Trap Logic: The look-alike is fungal granulomatous lymphadenitis, particularly cryptococcosis or histoplasmosis, distinguished by fungal stains identifying yeast forms rather than acid-fast bacilli. Another look-alike is other bacterial granulomatous disease including some Actinomyces and Nocardia species distinguished by bacterial morphology and specific staining.

Zoonotic/Reportable Flag: Mycobacterial disease is zoonotic with substantial public health implications. Elephant tuberculosis and captive artiodactyl bovine tuberculosis require coordinated regulatory response through USDA APHIS and state animal health authorities. Occupational health follow-up for personnel with case exposure is standard. Institutional biosafety protocols require immediate implementation upon suspect diagnosis.

Hematopoietic Neoplasia

Lymphoma Across Taxa

Lymphoma across taxa is one of the more common neoplastic entities recognized in captive and free-ranging wildlife pathology. The disease presents with variable anatomic distributions: multicentric lymphoma affecting multiple lymphoid organs simultaneously, alimentary lymphoma with predominant gastrointestinal involvement, mediastinal lymphoma with thymic or mediastinal lymph node primary involvement, and cutaneous lymphoma with primary skin involvement. Lymphoma has been documented in captive nonhuman primates at recognizable prevalence with viral associations in some cases (simian virus infections have been associated with lymphoma in some captive nonhuman primate populations), in captive ferrets at high prevalence, in captive avian species with species-specific patterns including retroviral-associated lymphoma, in captive reptiles with documented case series, and across other captive species. Histopathologic characterization with immunohistochemistry for T-cell markers (CD3) and B-cell markers (CD20, PAX5) supports the diagnosis and, in some species, has prognostic implications.

Retroviral-Associated Hematopoietic Disease

Retroviral-associated hematopoietic disease in captive species includes feline leukemia virus and feline immunodeficiency virus in captive felid populations with documented species-specific patterns, simian retroviruses in captive nonhuman primates including simian type D retrovirus and simian immunodeficiency virus, reticuloendotheliosis virus and avian leukosis virus in captive avian species, and other retroviral entities in various captive species. Retroviral disease produces both hematopoietic neoplasia (lymphoma and leukemia) and non-neoplastic disease including immunosuppression and specific end-organ pathology. Recognition of retroviral disease requires serology, viral culture, or molecular characterization complemented by histopathologic characterization of associated pathology.

Leukemia and Myeloproliferative Disease

Leukemia and myeloproliferative disease across taxa includes acute lymphoid leukemia, acute myeloid leukemia, chronic lymphocytic leukemia, and chronic myeloproliferative disease. Recognition requires histopathologic characterization of bone marrow, spleen, and other affected tissues combined with flow cytometry when antemortem or fresh samples are available for characterization of the specific cellular lineage. Bone marrow effacement with monomorphic neoplastic cell populations distinguishes leukemia from reactive marrow changes. Species-specific leukemia patterns and predispositions are documented across captive species.

Applied Case: Multicentric Lymphoma in a Captive Ferret

A 6-year-old female captive ferret (Mustela putorius furo) had been under veterinary care for progressive weight loss, palpable peripheral lymphadenopathy, and reduced activity over several months. Antemortem clinical assessment including complete blood count and biochemistry, thoracic and abdominal imaging, and lymph node cytology had returned a diagnosis of multicentric lymphoma. Palliative supportive care was elected; the animal was humanely euthanized after progressive quality of life decline. Necropsy focused on characterization of the disease distribution and definitive histopathologic classification.

Systematic necropsy demonstrated generalized peripheral and internal lymphadenopathy with markedly enlarged mesenteric, submandibular, and popliteal lymph nodes; splenomegaly with mottled cut surface; hepatomegaly with pale patchy parenchymal changes; and mediastinal mass consistent with mediastinal lymph node involvement. Gastric wall thickening was noted with prominent mucosal changes suggesting alimentary tract lymphoma component. Histopathology confirmed multicentric lymphoma with T-cell immunophenotype by immunohistochemistry; the classification followed the World Health Organization lymphoma classification framework adapted for veterinary application. The final morphologic and etiologic diagnosis was multicentric T-cell lymphoma with hepatic, splenic, mediastinal, and gastrointestinal involvement.

Cross-taxa reasoning at case interpretation drew on the extensive documented literature of lymphoma in captive ferrets. Lymphoma is one of the most common neoplasms in captive ferrets with well-recognized clinical presentations, imaging findings, and histopathologic patterns. The species-specific predisposition has been characterized in the veterinary literature with documented associations to age, husbandry factors, and, in some cases, viral etiologies. The case illustrated the cross-taxa comparison approach: the disease pattern was recognizable against domestic species lymphoma reference; the histopathologic classification followed frameworks developed in domestic species; and the interpretive approach transported readily to the ferret without substantive modification. Institutional response included the standard reporting pathway and contribution to the ongoing veterinary literature on ferret lymphoma.

THE COMPARATIVE NECROPSY PATTERN SYSTEM — Chapter 11 Endocrine, Reproductive, and Hematolymphatic Pattern Foundations

---

Diabetes Mellitus Pattern in Captive Nonhuman Primates and Captive Psittacines: Chronic hyperglycemia with metabolic consequences across captive species with species-specific predispositions. Anchor: pancreatic islet histopathology with immunohistochemistry. Trap: stress hyperglycemia discriminated by absence of chronic changes. Flag: institutionally documented for dietary and husbandry review.

Endometrial Hyperplasia and Pyometra Pattern in Captive Nonhuman Primates: Uterine cystic hyperplasia and purulent content in captive primates with chronic cyclicity without pregnancy. Anchor: gross and histopathologic characterization with bacterial culture. Trap: normal luteal phase changes discriminated by degree and inflammatory response. Flag: institutionally reportable for reproductive management review.

Granulomatous Lymphadenitis Pattern Signaling Mycobacterial Disease Across Taxa: Granulomatous lymph nodes with caseation and acid-fast bacilli across mammalian and avian taxa. Anchor: histopathology with acid-fast staining and mycobacterial culture. Trap: fungal granulomatous disease discriminated by fungal stains. Flag: zoonotic with regulatory reporting through USDA APHIS and state authorities.

Summary and Key Concepts

Endocrinopathies in non-domestic species include thyroid disease, adrenal disease (with notable captive ferret hyperadrenocorticism), diabetes mellitus across taxa, and pituitary and reproductive endocrine disease with species-specific presentations.

Reproductive pathology carries direct population-level management implications at Species Survival Plan facilities; endometrial hyperplasia and pyometra in captive nonhuman primates, uterine leiomyoma in aged great apes, and reproductive tract neoplasia are recurring recognitions.

Splenic and lymph node pathology serves as a sentinel indicator of systemic disease processes; reactive, infectious, and neoplastic changes provide diagnostic anchors for underlying disease characterization.

Granulomatous lymphadenitis with mycobacterial disease produces recognizable patterns across taxa with zoonotic and regulatory reporting implications requiring coordinated response.

Hematopoietic neoplasia across taxa includes lymphoma (most common) with variable anatomic distributions and immunophenotypes, leukemia and myeloproliferative disease, and retroviral-associated hematopoietic disease with species-specific patterns.

Ancillary diagnostic support for endocrine, reproductive, and hematolymphatic disease includes hormone assays, immunohistochemistry for specific cellular lineage markers, flow cytometry for hematopoietic neoplasia characterization, and molecular characterization of retroviral and other pathogens.

CHAPTER 12: VIRAL DISEASES OF WILDLIFE AND ZOO ANIMALS

Learning Objectives

1. Recognize herpesvirus disease patterns across wildlife and zoo taxa with attention to species-specific etiologic agents and clinical presentations.
2. Identify poxvirus, adenovirus, and circovirus disease patterns across affected species.
3. Interpret morbillivirus and related paramyxovirus disease patterns in wildlife populations with attention to unusual mortality events.
4. Recognize retrovirus disease patterns in captive and free-ranging non-domestic species.
5. Apply the Comparative Necropsy Pattern callout structure to viral disease recognition across taxa.
6. Coordinate ancillary viral diagnostics including polymerase chain reaction, viral isolation, immunohistochemistry, and next-generation sequencing approaches.

Viral diseases of wildlife and zoo animals constitute a substantial component of the diagnostic workload in the discipline. Viral disease patterns range from peracute mortality events with characteristic gross findings (elephant endotheliotropic herpesvirus in juvenile elephants, ranavirus in ectothermic vertebrates, avian influenza in poultry and wildlife) to chronic disease with slow progression (retroviruses in some captive populations) to intermediate patterns with variable clinical presentations. The pathologist working viral cases carries the interpretive burden of recognizing viral patterns from gross morphology and cytology in real time, directing appropriate ancillary workup to characterize the specific etiologic agent, and communicating findings through appropriate institutional and regulatory channels. This chapter addresses viral disease across the taxonomic breadth encountered in wildlife and zoo pathology practice with attention to the recurring patterns that support recognition across species.

The chapter organizes viral disease into four operational domains reflecting virus family or virus type organization. Herpesviruses across taxa demonstrate the wide taxonomic range and pattern diversity of this virus family. Poxviruses, adenoviruses, and circoviruses represent additional DNA virus families with characteristic disease patterns. Morbilliviruses and related paramyxoviruses address the paramyxovirus family diseases including cetacean morbillivirus and phocine distemper virus. Retroviruses complete the chapter with attention to the RNA retrovirus family diseases documented in captive and free-ranging species.

Herpesviruses Across Taxa

Alphaherpesviruses

Alphaherpesviruses across non-domestic species include a wide range of species-specific viruses with variable clinical significance and pathogenicity. Herpes B (Macacine alphaherpesvirus 1) in macaques is the paradigmatic example of a virus with limited pathogenicity in the natural host but catastrophic zoonotic potential; the virus produces mild oral vesicular disease in macaques but has near-uniformly fatal encephalitic potential in human infections requiring immediate post-exposure prophylaxis in exposed humans. Elephant endotheliotropic herpesvirus (elephantid herpesviruses 1-8) produces acute hemorrhagic disease in juvenile Asian and African elephants with characteristic multifocal necrosis in liver, heart, and other organs; the disease is documented as a leading cause of mortality in captive elephant calves. Owl herpesvirus, falconid herpesvirus, and psittacid herpesviruses (Pacheco disease) produce multifocal hepatic necrosis in their respective avian host species. Chelonid herpesviruses produce fibropapillomatosis in free-ranging sea turtles and stomatitis-rhinitis-conjunctivitis syndrome in captive tortoises. Recognition of alphaherpesvirus disease requires species-specific molecular characterization complemented by histopathologic identification of characteristic intranuclear inclusion bodies.

Betaherpesviruses and Gammaherpesviruses

Betaherpesviruses and gammaherpesviruses in non-domestic species produce more varied disease patterns than the alphaherpesvirus group. Some betaherpesviruses and gammaherpesviruses cause latent infections with periodic reactivation producing clinical disease under stress or immunosuppression. Simian gammaherpesviruses in captive nonhuman primates have been associated with lymphoproliferative disease. Marine mammal gammaherpesviruses have been characterized as causes of specific disease presentations including cetacean gammaherpesvirus infections. Recognition of these viruses requires molecular characterization and, in cases with lymphoproliferative disease, immunohistochemistry for characterization of neoplastic cell populations.

Emerging Herpesvirus Disease Recognition

Emerging herpesvirus disease recognition in non-domestic species reflects the ongoing discovery of new herpesvirus species associated with clinical disease. Molecular characterization of clinical specimens using consensus herpesvirus polymerase chain reaction primers has identified numerous novel herpesviruses across taxa in the past two decades. Some newly recognized viruses have been associated with specific clinical presentations; others have been identified as incidental findings without clear disease association. The interpretive challenge in emerging herpesvirus recognition includes distinguishing incidental viral presence from causative disease association, requiring integration of molecular findings with histopathologic characterization of associated disease.

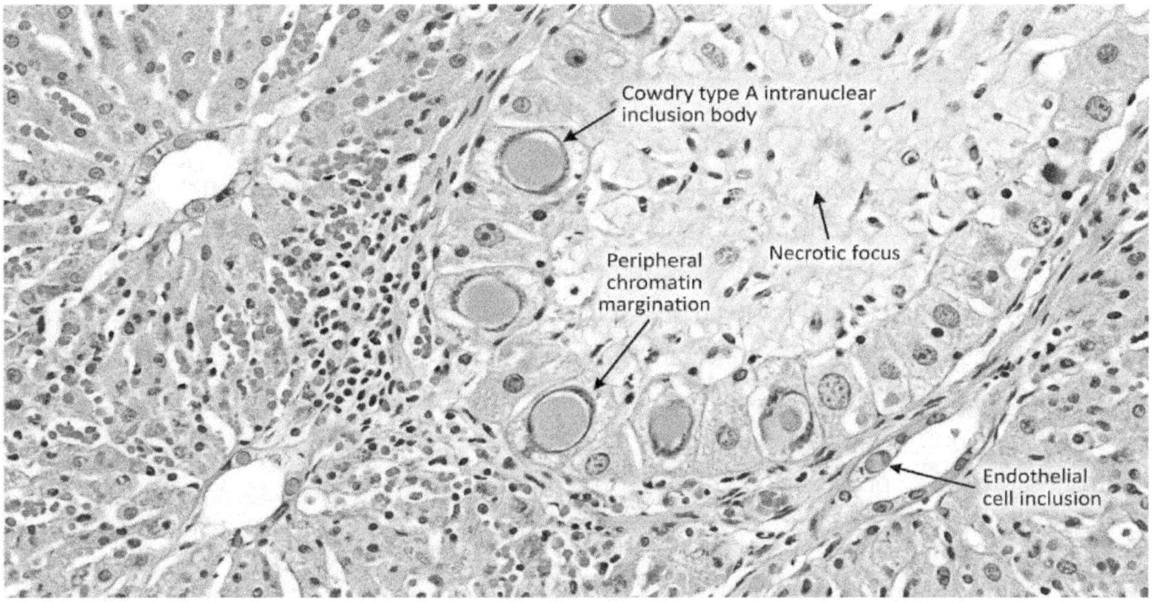

THE COMPARATIVE NECROPSY PATTERN SYSTEM — Multifocal Hepatic Necrosis Pattern Signaling Herpesvirus Disease Across Taxa

---

The Pattern: Multifocal to coalescing hepatic necrosis with characteristic Cowdry type A intranuclear inclusion bodies in hepatocytes at foci margins, indicating alphaherpesvirus disease in the affected species.

Cross-Taxa Signature: Recognized across an unusually wide taxonomic range: nonhuman primates (herpes B in macaques, callitrichid herpesvirus in marmosets), elephants (elephant endotheliotropic herpesvirus in juvenile calves), captive avian species (psittacid herpesvirus 1, falconid herpesvirus, owl herpesvirus across affected species), captive reptiles (chelonid herpesviruses in chelonians), and other captive species with characterized species-specific herpesviruses. The gross morphology of multifocal necrosis with characteristic inclusion bodies is remarkably consistent across taxonomic classes despite the substantial evolutionary distance between affected host species.

Diagnostic Anchor: Cowdry type A intranuclear inclusion bodies (eosinophilic, glassy, with peripheral chromatin margination) in hepatocytes at the periphery of necrotic foci, confirmed by immunohistochemistry or polymerase chain reaction targeting the taxon-appropriate herpesvirus species.

Trap Logic: The look-alike is bacterial hepatic necrosis without inclusion bodies but with neutrophil-rich exudate and gram-stainable bacteria within necrotic tissue. Discrimination: bacterial necrosis demonstrates gram-stainable organisms and neutrophil-rich response; herpesvirus disease demonstrates inclusion bodies with lymphocytic-dominant response.

Zoonotic/Reportable Flag: Herpes B (Macacine alphaherpesvirus 1) is a hard-stop biosafety concern requiring immediate consultation with institutional biosafety, occupational health, and public health authorities upon suspect diagnosis. Elephant endotheliotropic herpesvirus disease is institutionally reportable at Species Survival Plan facilities. Other herpesvirus diseases are generally not zoonotic.

Poxviruses, Adenoviruses, and Circoviruses

Poxvirus Disease Across Taxa

Poxvirus disease across non-domestic species includes avian pox in numerous avian species with characteristic proliferative dermatologic lesions, particularly affecting non-feathered skin including feet, eyelids, and beak base; monkeypox and related orthopoxviruses in captive nonhuman primates with characteristic cutaneous and mucosal vesicular disease; parapoxviruses in captive artiodactyls with characteristic proliferative lesions; and species-specific poxviruses in various captive species. Avian pox disease demonstrates recognizable histopathologic patterns including epidermal hyperplasia with intracytoplasmic eosinophilic viral inclusion bodies (Bollinger bodies) confirming the diagnosis. Recognition of avian pox in captive collections has population-level implications because the disease can spread readily among susceptible birds under captive conditions.

Adenovirus Disease Patterns

Adenovirus disease patterns across taxa include canine adenovirus 1 (infectious canine hepatitis) in captive wild carnivores producing hepatic necrosis with characteristic intranuclear inclusion bodies; avian adenoviruses in captive avian species including psittacine adenoviruses, falconid adenovirus, and species-specific patterns in gallinaceous birds; reptile adenoviruses particularly prominent in bearded dragons and other agamid lizards producing characteristic enteric disease with intranuclear inclusion bodies in enterocytes; and species-specific adenoviruses across various captive species. Recognition requires histopathologic identification of intranuclear inclusion bodies complemented by molecular characterization or immunohistochemistry.

Circovirus Disease Recognition

Circovirus disease recognition in non-domestic species has expanded substantially in recent decades with characterization of numerous circoviruses across avian, mammalian, and fish species. Beak and feather disease virus (psittacine circovirus) produces characteristic dermatologic and feather disease in captive psittacines with substantial population-level impact in some collections. Avian circoviruses in other bird species produce variable disease patterns. Porcine circovirus 2-like viruses in wild suids and captive artiodactyls produce documented disease. Fish circoviruses have been characterized in captive fish populations. Recognition of circovirus disease requires molecular characterization complemented by histopathologic identification of associated pathology.

Applied Case: Avian Pox Outbreak in a Passerine Rehabilitation Facility

A wildlife rehabilitation facility housing multiple passerine species experienced sudden onset of dermatologic lesions affecting multiple individuals across several species during a summer period. Clinical presentation included characteristic proliferative lesions on non-feathered skin regions including feet, eyelids, and cere areas, with some individuals demonstrating progression to systemic disease. Comprehensive necropsy was performed on cases with progression to mortality. Necropsy findings included proliferative dermatologic lesions with characteristic gross appearance including nodular growths and, in some individuals, ulcerated lesions with associated infection. Histopathology confirmed the diagnosis with characteristic epidermal hyperplasia containing prominent intracytoplasmic eosinophilic viral inclusion bodies (Bollinger bodies) pathognomonic for avian pox. Molecular characterization identified the specific avian poxvirus strain. Institutional response addressed vector management given the recognized role of mosquitoes and other biting arthropods in avian pox transmission, quarantine of affected individuals, and coordinated reporting through state wildlife health authorities for regional avian pox surveillance.

Retroviral Disease Recognition and Regulatory Considerations

Retroviral disease recognition in captive collections carries substantial implications for both individual case management and population-level program management. Screening protocols at Species Survival Plan facilities managing susceptible species typically include retroviral testing at appropriate life stages and before transfer between institutions. Endemic retroviral infection in some captive populations complicates program management by requiring careful monitoring of disease progression and by potentially limiting genetic exchange opportunities across institutions. Regulatory considerations for retroviral disease vary by specific virus and by jurisdiction; some retroviral diseases carry specific regulatory reporting requirements while others are managed primarily through institutional protocols. Coordinated species-level surveillance through Species Survival Plan structures supports characterization of retroviral disease epidemiology and informs management recommendations for affected populations. Recognition of retroviral disease at necropsy contributes to individual case understanding and to population-level surveillance datasets.

THE COMPARATIVE NECROPSY PATTERN SYSTEM — Beak and Feather Disease Pattern in Captive Psittacines

---

The Pattern: Progressive feather dystrophy with abnormal feather formation, beak abnormalities with characteristic overgrowth or necrosis, and, in severely affected individuals, systemic immunosuppression with secondary infectious disease in captive psittacines infected with beak and feather disease virus.

Cross-Taxa Signature: Recognized across captive psittacine species with variable species susceptibility; some species demonstrate high susceptibility (cockatoos, African grey parrots, some macaws) while other species demonstrate relative resistance. The disease is documented at high prevalence in some captive collections and represents a leading concern for psittacine collection management. Free-ranging populations of some Australian psittacine species have documented endemic infection.

Diagnostic Anchor: Molecular characterization by polymerase chain reaction targeting beak and feather disease virus DNA confirms the etiology. Histopathologic characterization of feather follicles and epidermis demonstrates characteristic changes including intracytoplasmic and intranuclear viral inclusion bodies within basophilic staining. Antemortem confirmation supports individual and population-level management.

Trap Logic: The look-alike is polyomavirus infection in psittacines with similar dermatologic and feather disease manifestations distinguished by molecular characterization. Another look-alike is chronic malnutrition or husbandry-related feather disease distinguished by molecular testing.

Zoonotic/Reportable Flag: Not zoonotic. Institutionally reportable at collections managing susceptible psittacine species; collection-level surveillance and quarantine protocols apply upon confirmed detection.

Morbilliviruses and Related Paramyxoviruses in Wildlife

Cetacean Morbillivirus

Cetacean morbillivirus has produced documented unusual mortality events in bottlenose dolphins across multiple geographic regions with characteristic pathology and coordinated surveillance response through the NOAA Fisheries Marine Mammal Health and Stranding Response Program. The pathologic pattern includes interstitial pneumonia with multinucleate giant cells (syncytia) demonstrating characteristic intracytoplasmic and intranuclear viral inclusion bodies, meningoencephalitis with similar syncytia in central nervous system tissue, and immunosuppression with secondary infectious disease in affected individuals. The disease is a leading cause of documented unusual mortality events in cetacean populations and has substantial conservation implications for affected species.

Phocine Distemper Virus

Phocine distemper virus produced substantial documented unusual mortality events in harbor seal populations across the North Atlantic during epidemic periods in 1988 and 2002 with subsequent smaller outbreaks documented in various regions. The pathology parallels the cetacean morbillivirus pattern with interstitial pneumonia, meningoencephalitis, and characteristic syncytia and viral inclusion bodies. The disease is a well-characterized cause of population-level pinniped mortality with documented ecological and conservation implications. Coordinated surveillance through the marine mammal stranding network permits detection of outbreak events and characterization of viral epidemiology across affected populations.

Terrestrial Morbilliviruses and Related Paramyxoviruses

Terrestrial morbilliviruses and related paramyxoviruses include canine distemper virus with substantial wildlife species susceptibility including outbreak potential in wild carnivore populations, historical rinderpest with documented captive artiodactyl impact before eradication, peste des petits ruminants with implications for captive artiodactyl collections in regions with endemic disease, and Newcastle disease virus in captive avian populations with substantial regulatory reporting implications. The pattern of morbillivirus disease across mammalian taxa demonstrates consistent syncytia formation with characteristic viral inclusion bodies; the specific virus requires species-specific molecular characterization.

Applied Case: Canine Distemper Virus in a Captive Amur Leopard Cub

A 6-month-old male Amur leopard (Panthera pardus orientalis) cub housed in a Species Survival Plan managed collection developed acute onset neurologic clinical signs including seizures, ataxia, and behavioral changes. Antemortem workup identified findings consistent with viral encephalitis; molecular testing for canine distemper virus returned positive. The cub was humanely euthanized after progressive neurologic decline. Necropsy focused on characterization of the disease distribution and confirmation of the antemortem diagnosis. Systematic necropsy demonstrated the characteristic morbillivirus pathology pattern including interstitial pneumonia with multinucleate giant cells and viral inclusion bodies, and meningoencephalitis with similar syncytia in central nervous system tissue. Cross-taxa reasoning at case interpretation drew on the extensive documented literature of canine distemper virus in wild carnivores. The disease has documented substantial wildlife impact including outbreak potential in wild carnivore populations, susceptibility of multiple carnivore families beyond canids, and, particularly relevant to this case, documented susceptibility of captive large felids to the disease with historical outbreaks in captive lion and tiger populations. Institutional response addressed collection biosafety, exposure risk assessment for other susceptible individuals, and coordination with Species Survival Plan authorities regarding the case implications.

Retroviruses in Non-Domestic Species

Feline Leukemia Virus and Feline Immunodeficiency Virus Analogs

Feline leukemia virus and feline immunodeficiency virus analogs in captive and free-ranging non-domestic felids include feline leukemia virus infection in some captive large felid populations with documented pathology comparable to domestic felid disease, feline immunodeficiency virus lineages in various wild felid species with substantial genetic diversity documented across species, and species-specific retroviruses in various captive felid species. Recognition of feline retroviral disease in captive collections has population-level management implications; screening protocols and surveillance programs support prevention of introduction and management of endemic infection.

Simian Retroviruses

Simian retroviruses in captive and free-ranging nonhuman primates include simian immunodeficiency virus (SIV) with substantial documented natural infection in many African primate species without disease and with lentiviral disease in some captive contexts, simian type D retrovirus with associated disease in captive nonhuman primate populations, simian foamy virus with substantial natural infection prevalence but limited associated disease, and simian T-lymphotropic virus with associated lymphoproliferative disease. Recognition requires molecular or serologic characterization and, in cases with associated disease, histopathologic characterization of the specific disease patterns.

Avian and Other Retroviral Disease

Avian retroviral disease includes reticuloendotheliosis virus with characteristic lymphoproliferative disease in captive and wild avian species, avian leukosis virus with associated tumor formation in captive gallinaceous birds, and species-specific retroviruses in various avian species. Marine mammal retroviruses have been characterized in some cetacean species. Reptile retroviruses have been documented in some captive species. Recognition of avian and other retroviral disease supports population-level management at collections with documented endemic infection.

Applied Case: Pacheco Disease Outbreak in a Mixed Psittacine Collection

A mixed psittacine collection experienced sudden mortality events affecting multiple individuals across several species over a two-week period. Antemortem clinical signs were minimal in affected individuals; most animals were found deceased with no significant premortem observation. Comprehensive necropsy was performed on multiple case submissions with attention to identification of a common etiologic agent given the outbreak pattern. Necropsy of representative cases demonstrated the classical pattern of Pacheco disease: multifocal to coalescing hepatic necrosis with pale to red-tinged foci distributed randomly throughout both hepatic lobes; splenic necrotic foci with similar distribution; and, in some cases, bursal, thymic, and pancreatic involvement with similar necrotic pattern. Cross-taxa reasoning at case interpretation drew on the extensive documented literature of Pacheco disease in captive psittacine collections. Psittacid herpesvirus 1 produces the disease with characteristic peracute presentation and, in outbreak settings, substantial mortality across susceptible species. Recognition of the pattern in the initial cases prompted collection-wide surveillance and quarantine protocol implementation. Molecular characterization confirmed psittacid herpesvirus 1 with genotype identification supporting epidemiologic characterization. The outbreak was ultimately controlled through coordinated case management, quarantine of affected areas, and treatment of exposed but clinically healthy individuals with appropriate antiviral protocols.

Applied Case: Ranavirus in a Captive Chelonian Collection

A collection of captive box turtles experienced substantial mortality with characteristic clinical signs including oral and nasal exudate, conjunctivitis, and, in advanced cases, systemic disease with mortality. Necropsy demonstrated the classical pattern of ranavirus disease: multifocal hepatic and splenic necrosis with characteristic intracytoplasmic basophilic viral inclusion bodies on histopathology; oral and pharyngeal mucosal necrosis with associated inflammatory response; and, in advanced cases, systemic involvement including hemorrhagic disease. Cross-taxa reasoning drew on the documented literature of ranavirus disease across chelonian species and across ectothermic vertebrates broadly. Frog virus 3-like ranaviruses have been documented across North American chelonian species with characterization of the disease patterns and epidemiology. Molecular confirmation with polymerase chain reaction targeting the ranavirus major capsid protein gene supported the diagnosis. Institutional response addressed collection biosecurity review, quarantine of affected animals, environmental sanitation, and coordinated reporting through the state wildlife health veterinarian and USDA APHIS as appropriate for the World Organisation for Animal Health-notifiable disease designation.

Molecular Diagnostic Approaches to Viral Disease

Molecular diagnostic approaches to viral disease in non-domestic species include polymerase chain reaction with virus-specific primers, consensus polymerase chain reaction with family-specific primers permitting detection of novel viral species within a virus family, next-generation sequencing with metagenomic approaches permitting unbiased characterization of viral sequences in clinical specimens, and immunohistochemistry with virus-specific antibodies. Each approach has interpretive strengths and limitations. Virus-specific polymerase chain reaction requires prior knowledge of the target virus but provides high sensitivity and specificity when appropriately validated. Consensus polymerase chain reaction permits detection of novel viruses within a family but may have lower sensitivity than species-specific assays. Metagenomic next-generation sequencing permits unbiased characterization but requires bioinformatic interpretation and consideration of contamination sources. Immunohistochemistry provides definitive characterization at the tissue level but requires appropriate species-cross-reactive antibodies. Integration of multiple approaches supports comprehensive viral disease characterization.

Applied Case: Systematic Metagenomic Investigation of Undiagnosed Mortality

A captive collection of an unusual bird species experienced repeated mortality events over a two-year period with no consistent etiologic diagnosis despite standard workup. Fresh-frozen tissue samples from multiple cases were submitted for metagenomic next-generation sequencing at a reference research laboratory. Metagenomic analysis identified sequences consistent with a previously uncharacterized herpesvirus with substantial homology to known avian herpesviruses. Follow-up molecular characterization using virus-specific primers designed against the metagenomic sequences confirmed the presence of the novel virus in multiple affected individuals with corresponding histopathologic changes including hepatic necrosis with intranuclear inclusion bodies. The identification of the novel virus permitted implementation of specific molecular surveillance across the collection and management interventions to reduce transmission. The case illustrated the utility of metagenomic approaches for cases refractory to standard viral diagnostic workup and the ongoing recognition of novel viral pathogens in captive collections through molecular approaches. Integration of metagenomic characterization with histopathologic correlation supports the interpretive distinction between clinically significant viral infection and incidental viral presence.

THE COMPARATIVE NECROPSY PATTERN SYSTEM — Cetacean Morbillivirus Pattern in Stranded Bottlenose Dolphins

The Pattern: Interstitial pneumonia with multinucleate giant cells (syncytia) demonstrating characteristic intracytoplasmic and intranuclear viral inclusion bodies, meningoencephalitis with similar syncytia in central nervous system tissue, and immunosuppression in stranded cetaceans during documented unusual mortality events.

Cross-Taxa Signature: Recognized across cetacean species with variable susceptibility; bottlenose dolphins have been the most commonly affected species in documented unusual mortality events. Cetacean morbillivirus is one of several marine mammal morbilliviruses including porpoise morbillivirus and dolphin morbillivirus. The pattern parallels other morbillivirus diseases including phocine distemper virus in pinnipeds, canine distemper virus in wild carnivores, and other morbilliviruses.

Diagnostic Anchor: Polymerase chain reaction targeting cetacean morbillivirus phosphoprotein gene confirms the etiology. Histopathologic recognition of characteristic syncytia and viral inclusion bodies supports the diagnosis. Immunohistochemistry with morbillivirus-specific antibodies demonstrates viral antigen in affected tissues.

Trap Logic: The look-alike is Brucella species infection with similar pulmonary and central nervous system pathology in cetaceans, distinguished by molecular and culture-based characterization. Another look-alike is other viral pneumonia in cetaceans distinguished by histopathologic patterns and molecular testing.

Zoonotic/Reportable Flag: Not directly zoonotic to humans. Reportable through the coordinated marine mammal stranding network to NOAA Fisheries; unusual mortality event declarations may follow detection during ongoing outbreak periods.

THE COMPARATIVE NECROPSY PATTERN SYSTEM — Chapter 12 Viral Disease Pattern Foundations

Multifocal Hepatic Necrosis Pattern Signaling Herpesvirus Disease Across Taxa: Multifocal necrosis with Cowdry type A intranuclear inclusions across primates, elephants, birds, and reptiles. Anchor: intranuclear inclusion body morphology. Trap: bacterial necrosis discriminated by neutrophil-rich response. Flag: herpes B in macaques is a hard-stop biosafety concern.

Beak and Feather Disease Pattern in Captive Psittacines: Progressive feather dystrophy and beak abnormalities from psittacine circovirus infection. Anchor: PCR for beak and feather disease virus. Trap: polyomavirus infection discriminated by molecular characterization. Flag: institutionally reportable for collection surveillance.

Cetacean Morbillivirus Pattern in Stranded Bottlenose Dolphins: Interstitial pneumonia with syncytia and meningoencephalitis in stranded cetaceans during unusual mortality events. Anchor: PCR for cetacean morbillivirus with immunohistochemistry. Trap: Brucella infection discriminated by molecular and culture characterization. Flag: reportable to NOAA Fisheries with potential UME declaration.

Summary and Key Concepts

Herpesviruses across taxa include alphaherpesviruses with characteristic multifocal necrosis pattern (elephant EEHV, primate herpes B, avian and reptile species-specific herpesviruses), betaherpesviruses and gammaherpesviruses with more varied disease patterns, and emerging herpesvirus recognition supported by molecular characterization.

Poxvirus disease includes avian pox with characteristic proliferative dermatologic lesions, monkeypox in captive primates, and species-specific patterns; adenovirus disease includes canine adenovirus 1, avian adenoviruses, and reptile adenoviruses with characteristic inclusion body patterns.

Circovirus disease includes beak and feather disease virus with substantial captive psittacine population impact and other circoviruses across taxa with expanding characterization.

Morbilliviruses in wildlife include cetacean morbillivirus with documented UME events, phocine distemper virus with pinniped population impact, and terrestrial morbilliviruses including canine distemper virus with substantial wildlife carnivore susceptibility.

Retroviruses in non-domestic species include feline leukemia virus and feline immunodeficiency virus analogs in captive felids, simian retroviruses in nonhuman primates, and avian retroviruses with associated lymphoproliferative disease.

Recognition of viral disease across taxa supports individual case management, collection-level biosafety, coordinated regulatory surveillance, and conservation-relevant surveillance for wildlife populations at risk of viral disease impact.

CHAPTER 13: HIGHLY PATHOGENIC AVIAN INFLUENZA AND CROSS-SPECIES SPILLOVER

Learning Objectives

1. Recognize highly pathogenic avian influenza pathology in avian reservoir species with attention to the H5N1 clade dominant since 2022.
2. Identify mammalian spillover disease pattern in marine mammals, mustelids, wild carnivores, and other affected mammals.
3. Apply appropriate diagnostic approach and biosafety protocols to HPAI-suspect wildlife necropsy cases.
4. Coordinate with USDA APHIS, state animal health authorities, and public health authorities during HPAI outbreaks.
5. Apply the Comparative Necropsy Pattern callout structure to HPAI recognition across affected species.
6. Recognize the emerging concerns regarding mammal-to-mammal transmission and implications for continued surveillance.

Highly pathogenic avian influenza has become the single most significant emerging infectious disease in wildlife pathology practice during the current decade. The panzootic that began with the 2022 introduction of H5N1 clade 2.3.4.4b viruses into wild bird populations across the Americas has produced sustained outbreak conditions across multiple continents, catastrophic mortality in several bird species, unprecedented mammalian spillover events including documented mammal-to-mammal transmission in farmed mink and expanded infection of marine mammals, and ongoing public health concerns about the pandemic potential of the virus. This chapter addresses the current understanding of highly pathogenic avian influenza pathology in wildlife and zoo pathology practice with attention to the recognition patterns, diagnostic approach, and coordinated regulatory response required for cases in the current disease context.

The chapter organizes highly pathogenic avian influenza pathology into four operational domains. Avian reservoir pathology addresses the disease patterns in affected wild and captive avian species. Mammalian spillover addresses the disease patterns in marine mammals, mustelids, wild carnivores, and other affected mammalian species. Diagnostic approach and biosafety cover the specific requirements for HPAI-suspect necropsy cases. Emerging strain surveillance since 2022 addresses the ongoing evolution of the viral panzootic and its implications for continued wildlife pathology practice.

Avian Reservoir Pathology

Waterfowl and Shorebird Reservoir Species

Waterfowl and shorebird species serve as the natural reservoir hosts for low-pathogenicity avian influenza viruses circulating in the North American wild bird ecosystem; historically, these hosts maintained low-pathogenicity avian influenza infection with limited pathologic consequence. The 2022 emergence of highly pathogenic H5N1 clade 2.3.4.4b viruses into these reservoir species produced substantial mortality in some waterfowl and shorebird populations with characteristic necropsy findings including multifocal to coalescing necrosis in liver, spleen, and other organs; hemorrhage in multiple tissue compartments; and, in some species, neurologic disease with meningoencephalitis and viral antigen detectable in neurons and glia. The pattern differs from the historical low-pathogenicity avian influenza in these species and reflects the substantial pathogenicity change of the current viral strain.

Colonial Nesting Seabirds and Raptors

Colonial nesting seabirds including gannets, terns, and gulls have experienced substantial mortality during the current HPAI panzootic with documented outbreak events at colonial nesting sites producing localized mass mortality. The seabird pathology pattern includes multifocal organ necrosis with prominent hepatic and splenic involvement, neurologic disease with meningoencephalitis, and, in some cases, pancreatic involvement. Raptor mortality has been documented across bald eagles, red-tailed hawks, great horned owls, peregrine falcons, and other raptor species with characteristic patterns including neurologic disease predominance in some species. The predatory feeding strategy of raptors places them at particular risk through consumption of infected prey species. Necropsy of raptor cases requires appropriate biosafety escalation.

Captive Avian Species and Zoo Collection Impact

Captive avian species at zoo collections and other managed facilities have experienced HPAI outbreaks with substantial collection-level impact during the current panzootic. Affected collections have implemented enhanced biosecurity protocols including indoor housing during high-risk periods, restricted visitor access to bird areas, and rapid response protocols for suspected cases. Zoo collection impact has included documented cases in a range of captive avian species with variable species susceptibility; some captive species have demonstrated substantial mortality while others have demonstrated apparent resistance. Recognition of HPAI in captive collections triggers coordinated response with USDA APHIS, state animal health authorities, and, at accredited facilities, Association of Zoos and Aquariums response protocols.

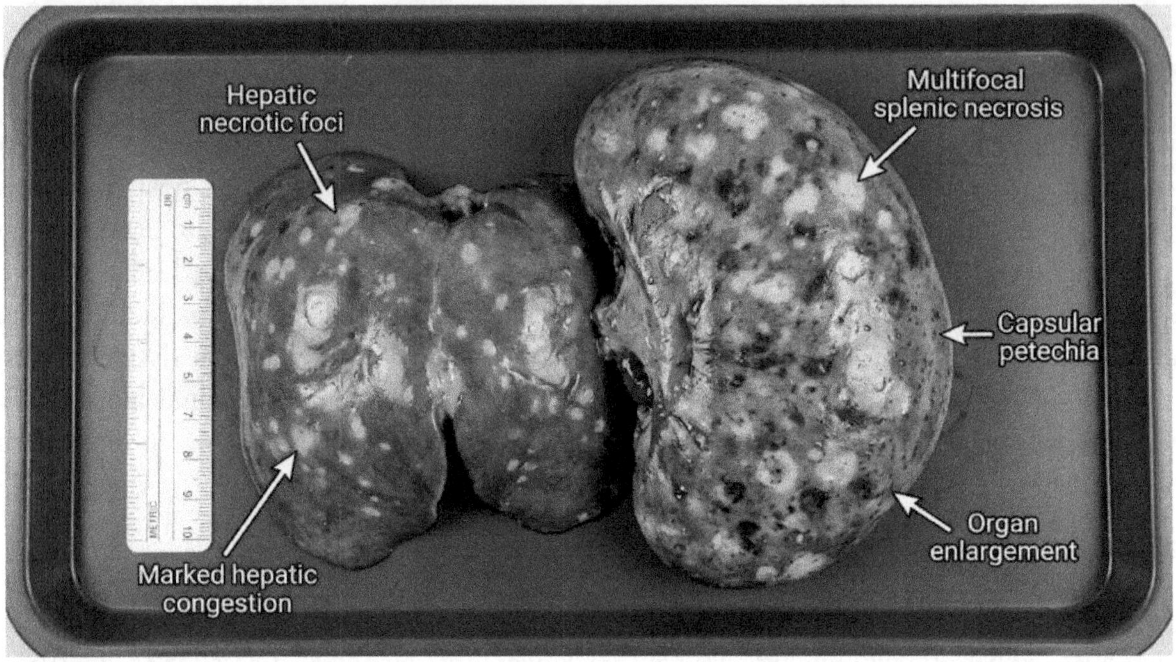

THE COMPARATIVE NECROPSY PATTERN SYSTEM — Multifocal Systemic Necrosis Pattern in HPAI-Affected Avian Species

The Pattern: Multifocal to coalescing necrosis in liver, spleen, and other visceral organs; hemorrhage in multiple tissue compartments including gastrointestinal mucosa, subcutaneous tissue, and body cavity serosal surfaces; and, in many species, neurologic disease with meningoencephalitis in avian species during documented HPAI outbreak periods.

Cross-Taxa Signature: Recognized across avian orders during the current H5N1 panzootic. Waterfowl and shorebirds demonstrate the pattern with substantial variability in species susceptibility. Colonial nesting seabirds including gannets, terns, and gulls have experienced localized outbreak events with high mortality. Raptors including bald eagles, red-tailed hawks, and great horned owls have demonstrated the disease with neurologic predominance in some species. Captive avian species have experienced outbreaks with collection-level implications.

Diagnostic Anchor: Real-time polymerase chain reaction targeting influenza A viral RNA with subsequent characterization of the H5 subtype confirms the diagnosis. Immunohistochemistry with influenza A-specific antibodies demonstrates viral antigen in affected tissues. Histopathologic recognition of the characteristic multifocal necrosis pattern supports the diagnostic direction before molecular confirmation.

Trap Logic: The look-alike is other systemic viral disease in avian species (Newcastle disease virus, some herpesvirus disease) with similar gross patterns distinguished by molecular characterization. Another look-alike is systemic bacterial disease with multiple organ involvement distinguished by culture and by histopathologic characterization of the specific inflammatory response.

Zoonotic/Reportable Flag: HPAI H5N1 is a federally reportable disease with substantial public health surveillance implications. Suspect cases require immediate notification of USDA APHIS Veterinary Services and state animal health authorities. Biosafety escalation to BSL-3 practices with appropriate personal protective equipment is required. Personnel exposure requires occupational health follow-up. Institutional biosafety officer notification precedes continued handling of suspect tissues.

Mammalian Spillover

Marine Mammal Spillover Events

Marine mammal spillover events during the current HPAI panzootic have been documented across pinniped species including harbor seals, gray seals, elephant seals, and sea lions. Substantial outbreaks with mass mortality events have been documented in several regions with characteristic pathology including multifocal necrosis in liver, spleen, and other organs; neurologic disease with meningoencephalitis and viral antigen detection in neurons and glial cells; and, in some cases, respiratory disease with interstitial pneumonia. The pattern reflects mammalian adaptation of the virus during the current panzootic and demonstrates the substantial cross-species transmission potential of the current H5N1 clade. Coordination with the NOAA Fisheries Marine Mammal Health and Stranding Response Program supports coordinated surveillance and response.

Mustelid and Wild Carnivore Spillover

Mustelid and wild carnivore spillover events have been documented across multiple species during the current panzootic. Farmed mink outbreaks in Spain and other locations have demonstrated documented mammal-to-mammal transmission with substantial implications for pandemic potential assessment. Wild carnivore infections including foxes, coyotes, bobcats, mountain lions, black bears, and other species have been documented across affected geographic regions with characteristic pathology including neurologic disease with meningoencephalitis, multifocal organ necrosis, and, in many cases, respiratory disease. The predatory feeding strategy of these species places them at particular risk through consumption of infected bird carrion or prey. Recognition patterns include the neurologic predominance in many mammalian spillover cases distinguishing them from typical bacterial or protozoal disease.

Applied Case: HPAI Spillover in a Wild Red Fox

A wild red fox (Vulpes vulpes) was recovered from a rural area with observed neurologic clinical signs including seizures and behavioral abnormalities. Given the ongoing regional HPAI outbreak in bird populations and the recognized risk of mammalian spillover, the state wildlife health veterinarian coordinated appropriate handling and submission. Necropsy was performed under strict biosafety protocols with attention to potential HPAI suspect status. External examination demonstrated appropriate body condition without external trauma. Coelomic necropsy demonstrated the characteristic multifocal necrosis pattern with hepatic, splenic, and other organ involvement. Brain examination demonstrated meningeal congestion. Sample collection prioritized potential HPAI diagnostic tissues; real-time polymerase chain reaction targeting influenza A viral RNA returned positive with subsequent H5 subtype characterization. Molecular characterization identified the H5N1 clade 2.3.4.4b consistent with the current panzootic strain. Regulatory response was immediate with notification of USDA APHIS and coordination with public health authorities regarding potential human exposure to the individual and to the recovered environment. Biosafety review at the diagnostic laboratory addressed personnel exposure follow-up.

Diagnostic Approach and Reportability

Case Receipt and Biosafety Escalation

Case receipt and biosafety escalation for HPAI-suspect wildlife cases begins at submission with recognition of species and epidemiologic context. Cases with elevated risk indicators (species with recognized susceptibility submitted from regions with active HPAI circulation, cases with neurologic clinical signs, cases with characteristic gross appearance suggesting HPAI) are escalated to BSL-3 practices immediately at receipt. Personal protective equipment includes N95 or higher respiratory protection or powered air-purifying respirator, disposable coveralls, cut-resistant gloves beneath examination gloves, eye protection, and containment technique that minimizes aerosol generation. Institutional biosafety officer notification precedes continued handling. Personnel exposure documentation supports subsequent occupational health follow-up if warranted.

Regulatory Reporting Pathway

Regulatory reporting pathway for HPAI-suspect wildlife cases follows the coordinated state and federal surveillance protocols. State wildlife health veterinarian notification typically precedes diagnostic confirmation for cases with elevated suspect status. USDA APHIS Veterinary Services notification is required for suspect and confirmed cases with specific reporting timelines. The National Veterinary Services Laboratories provides confirmation testing for suspect cases and coordinates the ongoing federal surveillance response. State agriculture and health authorities may have parallel reporting requirements. Coordinated communication between diagnostic laboratories, state and federal authorities, and, in cases with human exposure, public health authorities supports appropriate response.

Sample Submission and Reference Testing

Sample submission for HPAI-suspect cases requires attention to biosafety-appropriate packaging following Category A infectious substance shipping regulations, specific sample selection with fresh-frozen brain, lung, spleen, and other tissues as appropriate, appropriate transport medium for samples destined for viral isolation, and coordination with the receiving laboratory before submission. Reference testing at approved laboratories provides definitive characterization including subtype identification, pathotype characterization, and, when applicable, genetic characterization supporting the ongoing molecular epidemiology of the panzootic. Turnaround time varies by laboratory and by testing volume but expedited processing is typically available for suspect cases with public health implications.

Emerging Strain Surveillance Since 2022

Panzootic Evolution and Geographic Spread

The panzootic evolution and geographic spread of H5N1 clade 2.3.4.4b viruses since 2022 has produced sustained outbreak conditions across the Americas, Europe, Asia, and Africa with variable disease impact across affected regions. Wild bird surveillance networks have documented the ongoing viral circulation with characterization of specific strain lineages, genetic reassortment events, and mammalian adaptation markers. Wildlife pathology contributions to this surveillance include case-based genetic characterization of viral strains from affected animals, contributing to the ongoing molecular epidemiology of the disease. The current situation is unprecedented in the sustained mammalian spillover documented across multiple species and geographic regions.

Mammal-to-Mammal Transmission Recognition

Mammal-to-mammal transmission recognition is a critical component of ongoing HPAI surveillance during the current panzootic. Documented mammal-to-mammal transmission events including the farmed mink outbreaks in Spain in 2022 and subsequent similar events have raised substantial concerns about the pandemic potential of the virus. Recognition of mammal-to-mammal transmission requires epidemiologic characterization of case clusters combined with genetic characterization of viral isolates from affected individuals; genetic evidence of mammalian adaptation markers in isolates from mammalian cases supports the recognition of mammalian transmission. Ongoing surveillance for mammal-to-mammal transmission across wildlife and captive populations remains a public health priority.

Ongoing Surveillance and Continued Vigilance

Ongoing surveillance and continued vigilance for HPAI in wildlife pathology practice includes maintenance of appropriate biosafety practices for suspect cases regardless of the current outbreak intensity, contribution to coordinated surveillance datasets through appropriate case reporting, integration with the broader One Health surveillance framework, and preparation for potential expansion of the disease impact including further mammalian adaptation. Wildlife pathology plays a critical sentinel role in the ongoing surveillance for HPAI and other emerging infectious diseases; case-by-case recognition contributes to the coordinated response that supports both animal and human health protection.

THE COMPARATIVE NECROPSY PATTERN SYSTEM — Meningoencephalitis Pattern Signaling HPAI Mammalian Spillover

The Pattern: Neurologic disease with meningoencephalitis, multifocal organ necrosis, and characteristic pathology in a mammalian species with epidemiologic exposure to HPAI-infected birds during documented outbreak periods.

Cross-Taxa Signature: Recognized across multiple mammalian taxa during the current panzootic including marine mammals (harbor seals, gray seals, elephant seals, sea lions), wild carnivores (foxes, coyotes, mountain lions, black bears), mustelids (mink, otters, fishers), and other mammalian species with exposure to infected birds or prey. The pattern is unified across species by the epidemiologic context and by the characteristic neurologic and multifocal necrosis distribution.

Diagnostic Anchor: Real-time polymerase chain reaction targeting influenza A viral RNA with H5 subtype characterization from brain, lung, or other affected tissue. Immunohistochemistry demonstrating viral antigen in neurons and glial cells supports the neurologic component of the disease.

Trap Logic: The look-alike in a wild carnivore is rabies with similar neurologic clinical presentation distinguished by molecular characterization. Another look-alike is bacterial septicemia with disseminated intravascular coagulation distinguished by absence of viral antigen and by different histopathologic patterns.

Zoonotic/Reportable Flag: HPAI mammalian spillover is a federally reportable condition with substantial public health surveillance implications. Immediate notification of USDA APHIS, state animal health authorities, and, when human exposure is documented, public health authorities is required. Biosafety escalation to BSL-3 with appropriate PPE is required for continued handling.

THE COMPARATIVE NECROPSY PATTERN SYSTEM — Chapter 13 HPAI Pattern Foundations

---

Multifocal Systemic Necrosis Pattern in HPAI-Affected Avian Species: Multifocal necrosis with hemorrhage and neurologic disease across waterfowl, shorebirds, seabirds, raptors, and captive species during the current panzootic. Anchor: influenza A PCR with H5 subtyping. Trap: Newcastle disease and other viral disease discriminated by molecular characterization. Flag: federally reportable with immediate USDA APHIS notification.

Meningoencephalitis Pattern Signaling HPAI Mammalian Spillover: Neurologic and multifocal organ disease in mammals exposed to HPAI-infected birds during the current panzootic. Anchor: influenza A PCR with H5 subtyping and immunohistochemistry demonstrating viral antigen. Trap: rabies discriminated by molecular characterization. Flag: reportable with public health surveillance implications.

Summary and Key Concepts

Highly pathogenic avian influenza H5N1 clade 2.3.4.4b has produced sustained panzootic conditions since 2022 with catastrophic wild bird mortality, unprecedented mammalian spillover, and ongoing public health concerns.

Avian reservoir pathology includes waterfowl and shorebirds, colonial nesting seabirds with documented mass mortality events, raptors with elevated risk through prey consumption, and captive avian species with substantial collection-level impact.

Mammalian spillover has been documented across marine mammals, mustelids, wild carnivores, and other affected species with characteristic neurologic and multifocal organ pathology.

Diagnostic approach requires immediate biosafety escalation to BSL-3 practices, coordinated regulatory reporting through USDA APHIS and state authorities, and appropriate sample submission to reference laboratories.

Documented mammal-to-mammal transmission events including farmed mink outbreaks have raised substantial concerns about pandemic potential requiring ongoing surveillance and preparedness.

Wildlife pathology plays a critical sentinel role in ongoing HPAI surveillance through case-by-case recognition and contribution to coordinated One Health response.

CHAPTER 14: BACTERIAL DISEASES OF NON-DOMESTIC SPECIES

Learning Objectives

1. Recognize mycobacterial disease patterns across taxa including tuberculosis in captive elephants and artiodactyls and non-tuberculous mycobacteriosis in captive collections.
2. Identify brucellosis in wildlife reservoirs with attention to marine mammal brucellosis, ungulate brucellosis, and regulatory reporting requirements.
3. Interpret Salmonella, Yersinia, and other enteric bacterial pathogens across taxa including reptile Salmonella carriage and its zoonotic implications.
4. Recognize Erysipelothrix, Francisella, and emerging bacterial disease in wildlife and zoo populations.
5. Apply the Comparative Necropsy Pattern callout structure to bacterial disease recognition across taxa.
6. Coordinate ancillary bacterial diagnostics including culture, molecular characterization, and species identification appropriate to the anticipated pathogen.

Bacterial diseases of wildlife and zoo species constitute a large and varied differential covering pathogens of substantial regulatory concern (mycobacterial disease and brucellosis with specific reporting requirements), pathogens of substantial zoonotic significance (Salmonella species across taxa and several others), pathogens with catastrophic wildlife population impact (avian cholera in waterfowl, tularemia in lagomorphs, plague in prairie dogs and their predators), and pathogens with emerging or expanding geographic distribution. The pathologist working bacterial cases carries a substantial interpretive burden because the specific bacterial pathogen often cannot be identified from gross morphology alone and because appropriate ancillary workup requires knowledge of the anticipated differential given species, epidemiologic context, and gross findings. This chapter addresses the recurring bacterial disease patterns across taxa with attention to the specific pathogens most likely to be encountered and to the appropriate diagnostic and reporting response.

The chapter organizes bacterial disease into four operational domains. Mycobacterial disease across taxa addresses tuberculosis in captive elephants and artiodactyls, non-tuberculous mycobacteriosis in captive collections, and species-specific mycobacterial patterns. Brucellosis in wildlife reservoirs addresses the range of brucellosis in ungulate and marine mammal populations with attention to regulatory reporting requirements. Salmonella, Yersinia, and enteric bacterial pathogens address the enteric bacterial differential with attention to reptile Salmonella carriage and its zoonotic implications. Erysipelothrix, Francisella, and emerging bacterial disease completes the chapter with attention to the range of emerging bacterial patterns documented in wildlife and zoo pathology practice.

Mycobacterial Disease Across Taxa

Tuberculosis in Captive Elephants

Tuberculosis in captive elephants caused primarily by Mycobacterium tuberculosis represents one of the most extensively characterized bacterial diseases in captive wildlife populations. The disease has been documented in captive Asian and African elephants across multiple continents with substantial coordinated surveillance response including regular antemortem screening protocols, treatment protocols for confirmed cases, and detailed institutional response frameworks. Antemortem screening includes trunk wash microbiology, serologic testing with several available assays, and, in some cases, gastric lavage sampling. The disease produces the characteristic granulomatous lymphadenitis pattern with well-demarcated granulomas containing central caseation, epithelioid macrophage cuffs, multinucleate giant cells, and, in advanced disease, mineralization or cavitation. Recognition of tuberculosis at necropsy triggers coordinated regulatory response with USDA APHIS Veterinary Services, state animal health authorities, and, at accredited facilities, Association of Zoos and Aquariums response protocols. Occupational health follow-up for personnel with elephant contact history is standard given the recognized human-to-elephant and elephant-to-human transmission potential.

Bovine Tuberculosis in Wild and Captive Artiodactyls

Bovine tuberculosis caused by Mycobacterium bovis remains an important disease in wild and captive artiodactyl populations across multiple geographic regions. Wild cervid populations in specific regions of North America maintain endemic M. bovis infection with substantial implications for wildlife-livestock interface management; the Michigan bovine tuberculosis situation in free-ranging white-tailed deer represents a well-characterized example with sustained surveillance and management response over decades. Captive artiodactyl collections may develop tuberculosis through complex transmission dynamics including historical introduction, wildlife-domestic interface exposure, or nosocomial transmission within collections. Recognition of bovine tuberculosis in wild or captive artiodactyls triggers substantial regulatory response including notification of state animal health authorities and USDA APHIS Veterinary Services, potential coordinated response with agricultural authorities regarding livestock interface implications, and, in wild populations, coordinated wildlife management response.

Avian Mycobacteriosis

Avian mycobacteriosis caused by Mycobacterium avium complex organisms is documented across captive avian species including psittacines, waterfowl, ratites, and other collections. The disease produces characteristic granulomatous lesions distributed across visceral organs including liver, spleen, intestines, and, in advanced cases, extraparenchymal locations. Gross recognition includes multifocal firm nodular lesions with characteristic pale color and firm texture; histopathology demonstrates granulomatous inflammation with acid-fast bacilli identified by Ziehl-Neelsen staining. Recognition of avian mycobacteriosis in a captive collection has substantial collection-level implications including surveillance of other birds in the collection, potential environmental sampling for source identification, and occupational health considerations given the recognized zoonotic potential of M. avium complex organisms in immunocompromised humans.

Non-Tuberculous Mycobacteriosis in Reptiles, Fish, and Other Species

Non-tuberculous mycobacteriosis in reptiles, fish, and other captive species is caused by various environmental mycobacterial species including Mycobacterium chelonae, Mycobacterium abscessus, Mycobacterium fortuitum, and Mycobacterium marinum. Fish mycobacteriosis is particularly prominent in captive aquarium collections with recognized species predispositions. Reptile mycobacteriosis produces characteristic granulomatous lesions with acid-fast bacilli identifiable on histopathology. Species identification of the specific mycobacterial isolate is important because the environmental mycobacteria carry variable zoonotic potential and antimicrobial susceptibility profiles.

THE COMPARATIVE NECROPSY PATTERN SYSTEM — Granulomatous Visceral Pattern Signaling Mycobacterial Disease Across Taxa

The Pattern: Multifocal granulomatous lesions distributed across visceral organs including liver, spleen, lymph nodes, and lung with characteristic gross appearance of well-demarcated pale firm foci and histopathologic identification of acid-fast bacilli within granulomatous inflammatory response indicating mycobacterial disease.

Cross-Taxa Signature: Recognized across virtually every taxonomic group encountered in wildlife and zoo pathology including elephants (Mycobacterium tuberculosis), artiodactyls (Mycobacterium bovis), nonhuman primates (Mycobacterium tuberculosis and Mycobacterium bovis), captive avian species (Mycobacterium avium complex), captive reptiles (non-tuberculous mycobacteria including Mycobacterium chelonae and related species), captive fish (Mycobacterium marinum, Mycobacterium fortuitum, and others), and other captive species. The gross morphology of the granulomatous pattern is highly consistent across affected taxa; the specific mycobacterial species requires species-specific culture and molecular characterization.

Diagnostic Anchor: Histopathologic recognition of granulomatous architecture confirmed by acid-fast staining (Ziehl-Neelsen) demonstrating acid-fast bacilli. Mycobacterial culture on appropriate media with prolonged incubation (up to 12 weeks) supports the definitive species identification. Molecular characterization by polymerase chain reaction with mycobacterial-specific primers permits rapid identification of the specific mycobacterial species.

Trap Logic: The look-alike is fungal granulomatous disease with similar granulomatous morphology distinguished by fungal stains identifying yeast forms rather than acid-fast bacilli. Another look-alike is granulomatous disease of foreign body or other non-infectious origin distinguished by absence of infectious organisms on staining and culture.

Zoonotic/Reportable Flag: Mycobacterial disease carries substantial zoonotic and regulatory implications. Tuberculosis and bovine tuberculosis are federally reportable with coordinated USDA APHIS response required. Occupational health follow-up for exposed personnel is standard. Non-tuberculous mycobacteria carry variable zoonotic potential requiring case-specific assessment. Biosafety escalation for suspect cases precedes continued tissue handling.

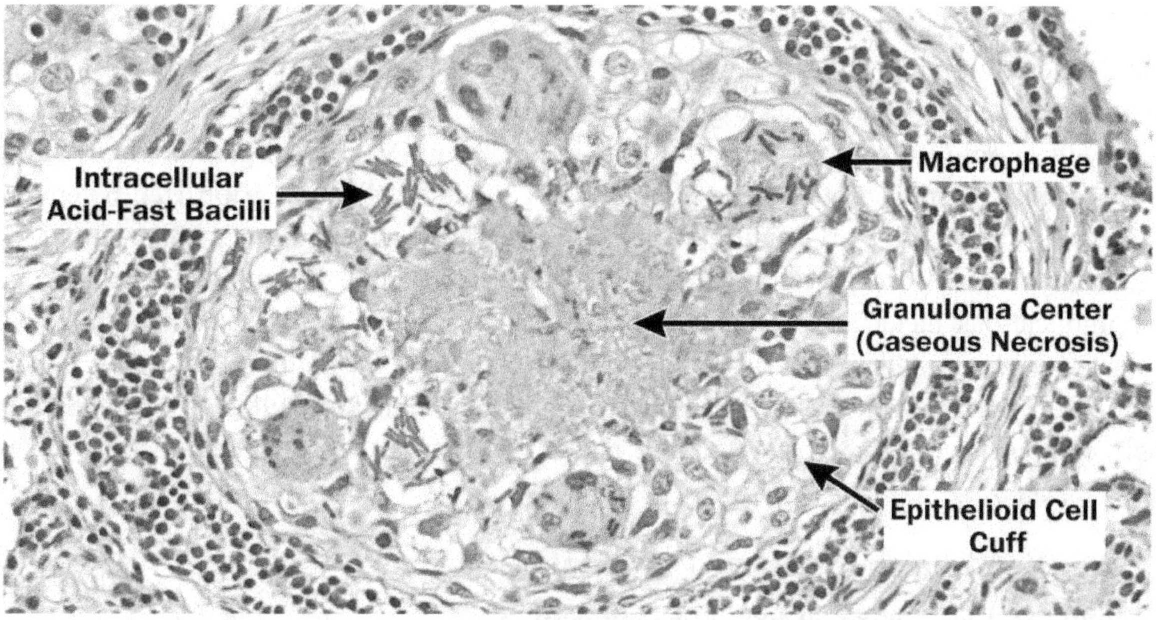

Brucellosis in Wildlife Reservoirs

Marine Mammal Brucellosis

Marine mammal brucellosis is caused primarily by Brucella pinnipedialis and Brucella ceti (formerly grouped as marine mammal Brucella species), which produce disease in pinniped and cetacean populations respectively. The disease produces characteristic pathology including placental infection with abortion in pregnant females, orchitis and epididymitis in males, meningoencephalitis with neurologic clinical signs in some individuals, and multifocal granulomatous lesions in various organs. The zoonotic potential of marine mammal Brucella species has been documented with human cases reported following occupational exposure. Recognition at necropsy triggers biosafety escalation and coordination with state animal health authority, NOAA Fisheries when marine mammals are involved, and, in cases with potential human exposure, public health authorities.

Ungulate Brucellosis and Yellowstone Ecosystem

Ungulate brucellosis primarily caused by Brucella abortus remains an important disease at the wildlife-livestock interface in specific regions of North America including the Greater Yellowstone Ecosystem where the disease is endemic in wild bison and elk populations with substantial implications for cattle brucellosis control. Coordinated management response includes surveillance in wild populations, hazing to reduce wildlife-cattle contact during vulnerable periods, and periodic testing and slaughter of individual animals in some management contexts. The disease produces characteristic reproductive pathology including placentitis with abortion and reproductive tract involvement in males. Recognition at necropsy triggers the coordinated regulatory response through USDA APHIS Veterinary Services and state agriculture authorities.

Applied Case: Brucella Ceti in a Stranded Harbor Porpoise

An adult female harbor porpoise (Phocoena phocoena) was recovered from a stranding site along the mid-Atlantic coast with observed neurologic clinical signs before death including disorientation and characteristic head-weaving. Given the marine mammal stranding context, comprehensive necropsy was performed with attention to the neurologic presentation. Systematic necropsy demonstrated meningeal congestion with prominent central nervous system involvement. Multifocal granulomatous lesions were identified in liver, spleen, and mesenteric lymph nodes. Sample collection prioritized potential Brucella diagnostic tissues; aerobic bacterial culture with Brucella-specific media returned characteristic organisms within 5 days; molecular characterization identified Brucella ceti. Institutional response addressed biosafety implications including personnel exposure follow-up and coordinated reporting through the NOAA Fisheries Marine Mammal Health and Stranding Response Program. Cross-taxa reasoning at case interpretation drew on the documented literature of marine mammal brucellosis with recognition of the neurologic component of Brucella ceti disease and the substantial zoonotic implications for personnel handling suspect cases.

Salmonella, Yersinia, and Enteric Bacterial Pathogens

Reptile Salmonella Carriage and Zoonotic Implications

Reptile Salmonella carriage is nearly ubiquitous in some reptile species with commensal-to-pathogenic transition depending on host and environmental factors. The zoonotic significance of reptile Salmonella carriage is substantial and independent of the individual reptile's disease status; human infection through pet reptile contact has been documented at recognizable incidence with specific attention to pediatric infections. The interpretive challenge at necropsy is distinguishing clinically significant Salmonella infection with associated enteric lesions from commensal carriage; culture confirmation without associated pathology represents the latter, while culture confirmation with enterocolitis or systemic disease represents the former. Institutional and public health messaging regarding reptile Salmonella is important for personnel handling reptile cases and for downstream educational communication.

Yersinia Species Disease Across Taxa

Yersinia species disease across taxa includes Yersinia pseudotuberculosis producing characteristic multifocal hepatic and splenic necrosis in captive avian species (particularly psittacines and waterfowl), captive nonhuman primates, and other captive mammals. The gross pattern includes multifocal pale to red-tinged necrotic foci with associated hepatosplenomegaly; histopathology demonstrates necrotic foci with gram-negative bacterial rods identifiable in tissue. Yersinia pestis (plague) produces catastrophic wildlife population impact in prairie dog populations and their predators including black-footed ferrets with substantial documented conservation impact; Yersinia enterocolitica is documented in some captive species with characteristic enteric disease patterns.

Clostridial and Other Enteric Bacterial Disease

Clostridial disease across taxa includes Clostridium piliforme (Tyzzer disease) producing characteristic periportal hepatic necrosis with filamentous bacterial organisms within hepatocytes visible by Warthin-Starry staining; Clostridium perfringens with associated enteric disease; Clostridium difficile with associated colitis; and Clostridium botulinum with characteristic botulinum toxin-mediated disease documented in waterfowl outbreaks. Escherichia coli enteric disease is documented across taxa with strain-specific virulence factors. Campylobacter species produce enteric disease in some captive species. Recognition of the specific enteric bacterial etiology requires appropriate culture direction and, in some cases, molecular characterization.

THE COMPARATIVE NECROPSY PATTERN SYSTEM — Multifocal Hepatic and Splenic Necrosis Signaling Yersinia Disease Across Taxa

The Pattern: Multifocal pale to red-tinged necrotic foci in liver and spleen with hepatosplenomegaly and, on histopathology, necrotic foci containing gram-negative bacterial rods indicating Yersinia species disease.

Cross-Taxa Signature: Recognized across captive avian species (Yersinia pseudotuberculosis in psittacines, waterfowl, and other captive birds), captive nonhuman primates (Yersinia pseudotuberculosis), captive mammals across various species, and wild rodents (Yersinia pestis in prairie dogs and other affected species). The gross morphology is transportable across taxa; the specific Yersinia species requires species-specific culture and molecular characterization.

Diagnostic Anchor: Aerobic bacterial culture of fresh liver, spleen, or affected tissue with identification of Yersinia species. Histopathologic recognition of necrotic foci with gram-negative bacterial rods on tissue Gram stain supports the diagnostic direction.

Trap Logic: The look-alike is herpesvirus disease with similar multifocal hepatic and splenic necrosis distinguished by histopathologic identification of intranuclear inclusion bodies characteristic of herpesvirus (absent in Yersinia disease). Another look-alike is Salmonella septicemia with similar gross pattern distinguished by culture identification of the specific bacterial species.

Zoonotic/Reportable Flag: Yersinia pseudotuberculosis is zoonotic with occupational exposure risk. Yersinia pestis is a select agent with substantial regulatory reporting requirements and biosafety implications; suspect plague cases require immediate coordination with state and federal public health authorities. Yersinia enterocolitica is zoonotic with lower biosafety implications.

Erysipelothrix, Francisella, and Emerging Bacterial Disease

Erysipelothrix Disease

Erysipelothrix rhusiopathiae disease is documented across marine mammal species (particularly cetaceans with recognized clinical significance), captive avian species (with turkey erysipelas as a well-characterized disease), and other captive species. The disease produces characteristic gross and histopathologic patterns including cutaneous lesions with characteristic distribution, systemic disease with visceral involvement, and, in some cases, septicemia with rapid progression. Zoonotic potential exists with occupational exposure risk documented. Recognition at necropsy prompts appropriate ancillary workup with aerobic bacterial culture on appropriate media.

Francisella Tularensis and Tularemia

Francisella tularensis produces tularemia with substantial wildlife population impact in lagomorph populations including cottontail rabbits, jackrabbits, and hares. The disease produces characteristic multifocal hepatic and splenic necrosis pattern with associated systemic disease. Recognition of tularemia carries substantial biosafety implications because Francisella tularensis is a select agent with extremely high infectivity through respiratory or contact exposure; suspect cases require immediate biosafety escalation, coordination with state and federal public health authorities, and appropriate personnel exposure follow-up. The disease has documented catastrophic population-level impact in some wildlife species during outbreak periods.

Emerging Bacterial Disease Recognition

Emerging bacterial disease recognition in wildlife pathology practice includes newly characterized bacterial pathogens with recognized wildlife disease associations, expanded geographic distribution of previously documented pathogens, and antimicrobial resistance patterns with implications for treatment and management. Streptococcus species with wildlife-specific patterns have been characterized in various captive and wild populations. Bartonella species have been documented in various wildlife hosts with variable disease implications. Coxiella burnetii (Q fever agent) is documented in some wildlife populations with substantial zoonotic implications. Novel bacterial pathogens continue to be recognized through molecular characterization approaches supporting ongoing wildlife pathology practice.

Applied Case: Avian Cholera Outbreak in a Waterfowl Population

A wildlife management area recorded substantial waterfowl mortality during a fall migration period with hundreds of affected individuals across several species including mallards, pintails, and Canada geese. Field necropsy protocols were implemented by state wildlife health veterinarian coordination with representative specimens submitted to a coordinating laboratory for confirmatory diagnosis. Necropsy of representative specimens demonstrated the characteristic avian cholera pattern including multifocal hepatic necrotic foci with characteristic pale color and firm texture; hemorrhage in multiple tissue compartments including gastrointestinal mucosa and body cavity serosal surfaces; and, on histopathology, multifocal necrotic foci with abundant gram-negative bacterial cocci identifiable. Aerobic bacterial culture returned Pasteurella multocida growth within 48 hours with subsequent characterization of the specific serotype. Institutional response included coordination with the wildlife management area for carcass removal and appropriate disposal to reduce environmental contamination and continued transmission risk, coordination with state wildlife authorities for surveillance across broader waterfowl populations, and characterization of the specific bacterial strain contributing to the ongoing surveillance dataset for avian cholera epidemiology in North American waterfowl.

THE COMPARATIVE NECROPSY PATTERN SYSTEM — Chapter 14 Bacterial Disease Pattern Foundations

---

Granulomatous Visceral Pattern Signaling Mycobacterial Disease Across Taxa: Multifocal granulomatous lesions with acid-fast bacilli across mammalian, avian, reptile, and fish taxa. Anchor: histopathology with acid-fast staining and mycobacterial culture. Trap: fungal granulomatous disease discriminated by fungal stains. Flag: tuberculosis and bovine tuberculosis federally reportable with zoonotic implications.

Multifocal Hepatic and Splenic Necrosis Signaling Yersinia Disease Across Taxa: Multifocal necrotic foci with gram-negative bacterial rods across captive birds, primates, mammals, and wild rodents. Anchor: bacterial culture with species identification. Trap: herpesvirus disease discriminated by intranuclear inclusions. Flag: Yersinia pestis is a select agent requiring public health coordination.

Summary and Key Concepts

Mycobacterial disease across taxa includes tuberculosis in captive elephants, bovine tuberculosis in wild and captive artiodactyls, avian mycobacteriosis in captive avian collections, and non-tuberculous mycobacteriosis in reptiles, fish, and other captive species with substantial zoonotic and regulatory implications.

Brucellosis in wildlife reservoirs includes marine mammal brucellosis with recognized zoonotic potential, ungulate brucellosis at the wildlife-livestock interface, and other Brucella species disease across affected populations.

Salmonella, Yersinia, and enteric bacterial pathogens across taxa include the substantial zoonotic significance of reptile Salmonella carriage, Yersinia disease across avian and mammalian taxa including the plague concern in prairie dogs and predators, and clostridial and other enteric bacterial disease.

Erysipelothrix, Francisella, and emerging bacterial disease include the substantial biosafety implications of Francisella tularensis as a select agent, Erysipelothrix disease across marine mammals and other affected species, and ongoing recognition of novel and emerging bacterial pathogens through molecular characterization.

Recognition of bacterial disease patterns at necropsy triggers appropriate ancillary workup with culture and molecular characterization, coordinated regulatory reporting where applicable, and appropriate biosafety and occupational health response.

Wildlife bacterial disease recognition contributes to individual case management, collection-level biosafety, coordinated regulatory surveillance for reportable diseases, and public health surveillance for zoonotic pathogens with human exposure implications.

CHAPTER 15: FUNGAL AND OOMYCETE DISEASES

Learning Objectives

1. Recognize chytridiomycosis in amphibian populations caused by Batrachochytrium dendrobatidis and B. salamandrivorans with attention to conservation implications.
2. Identify aspergillosis patterns across captive avian and mammalian species with attention to species predispositions.
3. Recognize white-nose syndrome in bats caused by Pseudogymnoascus destructans with attention to the ongoing population-level impact.
4. Distinguish systemic mycoses including cryptococcosis, histoplasmosis, coccidioidomycosis, and blastomycosis with species-specific patterns.
5. Apply the Comparative Necropsy Pattern callout structure to fungal disease recognition across taxa.
6. Coordinate ancillary fungal diagnostics including mycologic culture, histopathologic special stains, and molecular characterization.

Fungal and oomycete diseases in wildlife and zoo pathology practice have gained substantial prominence over the past three decades with the emergence of catastrophic fungal panzootics affecting amphibian populations (chytridiomycosis) and North American bat populations (white-nose syndrome). These diseases have produced documented conservation impact at a scale exceeding many bacterial and viral pathogens and have driven substantial coordinated surveillance response including active biosecurity to prevent further introduction of pathogens into naive populations. The chapter addresses fungal disease recognition across the taxonomic breadth encountered in wildlife and zoo pathology practice with attention to the specific pathogens and to the ongoing surveillance response required for cases in current disease context.

The chapter organizes fungal and oomycete disease into four operational domains. Chytridiomycosis addresses the two documented Batrachochytrium species with substantial amphibian conservation implications. Aspergillosis across avian and mammalian taxa covers the range of Aspergillus disease documented in captive collections. White-nose syndrome addresses the Pseudogymnoascus destructans disease that has produced substantial North American bat population decline. Systemic mycoses and emerging fungal disease completes the chapter with attention to the broader range of fungal disease documented in wildlife and zoo pathology practice.

Chytridiomycosis: Batrachochytrium Dendrobatidis and B. Salamandrivorans

Batrachochytrium Dendrobatidis

Batrachochytrium dendrobatidis produces chytridiomycosis in amphibian populations across the globe with documented catastrophic impact including species-level extinctions in some Neotropical and Australian amphibian species during the panzootic emergence beginning in the late twentieth century. The disease produces characteristic epidermal thickening with hyperkeratosis of skin covering the digits and body, and, on histopathology, fungal thalli within the epidermal keratin layer are the pathognomonic finding. The species has been characterized as a globally distributed pathogen with genetic diversity documented across geographic regions supporting molecular epidemiologic characterization of the panzootic dynamics. Anuran species have been most severely affected with catastrophic population decline in some Neotropical and Australian species. Caudate species demonstrate variable susceptibility with some species substantially affected.

Batrachochytrium Salamandrivorans

Batrachochytrium salamandrivorans emerged as a distinct threat to caudate amphibians (salamanders and newts) with initial recognition in European caudate populations in 2013 producing substantial documented mortality including local population extinctions. The species demonstrates predilection for caudate amphibians with somewhat different clinical and pathologic presentation than B. dendrobatidis; the lesions are typically more prominent with cutaneous ulceration in advanced disease. Active biosecurity surveillance across North America aims to prevent introduction of B. salamandrivorans into the substantial North American caudate biodiversity given the potential catastrophic conservation impact of introduction. Import restrictions on amphibian trade have been implemented in several jurisdictions to reduce introduction risk.

Diagnostic Approach and Conservation Response

Diagnostic approach to chytridiomycosis includes histopathologic identification of fungal thalli within the epidermal keratin layer, molecular characterization by polymerase chain reaction targeting Batrachochytrium-specific sequences with species-level identification distinguishing B. dendrobatidis from B. salamandrivorans, and skin swab sampling for antemortem screening in living amphibians. Conservation response includes coordinated surveillance across amphibian populations, biosecurity protocols for reintroduction and translocation programs, treatment protocols for confirmed cases including antifungal therapy and elevated temperature exposure, and, for particularly vulnerable species, captive assurance colony maintenance to prevent species-level extinction.

Figure 15.1: Chytridiomycosis in a Frog: Fungal Thalli in Epidermis at 40× Magnification

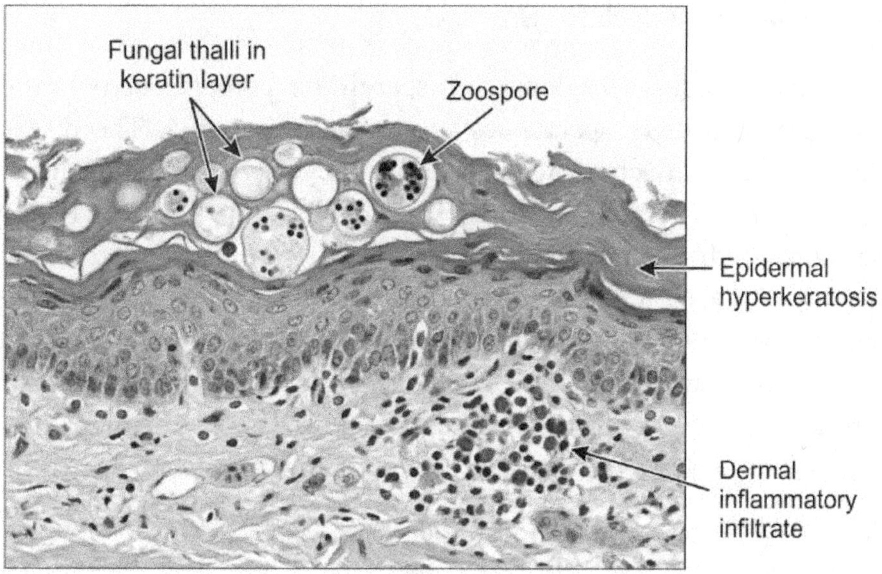

THE COMPARATIVE NECROPSY PATTERN SYSTEM — Chytridiomycosis Pattern in Free-Ranging and Captive Amphibians

The Pattern: Amphibian carcass with characteristic epidermal thickening, hyperkeratosis of skin covering the digits and body, and, on histopathology, fungal thalli within the epidermal keratin layer indicating chytridiomycosis.

Cross-Taxa Signature: Recognized across amphibian species with variable susceptibility; anuran species have been most severely affected by B. dendrobatidis with catastrophic population declines documented in some Neotropical and Australian species. Caudate amphibians demonstrate additional susceptibility to B. salamandrivorans with substantial European mortality documented and ongoing biosecurity surveillance to prevent North American introduction.

Diagnostic Anchor: Histopathologic demonstration of fungal thalli within the epidermal keratin layer with characteristic morphology. Molecular confirmation by polymerase chain reaction targeting Batrachochytrium-specific sequences with species-level identification confirms the diagnosis and distinguishes the two species.

Trap Logic: The look-alike is normal epidermal thickening in some amphibian species during specific physiologic states (breeding season in some species, environmental adaptation) distinguished by absence of fungal thalli. Another look-alike is other fungal skin disease in amphibians distinguished by the specific chytrid morphology.

Zoonotic/Reportable Flag: Chytridiomycosis is a World Organisation for Animal Health-notifiable disease requiring reporting through state and federal wildlife health authorities. Not zoonotic. Detection triggers biosecurity review of the affected population or collection, source investigation, and coordinated conservation response.

Aspergillosis Across Avian and Mammalian Taxa

Aspergillus Fumigatus and Related Species

Aspergillus fumigatus produces the dominant aspergillosis pathogen across captive avian populations with A. flavus, A. niger, and other species less commonly identified. The disease is documented at high prevalence in captive psittacines with African grey parrots documented at particularly elevated susceptibility. Captive raptors demonstrate substantial susceptibility with aspergillosis as one of the leading causes of morbidity and mortality in rehabilitation facilities. Waterfowl demonstrate susceptibility particularly during periods of stress or immunosuppression. The disease produces characteristic multifocal firm pulmonary nodules with air sac plaque and nodule formation; histopathology demonstrates granulomatous inflammation with fungal hyphae highlighted by Grocott-Gomori methenamine silver staining. Advanced cases demonstrate systemic involvement with hepatic, splenic, and other organ involvement. Aspergillus flavus and A. niger produce similar clinical and pathologic patterns.

Aspergillosis in Marine Mammals and Other Mammals

Aspergillosis in marine mammals has been documented across cetacean and pinniped species with characteristic pulmonary and, in some cases, disseminated disease. The species-specific predisposition and epidemiologic drivers of marine mammal aspergillosis are areas of ongoing characterization. Terrestrial mammalian aspergillosis is less common than avian aspergillosis but documented across various captive species with characteristic pulmonary and, less commonly, disseminated disease. Immunocompromised captive individuals demonstrate elevated susceptibility to opportunistic aspergillosis regardless of species.

Diagnostic Approach and Treatment Considerations

Diagnostic approach to aspergillosis includes gross recognition of characteristic pulmonary and air sac lesions with same-day cytology of impression smears from lesions demonstrating characteristic dichotomously branching septate fungal hyphae. Histopathology with special stains (Grocott-Gomori methenamine silver, periodic acid-Schiff) demonstrates the fungal hyphae with characteristic morphology. Mycologic culture on Sabouraud dextrose agar confirms the specific Aspergillus species. Molecular characterization by polymerase chain reaction with Aspergillus-specific primers provides species-level identification. Treatment considerations for captive collections include specific antifungal protocols with variable prognosis depending on disease extent, environmental management to reduce spore burden, and biosecurity considerations to prevent spread within collections.

THE COMPARATIVE NECROPSY PATTERN SYSTEM — Aspergillosis Pattern in Captive Avian Species

The Pattern: Multifocal firm pulmonary nodules with air sac plaque and nodule formation containing dichotomously branching septate fungal hyphae with associated granulomatous inflammatory response indicating aspergillosis in a captive avian species.

Cross-Taxa Signature: Recognized across captive avian orders with variable species susceptibility; African grey parrots and other psittacines demonstrate elevated susceptibility. Captive raptors demonstrate substantial susceptibility particularly during rehabilitation. Waterfowl demonstrate susceptibility particularly during stress. Ratites and other captive avian species demonstrate documented cases.

Diagnostic Anchor: Histopathologic demonstration of dichotomously branching septate fungal hyphae in tissue with associated granulomatous inflammation. Grocott-Gomori methenamine silver staining highlights the fungal hyphae. Culture with species identification confirms the specific Aspergillus species.

Trap Logic: The look-alike is other fungal disease including cryptococcosis (yeast forms rather than hyphae) and mucormycosis (broader non-septate hyphae). Discrimination: specific fungal morphology distinguishes Aspergillus from other fungal pathogens.

Zoonotic/Reportable Flag: Not zoonotic in most cases though occupational exposure in immunocompromised humans may pose risk. Institutionally reportable at collections with documented cases for husbandry review addressing ventilation, humidity, and spore burden.

White-Nose Syndrome in Bats

Pseudogymnoascus Destructans

Pseudogymnoascus destructans (formerly Geomyces destructans) is the causative agent of white-nose syndrome in North American bat populations with catastrophic population-level impact documented since first recognition in 2006 in New York. The disease produces characteristic white fungal growth on the muzzle, ears, and wing membranes of affected bats during hibernation with associated wing membrane damage, disrupted hibernation patterns, and, in advanced cases, mortality. Millions of bats have died from the disease across affected regions with substantial documented population declines in several bat species. The fungus grows optimally at cave hibernation temperatures and produces the characteristic disease during the winter hibernation period.

Diagnostic Approach and Pathology

Diagnostic approach to white-nose syndrome includes recognition of the characteristic gross appearance including white fungal growth on affected skin surfaces, ultraviolet fluorescence of affected wing membranes providing a characteristic diagnostic sign, and histopathologic identification of characteristic fungal cupping lesions in wing membrane histology. Molecular characterization by polymerase chain reaction targeting Pseudogymnoascus destructans-specific sequences confirms the diagnosis. Fresh tissue collection and fresh-frozen archival supports the ongoing coordinated surveillance response.

Applied Case: White-Nose Syndrome Surveillance in a Bat Hibernaculum

A state wildlife agency conducted routine surveillance at a bat hibernaculum with documented historical white-nose syndrome outbreaks; several bats were observed with clinical signs consistent with the disease and representative specimens were collected for confirmatory diagnosis. Necropsy of representative specimens demonstrated the characteristic gross appearance with white fungal growth on muzzle and wing membranes, poor body condition consistent with disrupted hibernation, and reduced brown adipose stores consistent with premature exhaustion of energy reserves. Ultraviolet illumination of wing membranes demonstrated characteristic orange-yellow fluorescence in affected areas providing rapid diagnostic support. Histopathology confirmed characteristic fungal cupping lesions in wing membrane tissue; molecular characterization confirmed Pseudogymnoascus destructans. Institutional response included coordinated reporting through the state wildlife health veterinarian and the coordinated white-nose syndrome surveillance network supporting the ongoing management response to the panzootic. The case contributed to the surveillance dataset supporting characterization of population-level impact and management response.

Systemic Mycoses and Emerging Fungal Disease

Cryptococcosis

Cryptococcosis caused by Cryptococcus neoformans and Cryptococcus gattii is documented across captive avian species (particularly psittacines with recognized susceptibility), captive mammals including nonhuman primates and marine mammals, and, less commonly, other captive species. The disease produces characteristic gross and histopathologic patterns including central nervous system involvement with meningitis or meningoencephalitis, pulmonary disease with nodular lesions, and, in disseminated disease, systemic organ involvement. Recognition includes histopathologic identification of characteristic yeast forms with prominent capsules highlighted by mucicarmine or Grocott-Gomori methenamine silver staining. Cryptococcus gattii has emerged as a substantial concern in the Pacific Northwest with documented outbreaks affecting both humans and various wildlife species.

Endemic Systemic Mycoses

Endemic systemic mycoses in geographic regions of North America include coccidioidomycosis (Coccidioides immitis and C. posadasii) in the American Southwest and Central and South America, histoplasmosis (Histoplasma capsulatum) in the Ohio and Mississippi River valleys and other endemic regions, and blastomycosis (Blastomyces dermatitidis) in similar endemic geographic distribution. Each produces characteristic gross and histopathologic patterns with granulomatous inflammatory response and specific fungal morphology. Wildlife susceptibility varies by species with documented cases across various captive and free-ranging populations. Recognition of endemic systemic mycoses at necropsy contributes to characterization of wildlife susceptibility patterns and to the broader One Health surveillance for these pathogens.

Emerging and Novel Fungal Disease Recognition

Emerging and novel fungal disease recognition in wildlife pathology continues as ongoing surveillance and molecular characterization identify newly recognized fungal pathogens. Ophidiomycosis (snake fungal disease) caused by Ophidiomyces ophiodiicola has emerged as a substantial concern in North American snake populations with expanding geographic distribution and characterized dermatologic disease. Novel fungal pathogens continue to be characterized in various wildlife populations. The interpretive challenge in emerging fungal disease recognition parallels other emerging infectious disease recognition including distinguishing incidental fungal presence from causative disease association, requiring integration of molecular findings with histopathologic characterization of associated disease.

THE COMPARATIVE NECROPSY PATTERN SYSTEM — Chapter 15 Fungal Disease Pattern Foundations

Chytridiomycosis Pattern in Free-Ranging and Captive Amphibians: Amphibian epidermal thickening with fungal thalli indicating Batrachochytrium infection. Anchor: histopathologic and molecular characterization with species-level identification. Trap: normal breeding-season epidermal changes discriminated by absent fungal thalli. Flag: WOAH-notifiable amphibian disease with conservation implications.

Aspergillosis Pattern in Captive Avian Species: Multifocal pulmonary nodules and air sac plaques with dichotomously branching septate fungal hyphae across captive avian orders. Anchor: histopathology with GMS staining and mycologic culture. Trap: other fungal disease discriminated by fungal morphology. Flag: institutionally reportable for husbandry review.

Summary and Key Concepts

Chytridiomycosis caused by Batrachochytrium dendrobatidis and B. salamandrivorans produces catastrophic amphibian population impact with documented species-level extinctions and ongoing biosecurity surveillance to prevent further pathogen spread.

Aspergillosis across captive avian and mammalian species with African grey parrots, captive raptors, and other affected species demonstrating recurring recognition of pulmonary and air sac nodular disease.

White-nose syndrome caused by Pseudogymnoascus destructans produces substantial North American bat population decline with characteristic clinical and pathologic patterns supporting coordinated surveillance response.

Systemic mycoses including cryptococcosis, coccidioidomycosis, histoplasmosis, and blastomycosis produce documented wildlife disease in various geographic regions with implications for One Health surveillance.

Emerging fungal disease including snake fungal disease and novel fungal pathogens continues to be recognized through ongoing surveillance and molecular characterization.

Fungal disease recognition at necropsy triggers appropriate ancillary workup with culture, histopathologic special stains, and molecular characterization supporting individual case management and coordinated surveillance response.

CHAPTER 16: PARASITIC DISEASES OF WILDLIFE AND ZOO ANIMALS

Learning Objectives

1. Recognize protozoal disease patterns across taxa including toxoplasmosis, sarcocystosis, and trypanosomiasis.
2. Identify nematode parasitism patterns across mammalian, avian, and reptile taxa.
3. Interpret trematode, cestode, and acanthocephalan parasitism with attention to species-specific hosts and life cycles.
4. Recognize arthropod parasites and vector-borne disease in wildlife populations.
5. Apply the Comparative Necropsy Pattern callout structure to parasitic disease recognition across taxa.
6. Coordinate ancillary parasitologic diagnostics including morphologic identification, molecular characterization, and serologic testing.

Parasitic diseases of wildlife and zoo animals cover an extraordinary range of pathogens from single-celled protozoa through metazoan helminths through arthropod ectoparasites, each producing characteristic disease patterns across taxa. The pathologist working parasitic cases requires familiarity with the major parasitic groups and their characteristic gross and histopathologic recognition, appropriate ancillary diagnostic direction for parasite identification, and understanding of the epidemiologic and conservation implications of parasitic disease in wildlife populations. Parasitism carries dual interpretive weight because parasites contribute to individual case pathology and because parasitic community composition provides insight into wildlife-environment interactions relevant to ecological surveillance.

The chapter organizes parasitic disease into four operational domains. Protozoal disease addresses toxoplasmosis, sarcocystosis, trypanosomiasis, and other protozoal infections across taxa. Nematode parasitism covers gastrointestinal, tissue-migrant, and specialized nematode infections. Trematodes, cestodes, and acanthocephalans address the helminth parasitism differential. Arthropod parasites and vector-borne disease completes the chapter with attention to ectoparasitism and its role in wildlife health surveillance.

Protozoal Disease: Toxoplasmosis, Sarcocystosis, Trypanosomiasis

Toxoplasma Gondii Infection Across Taxa

Toxoplasma gondii infection is documented across an unusually wide range of vertebrate hosts because the parasite has felid definitive hosts producing oocysts through fecal shedding with subsequent infection of intermediate hosts across mammalian, avian, and other vertebrate classes. Clinical toxoplasmosis in captive species is prominent in immunocompromised individuals and in species with particular susceptibility. Captive marsupials demonstrate substantial susceptibility with documented mortality events in captive collections. Captive nonhuman primates demonstrate variable susceptibility with New World primates generally more susceptible than Old World primates. Sea otters demonstrate substantial disease susceptibility with documented associations to freshwater outflow contamination and to fecal oocyst delivery to marine environments. The pathology of toxoplasmosis includes multifocal necrosis in various organs with characteristic tissue cyst formation identifiable on histopathology and, in acute disease, characteristic tachyzoite forms with associated inflammatory response.

Sarcocystis Species Infection

Sarcocystis species infection is documented across a wide range of wildlife taxa with substantial species diversity and complex life cycles involving predator definitive hosts and prey intermediate hosts. Wildlife sarcocystosis produces characteristic tissue cyst formation in muscle tissue of intermediate hosts, and, in some species, encephalitic disease in aberrant hosts. Sarcocystis neurona produces equine protozoal myeloencephalitis in horses with opossum as definitive host; wildlife susceptibility to related sarcocystoses has been documented across various species. Recognition of Sarcocystis infection at necropsy contributes to characterization of parasitic community composition in wildlife populations.

Trypanosome Infections in Wildlife

Trypanosome infections in wildlife include Trypanosoma cruzi (Chagas disease agent) documented in various wild mammalian reservoirs across the Americas with substantial One Health implications for human disease transmission, African trypanosomes with substantial wildlife disease impact in endemic regions, and other trypanosome species documented across various host taxa. Recognition of trypanosome infection at necropsy contributes to characterization of the parasitic disease burden in wildlife populations and to the broader One Health surveillance framework for vector-borne parasitic disease.

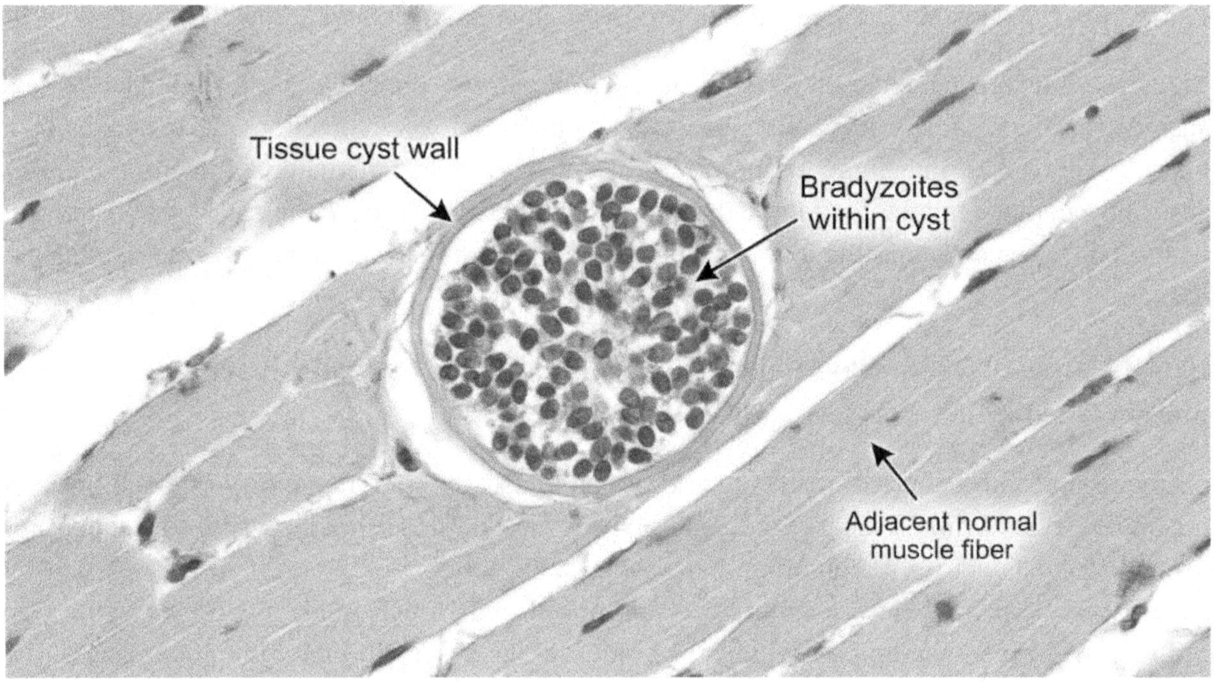

THE COMPARATIVE NECROPSY PATTERN SYSTEM — Multifocal Toxoplasma Necrosis Pattern in Captive Marsupials and New World Primates

---

The Pattern: Multifocal necrosis in various organs including liver, spleen, lung, and central nervous system with characteristic tissue cyst formation and, in acute disease, tachyzoite forms with associated inflammatory response indicating Toxoplasma gondii infection.

Cross-Taxa Signature: Recognized across captive marsupials with substantial documented susceptibility, New World primates (particularly callitrichids and other susceptible species), sea otters with documented environmental transmission, and other susceptible captive species. The gross and histopathologic patterns are broadly consistent across affected taxa.

Diagnostic Anchor: Histopathologic identification of characteristic tissue cyst forms with terminal-end bradyzoite morphology and, in acute disease, tachyzoite forms with associated inflammatory response. Immunohistochemistry with Toxoplasma-specific antibodies demonstrates parasite antigen in affected tissues. Molecular characterization by polymerase chain reaction confirms the etiology.

Trap Logic: The look-alike is other systemic protozoal disease including Sarcocystis and Neospora species distinguished by parasite morphology and molecular characterization. Another look-alike is bacterial or viral systemic disease distinguished by absence of parasitic organisms and by different histopathologic patterns.

Zoonotic/Reportable Flag: Toxoplasma gondii is zoonotic with substantial public health implications particularly for immunocompromised humans and pregnant women. Occupational exposure through necropsy of infected wildlife supports appropriate personnel awareness. Not typically regulatorily reportable but institutionally documented for surveillance.

Nematode Parasitism Across Taxa

Gastrointestinal Nematode Parasitism

Gastrointestinal nematode parasitism is documented across virtually all wildlife and zoo taxa with substantial species diversity and clinical significance varying by host susceptibility, parasite burden, and environmental factors. Common gastrointestinal nematode groups include ascarids (Toxocara, Baylisascaris, and other species) with substantial documented disease across captive and wild hosts, strongyles including trichostrongyles in captive ruminants with well-characterized disease patterns, hookworms (Ancylostoma, Uncinaria species) in captive carnivores and other affected species, and whipworms (Trichuris species) with documented disease across various hosts. Baylisascaris procyonis specifically warrants attention because of its recognized potential for aberrant migration in non-raccoon hosts producing severe neurologic disease and its zoonotic significance.

Tissue-Migrant Nematode Parasitism

Tissue-migrant nematode parasitism includes several notable disease-causing species. Parelaphostrongylus tenuis produces cerebrospinal parelaphostrongylosis in aberrant hosts including moose, elk, and captive artiodactyls of many species. Angiostrongylus cantonensis produces eosinophilic meningitis in various host species. Onchocerca species and related filarial worms produce characteristic tissue disease. Dirofilaria immitis (heartworm) affects captive wildlife with characteristic pulmonary and cardiac pathology. Recognition of tissue-migrant nematode disease requires histopathologic characterization of parasitic tract lesions and parasite identification from tissue sections.

Specialized Nematode Infections

Specialized nematode infections include lungworm infections in various species (Metastrongylus in suids, Dictyocaulus and Muellerius in ungulates, Angiostrongylus in various hosts), heartworm as noted, and various species-specific nematodes with characteristic patterns. Aelurostrongylus species in captive felids produce pulmonary disease. Trichuris species in captive nonhuman primates produce colonic disease. Species identification of nematode parasites contributes to characterization of the parasitic community in wildlife populations.

Trematodes, Cestodes, and Acanthocephalans

Trematode Parasitism

Trematode parasitism includes the hepatic trematodes with substantial wildlife disease documented, blood flukes (Schistosoma species and related trematodes) with documented wildlife disease and substantial One Health implications, intestinal trematodes across various taxa, and pulmonary trematodes (Paragonimus species) documented in some captive species. Fasciola hepatica and F. gigantica produce characteristic hepatic pathology including bile duct dilation and hemorrhagic migration tracts. Recognition of trematode parasitism at necropsy requires parasite recovery and morphologic or molecular identification.

Cestode Parasitism

Cestode parasitism includes taeniid cestodes with mammalian definitive hosts and characteristic wildlife intermediate host disease, Echinococcus species producing characteristic hydatid disease with substantial One Health implications, various fish tapeworms in captive fish and their piscivorous predators, and other cestode groups with documented wildlife disease. Cystic hydatid disease produces characteristic cystic lesions containing daughter cysts and protoscolices with substantial recognition value at necropsy. Alveolar echinococcosis (Echinococcus multilocularis) produces characteristic multifocal lesions with substantial documented disease in various wildlife hosts. Recognition contributes to One Health surveillance for these zoonotically important parasites.

Acanthocephalan and Other Helminth Parasitism

Acanthocephalan parasitism (thorny-headed worms) is documented across various wildlife taxa with characteristic gastrointestinal wall attachment producing focal inflammatory lesions. Various species-specific acanthocephalans have been documented in captive fish, birds, and mammals. Recognition of acanthocephalan parasitism at necropsy requires parasite recovery with morphologic identification.

THE COMPARATIVE NECROPSY PATTERN SYSTEM — Cerebrospinal Parelaphostrongylosis Pattern in Aberrant Cervid Hosts

The Pattern: Central nervous system disease in moose, elk, or captive artiodactyls with histopathologic identification of parasitic tract lesions in cerebrum and spinal cord and, in some cases, larval nematode sections in tissue indicating cerebrospinal parelaphostrongylosis from Parelaphostrongylus tenuis infection.

Cross-Taxa Signature: Recognized in aberrant hosts including moose, elk, caribou, and captive artiodactyls of many species. White-tailed deer serve as the normal definitive host without producing significant clinical disease. Aberrant host disease reflects larval migration through the central nervous system in hosts unable to complete the normal life cycle. The geographic distribution of the parasite in white-tailed deer determines the geographic risk zone for aberrant host disease.

Diagnostic Anchor: Histopathologic identification of parasitic tract lesions with characteristic inflammatory response including eosinophils and, in some sections, identifiable larval nematode structures. Molecular characterization by polymerase chain reaction with Parelaphostrongylus-specific primers supports the etiologic identification.

Trap Logic: The look-alike is other tissue-migrant nematode disease including Angiostrongylus infection and other filarial migrations distinguished by parasite morphology and molecular characterization. Another look-alike is other neurologic disease distinguished by absence of parasitic tract lesions.

Zoonotic/Reportable Flag: Not zoonotic. Institutionally significant at collections managing susceptible artiodactyl species in regions with sympatric white-tailed deer populations; preventive antiparasitic management and, where feasible, minimizing contact between the collection and wild white-tailed deer populations, support disease prevention.

Arthropod Parasites and Vector-Borne Disease

Ectoparasitism and Ectoparasite Identification

Ectoparasitism in wildlife populations includes tick, flea, louse, and mite infestations with substantial variation in host-parasite specificity. Ectoparasite identification at necropsy contributes to characterization of parasitic communities and to vector-borne disease surveillance because ectoparasite species identification provides information about the vector species present in the environment. Standardized ectoparasite collection at necropsy supports contribution to broader parasitic and vector-borne disease surveillance datasets. Individual case ectoparasitism may or may not contribute to clinical significance;

heavy ectoparasite burdens can produce documented anemia, dermatologic disease, and, in some cases, systemic debilitation from chronic parasitism.

Vector-Borne Disease Transmission

Vector-borne disease transmission through arthropod vectors produces substantial wildlife disease burden. Tick-borne diseases including Lyme disease (Borrelia burgdorferi), anaplasmosis, ehrlichiosis, and various tick-borne viral diseases affect wildlife populations. Flea-borne diseases including plague (Yersinia pestis) produce substantial wildlife disease. Mosquito-borne diseases including West Nile virus and equine encephalitis viruses affect wildlife. Recognition of vector-borne disease at necropsy requires ancillary workup with molecular or serologic characterization of the specific pathogens complemented by ectoparasite collection supporting vector identification.

Applied Case: Sarcoptic Mange Outbreak in a Wild Vulpine Population

A state wildlife agency conducted surveillance during a documented sarcoptic mange outbreak affecting the wild red fox population across multiple counties. Representative case submissions to a diagnostic laboratory permitted characterization of the disease pattern and confirmation of the etiologic organism. Necropsy of representative specimens demonstrated the characteristic pattern including extensive alopecia with hyperkeratotic thickened skin, poor body condition, and, on histopathology, characteristic mite infestation with associated inflammatory response. Skin scrapings demonstrated numerous Sarcoptes scabiei var. canis mites confirming the etiologic diagnosis. Institutional response included coordinated reporting through the state wildlife health veterinarian, characterization of the outbreak dynamics across the affected population, and consideration of population-level management interventions. The case series reinforced the recognition of sarcoptic mange as a substantial recurring cause of wildlife morbidity in wild carnivore populations with periodic outbreak dynamics.

THE COMPARATIVE NECROPSY PATTERN SYSTEM — Chapter 16 Parasitic Disease Pattern Foundations

---

Multifocal Toxoplasma Necrosis Pattern in Captive Marsupials and New World Primates: Multifocal necrosis with tissue cysts and tachyzoites across susceptible captive species. Anchor: histopathologic identification with immunohistochemistry and PCR confirmation. Trap: other systemic protozoal disease discriminated by parasite morphology. Flag: zoonotic with occupational exposure implications.

Cerebrospinal Parelaphostrongylosis Pattern in Aberrant Cervid Hosts: Central nervous system parasitic tract lesions in moose, elk, and captive artiodactyls with sympatric white-tailed deer. Anchor: histopathologic identification of parasitic tracts and molecular characterization. Trap: other tissue-migrant nematode disease discriminated by parasite morphology. Flag: institutionally significant for susceptible species collection management.

Summary and Key Concepts

Protozoal disease across taxa includes toxoplasmosis with substantial susceptibility in marsupials, New World primates, and sea otters; sarcocystosis with complex predator-prey life cycles; and trypanosomiasis with One Health implications.

Nematode parasitism includes gastrointestinal, tissue-migrant, and specialized nematode infections with recurring recognition of Baylisascaris zoonotic potential and Parelaphostrongylus aberrant host disease in cervids and captive artiodactyls.

Trematode, cestode, and acanthocephalan parasitism includes hepatic trematodes, hydatid disease with One Health implications, and various species-specific patterns across wildlife populations.

Arthropod parasites and vector-borne disease include ectoparasitism contributing to vector-borne disease surveillance and various tick-borne, flea-borne, and mosquito-borne pathogens with substantial wildlife disease burden.

Parasitic disease recognition at necropsy requires appropriate ancillary workup with morphologic identification, molecular characterization, and, where applicable, serologic testing supporting individual case characterization and broader surveillance.

Wildlife parasitic disease surveillance contributes to characterization of parasitic communities, monitoring for zoonotic and conservation-relevant parasites, and integration with One Health surveillance frameworks.

CHAPTER 17: PRION DISEASES AND TRANSMISSIBLE SPONGIFORM ENCEPHALOPATHIES

Learning Objectives

1. Recognize chronic wasting disease in cervids with attention to updated strain distribution since first identification.
2. Identify scrapie-related prion disease in wildlife and captive artiodactyl populations.
3. Apply appropriate diagnostic approach to suspected transmissible spongiform encephalopathy cases including tissue submission and testing protocols.
4. Coordinate reporting through state and federal animal health authorities for confirmed and suspect cases.
5. Recognize the biosafety and environmental persistence considerations that distinguish prion disease from other infectious disease.
6. Apply the Comparative Necropsy Pattern callout structure to prion disease recognition.

Prion diseases and transmissible spongiform encephalopathies occupy a distinct category in wildlife and zoo animal pathology because of the unique properties of the prion agents including their environmental persistence, their resistance to standard decontamination methods, and their substantial regulatory reporting requirements. Chronic wasting disease in cervids has emerged over the past six decades as the dominant transmissible spongiform encephalopathy of wildlife with expanding geographic and taxonomic distribution and substantial coordinated surveillance response. The chapter addresses the current understanding of prion disease in wildlife pathology practice with attention to the diagnostic and regulatory response required for suspect and confirmed cases.

The chapter organizes prion disease into three operational domains. Chronic wasting disease in cervids addresses the dominant wildlife prion disease with its updated strain distribution. Scrapie-related prion disease in wildlife covers the additional prion diseases documented in wildlife and captive populations. Diagnostic approach and reportability addresses the specific requirements for suspect and confirmed cases.

Chronic Wasting Disease in Cervids: Updated Strain Distribution

Geographic Distribution and Taxonomic Range

The geographic distribution of chronic wasting disease has expanded substantially since first identification in the late 1960s in captive cervids at a research facility in Colorado. Free-ranging cervid disease has been documented across much of North America with subsequent identification in Scandinavia and other regions. The taxonomic range of affected cervid species has similarly expanded with documented disease in mule deer, white-tailed deer, elk, moose, reindeer, and additional cervid species. Recent identification in reindeer in Scandinavia demonstrated species susceptibility not previously recognized and expanded the geographic distribution of the disease into new regions. Ongoing surveillance across North America and Europe supports characterization of the current disease distribution and identification of new geographic expansion.

Strain Diversity and Molecular Characterization

Strain diversity in chronic wasting disease has been increasingly characterized through molecular methods including strain typing and biochemical characterization. Multiple strains of the disease have been recognized with variable pathogenicity, geographic distribution, and species susceptibility patterns. Some strains demonstrate enhanced transmissibility or altered species range compared to others. Ongoing molecular characterization supports epidemiologic understanding of the disease dynamics and permits identification of new strain emergence. The molecular characterization has become a routine component of the coordinated surveillance response supporting broader understanding of the disease.

Clinical and Pathologic Recognition

Clinical presentation of chronic wasting disease includes progressive weight loss over months to years, behavioral abnormalities including reduced fear response and altered social interactions, progressive neurologic dysfunction with reduced coordination and, in advanced disease, difficulty ambulating and swallowing, and, in terminal disease, characteristic emaciation with associated systemic decline. Pathologic recognition at necropsy includes the poor body condition consistent with chronic disease, and, on histopathology of specific tissues including the obex region of the brainstem and the retropharyngeal lymph nodes, characteristic pathologic prion protein accumulation identified by immunohistochemistry. The characteristic spongiform change in central nervous system tissue reflects the underlying pathology at the cellular level.

THE COMPARATIVE NECROPSY PATTERN SYSTEM — Chronic Wasting Disease Pattern in Free-Ranging and Captive Cervids

The Pattern: Cervid carcass with characteristic clinical history including progressive weight loss and behavioral abnormalities, poor body condition at postmortem examination, and diagnostic tissue submission for prion testing on obex and retropharyngeal lymph node.

Cross-Taxa Signature: Recognized in cervid species including mule deer, white-tailed deer, elk, moose, reindeer, and additional species with expanding taxonomic distribution documented since first identification. Geographic distribution across North America and Europe continues to expand with ongoing surveillance.

Diagnostic Anchor: Immunohistochemistry or enzyme-linked immunosorbent assay demonstration of pathologic prion protein accumulation in obex or retropharyngeal lymph node from the affected animal. Confirmation testing at reference laboratories for regulatory submission.

Trap Logic: The look-alike is any other cause of progressive weight loss and neurologic decline in cervids, distinguished by prion testing. Other look-alikes include chronic mycobacterial disease and chronic parasitism which may produce similar body condition changes without the neurologic component.

Zoonotic/Reportable Flag: Chronic wasting disease is a reportable disease in the United States with state-specific and federal reporting pathways coordinated through USDA APHIS. While zoonotic potential to humans has not been established, precautionary handling guidance for hunters and consumers has been issued by public health authorities. All suspected cases require appropriate tissue submission through the coordinated surveillance network.

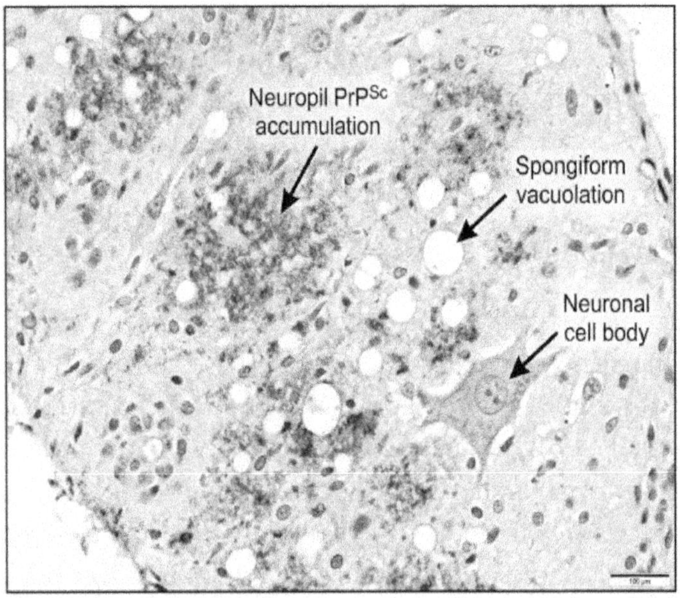

Figure 17.1: Chronic Wasting Disease in a White-Tailed Deer: Immunohistochemistry of Obex at 20× Magnification. (Caption text: Histopathological photomicrograph of brainstem obex region tissue showing prominent brown-staining pathologic prion protein accumulation throughout the neuropil; scattered spongiform vacuolation is present; neurons show variable immunohistochemical staining.)

Scrapie-Related Prion Disease in Wildlife

Wildlife Scrapie Documentation

Wildlife scrapie documentation is limited compared to the substantial captive artiodactyl disease documented during the historical bovine spongiform encephalopathy epidemic and captive ruminant scrapie surveillance. Wild ovid populations have had limited documented scrapie disease, and the natural history of scrapie in wild small ruminant populations continues to be characterized. Cross-species transmission of scrapie to captive artiodactyls at zoological institutions during the historical bovine spongiform encephalopathy epidemic period produced documented captive disease with subsequent surveillance response.

Bovine Spongiform Encephalopathy Historical Context

Bovine spongiform encephalopathy affected captive artiodactyls at zoological institutions during the historical epidemic period in the 1990s with documented disease in several captive artiodactyl species including exotic ungulates. The historical surveillance response established protocols for testing captive artiodactyls with clinical signs consistent with transmissible spongiform encephalopathy. While active testing volume has decreased substantially since the epidemic period, testing protocols remain in place for suspect cases at accredited zoological institutions and other captive artiodactyl facilities.

Feline Spongiform Encephalopathy

Feline spongiform encephalopathy affected captive felids during the historical bovine spongiform encephalopathy epidemic period with documented disease attributed to bovine spongiform encephalopathy prion exposure through food chain contamination. The historical surveillance response established protocols for testing captive felids with clinical signs consistent with transmissible spongiform encephalopathy. Contemporary case identification is uncommon reflecting the substantial reduction in exposure risk following historical intervention.

Diagnostic Approach and Reportability

Sample Collection and Handling

Sample collection and handling for suspected transmissible spongiform encephalopathy cases requires specific attention to tissue selection, biosafety practices during collection, and appropriate reference laboratory submission. Standard tissue submission for chronic wasting disease surveillance includes the obex region of the brainstem and the retropharyngeal lymph nodes with additional tissues including tonsils in some sampling protocols. Personal protective equipment appropriate to prion handling includes appropriate glove protection, and, where feasible, disposable instrument use during central nervous system tissue collection. Reusable instruments require specific decontamination protocols exceeding standard biological decontamination given the recognized resistance of prions to standard sterilization methods.

Reference Laboratory Submission

Reference laboratory submission for suspected transmissible spongiform encephalopathy cases follows the coordinated surveillance protocols established through USDA APHIS and state animal health authorities. National Veterinary Services Laboratories provide confirmation testing for suspect cases. Confirmatory testing methods include immunohistochemistry with prion-specific antibodies, enzyme-linked immunosorbent assay for pathologic prion protein, and, in some cases, additional confirmatory methods. Turnaround time varies by laboratory volume; expedited testing is available for cases with regulatory implications.

Coordinated Regulatory Response

Coordinated regulatory response to confirmed transmissible spongiform encephalopathy cases includes reporting through state animal health authority and USDA APHIS Veterinary Services with specific reporting timelines depending on the disease and jurisdiction. State-specific chronic wasting disease surveillance programs coordinate response including hunter education, testing infrastructure, carcass disposal protocols, and, in some jurisdictions, targeted removal of affected animals from wild populations. Institutional response at facilities with confirmed captive cases includes appropriate biosafety review, tissue archival requirements, and coordinated communication with regulatory partners regarding the case implications.

THE COMPARATIVE NECROPSY PATTERN SYSTEM — Chapter 17 Prion Disease Pattern Foundations

---

Chronic Wasting Disease Pattern in Free-Ranging and Captive Cervids: Cervid carcass with progressive neurologic decline and characteristic tissue submission for prion testing. Anchor: immunohistochemistry or ELISA for pathologic prion protein on obex and retropharyngeal lymph node. Trap: other chronic weight loss diseases discriminated by prion testing. Flag: reportable disease with coordinated USDA APHIS and state surveillance response.

Summary and Key Concepts

Chronic wasting disease in cervids has expanded substantially in geographic and taxonomic distribution since first identification with multiple strains characterized through molecular methods and ongoing surveillance response.

Scrapie-related prion disease in wildlife populations is limited in documentation while captive artiodactyl testing protocols established during the historical bovine spongiform encephalopathy epidemic remain in place.

Feline spongiform encephalopathy affected captive felids during the historical epidemic period with contemporary case identification uncommon reflecting substantial reduction in exposure risk.

Diagnostic approach includes specific tissue selection (obex and retropharyngeal lymph node for chronic wasting disease), biosafety practices during collection, and coordinated reference laboratory submission.

Coordinated regulatory response to confirmed transmissible spongiform encephalopathy cases follows established USDA APHIS and state animal health authority protocols with specific reporting requirements and management response.

Prion diseases occupy a distinct category among infectious diseases due to environmental persistence, resistance to standard decontamination, and substantial regulatory implications requiring coordinated response.

CHAPTER 18: NUTRITIONAL AND METABOLIC DISEASE

Learning Objectives

1. Recognize hypovitaminosis A and related vitamin deficiency patterns across captive species.
2. Identify metabolic bone disease patterns across taxa with attention to nutritional secondary hyperparathyroidism.
3. Interpret iron storage disease in captive frugivorous primates, black rhinoceros, and other predisposed species.
4. Recognize obesity, cardiovascular disease, and diet-related pathology in captive collections.
5. Apply the Comparative Necropsy Pattern callout structure to nutritional and metabolic disease recognition.
6. Coordinate ancillary nutritional and metabolic diagnostics including vitamin, mineral, and biochemical characterization.

Nutritional and metabolic disease in captive wildlife and zoo populations reflects the interpretive challenge of maintaining physiologic homeostasis in animals whose evolutionary dietary context differs substantially from their captive dietary provision. The disease patterns recognized in captive species include vitamin deficiencies from inadequate dietary provision, mineral imbalances from calcium-phosphorus dysregulation and other patterns, storage diseases from chronic dietary excess exceeding regulatory capacity, and lifestyle-related diseases including obesity and its cardiovascular consequences. The pathologist working nutritional and metabolic cases contributes both to individual case diagnostic conclusion and to population-level dietary management review at Species Survival Plan facilities where individual necropsy findings inform broader husbandry decisions.

The chapter organizes nutritional and metabolic disease into four operational domains. Hypovitaminosis A and related vitamin deficiencies addresses the vitamin deficiency patterns documented across captive species. Metabolic bone disease across taxa (referenced also in Chapter 10) addresses the calcium-phosphorus-related bone disease. Iron storage disease in managed populations covers the recurring interpretive challenge of dietary iron overload. Obesity, cardiovascular disease, and diet-related pathology completes the chapter with attention to the lifestyle-related disease patterns documented in captive collections.

Hypovitaminosis A and Related Vitamin Deficiencies

Hypovitaminosis A

Hypovitaminosis A is documented across captive species with inadequate dietary vitamin A provision producing characteristic clinical and pathologic patterns. Captive reptiles maintained on invertebrate-heavy diets without appropriate vitamin A supplementation develop hypovitaminosis A with characteristic squamous metaplasia of various epithelia including respiratory mucosa, renal collecting ducts, and reproductive tract epithelia. Captive fish including several species maintained on inadequate diets have documented vitamin A deficiency. Captive avian species with inadequate vitamin A demonstrate similar patterns. The gross and histopathologic recognition includes squamous metaplasia of affected epithelia, and the pattern is reversible with appropriate dietary correction if identified before advanced tissue damage. Recognition at necropsy triggers institutional dietary review addressing vitamin A content of the offered diet.

Hypovitaminosis D and Related Disease

Hypovitaminosis D produces rickets in growing captive animals and osteomalacia in adult animals with characteristic skeletal patterns. Recognition and management of hypovitaminosis D disease is addressed in Chapter 10. Hypovitaminosis E produces various species-specific patterns including capture myopathy potentiation in some ungulate species and steatitis in some captive fish species. Combined vitamin E and selenium deficiency produces characteristic patterns including white muscle disease in ungulates and other affected species. Recognition of specific vitamin deficiencies requires appropriate ancillary vitamin quantitation in tissue or serum with species-appropriate reference where available.

B Vitamins and Water-Soluble Vitamins

B vitamin deficiencies and other water-soluble vitamin deficiencies produce various species-specific patterns. Thiamine deficiency is documented in captive fish and captive fish-eating avian and mammalian species associated with consumption of thiaminase-containing fish species; recognition includes characteristic neurologic pathology. Riboflavin deficiency produces various patterns including cataracts in some avian species maintained on historically inadequate diets. Recognition of specific B vitamin deficiencies requires appropriate dietary review and, in some cases, targeted vitamin quantitation.

Metabolic Bone Disease Across Taxa

Nutritional Secondary Hyperparathyroidism

Nutritional secondary hyperparathyroidism from dietary calcium-phosphorus imbalance produces characteristic skeletal pathology across captive juvenile animals of many species with detailed coverage in Chapter 10. The disease remains one of the most common metabolic disorders in captive collections and requires institutional dietary review upon recognition.

Renal Secondary Hyperparathyroidism

Renal secondary hyperparathyroidism reflects chronic kidney disease with associated calcium-phosphorus dysregulation and characteristic secondary skeletal changes. The disease is documented in captive aged individuals of various species with chronic kidney disease. Recognition includes the primary renal disease with associated fibrous osteodystrophy or other secondary skeletal changes; the pattern distinguishes from nutritional secondary hyperparathyroidism by concurrent renal disease.

Metastatic Mineralization From Hypervitaminosis D

Hypervitaminosis D produces metastatic mineralization of soft tissues including kidneys, blood vessels, gastrointestinal tract, and lung with detailed coverage in Chapter 10. The condition is documented in captive psittacines and, less commonly, other captive species with iatrogenic or dietary vitamin D excess.

Iron Storage Disease in Managed Populations

Species-Specific Predisposition

Iron storage disease affects captive frugivorous primates (lemurs, marmosets, tamarins), black rhinoceros, tapirs, frugivorous bats, and several passerine species with detailed coverage in Chapter 6. The disease reflects chronic dietary iron overload in species with intestinal absorptive machinery adapted to iron-poor natural diets. Recognition and management of iron storage disease has substantial population-level implications at Species Survival Plan facilities.

Population-Level Management

Population-level management of iron storage disease includes coordinated dietary review across affected species, dietary tannin supplementation in some captive black rhinoceros programs, and coordinated Species Survival Plan surveillance supporting characterization of disease dynamics. Individual necropsy findings contribute to population-level management decisions.

Obesity, Cardiovascular Disease, and Diet-Related Pathology

Obesity in Captive Populations

Obesity in captive populations reflects the challenge of maintaining appropriate body condition in animals whose captive activity levels and dietary provision differ from their natural context. Documented obesity is prominent in captive nonhuman primates (particularly great apes and some cercopithecines), captive marine mammals, captive carnivores in some collections, and other captive species. The condition contributes to secondary disease including cardiovascular disease, diabetes mellitus, degenerative joint disease, and reduced reproductive success. Recognition at necropsy contributes to characterization of individual case clinical significance and to broader population-level management of body condition scoring and dietary provision.

Cardiovascular Disease Related to Diet

Cardiovascular disease related to diet includes atherosclerosis in captive psittacines associated with chronic dyslipidemia and dietary factors, cardiovascular disease in captive nonhuman primates with dietary contribution, and species-specific patterns documented in various captive populations. Recognition at necropsy contributes to the diet-cardiovascular disease association understanding across captive species.

Applied Case: Iron Storage Disease Population Surveillance in Captive Lemurs

A Species Survival Plan managed collection maintaining a substantial ring-tailed lemur population has coordinated iron storage disease surveillance across the collection through routine necropsy characterization of aged individuals and periodic antemortem screening including serum ferritin measurement and, in some individuals, liver biopsy under anesthesia when clinically warranted. Case review across recent years demonstrated consistent identification of dietary iron storage disease at necropsy in aged individuals with variable severity of associated hepatic pathology. Institutional response included ongoing dietary composition review with laboratory verification of iron content across offered diet components, consideration of dietary modification strategies including reduced iron content in offered diet components and dietary tannin supplementation, and coordinated Species Survival Plan surveillance supporting cross-institutional characterization of disease dynamics in the species. The case series illustrated the interpretive integration required across individual necropsy findings and population-level management: individual cases contribute to characterization of disease burden while population-level intervention supports prevention of future cases.

THE COMPARATIVE NECROPSY PATTERN SYSTEM — Nutritional and Metabolic Disease Pattern Recognition in Captive Populations

---

The Pattern: Recognition of characteristic nutritional deficiency, mineral imbalance, storage disease, or obesity-related pathology in captive species with dietary or husbandry factors contributing to the disease process.

Cross-Taxa Signature: Recognized across captive species with variable species-specific predispositions. Hypovitaminosis A affects captive reptiles and other affected species. Nutritional secondary hyperparathyroidism affects captive juvenile reptiles, birds, and mammals. Iron storage disease affects captive frugivorous primates, black rhinoceros, and other predisposed species. Obesity affects captive nonhuman primates, marine mammals, and various other captive species.

Diagnostic Anchor: Recognition of the characteristic gross and histopathologic pattern combined with dietary and husbandry history supports the diagnosis. Ancillary vitamin, mineral, or biochemical quantitation supports specific characterization.

Trap Logic: The look-alike is the primary infectious or neoplastic disease with secondary nutritional consequences, distinguished by primary disease identification. Another look-alike is age-related change with secondary metabolic consequences distinguished by specific disease pattern recognition.

Zoonotic/Reportable Flag: Not zoonotic or regulatorily reportable. Institutionally reportable at Species Survival Plan facilities for dietary and husbandry review supporting prevention of future cases.

Nutritional and Metabolic Disease Pattern Recognition in Captive Populations: Recognition of characteristic vitamin deficiency, mineral imbalance, storage disease, or lifestyle-related pathology in captive species with dietary contribution. Anchor: pattern recognition with dietary history. Trap: primary infectious or neoplastic disease with secondary nutritional consequences. Flag: institutionally reportable for population-level dietary and husbandry review.

Summary and Key Concepts

Hypovitaminosis A produces squamous metaplasia patterns in captive reptiles, fish, and other affected species; other vitamin deficiencies produce species-specific patterns requiring recognition and dietary review.

Metabolic bone disease across taxa includes nutritional secondary hyperparathyroidism, renal secondary hyperparathyroidism, and metastatic mineralization from hypervitaminosis D with detailed coverage in Chapter 10.

Iron storage disease in captive frugivorous primates, black rhinoceros, and other predisposed species has detailed coverage in Chapter 6 with substantial population-level management implications.

Obesity in captive populations contributes to secondary disease including cardiovascular disease, diabetes mellitus, and reduced reproductive success with recognition across captive nonhuman primates, marine mammals, and other affected species.

Diet-related cardiovascular disease includes atherosclerosis in captive psittacines and other species-specific patterns documented in captive populations.

Individual necropsy findings of nutritional and metabolic disease contribute to population-level dietary and husbandry management at Species Survival Plan facilities supporting prevention of future cases across affected species.

CHAPTER 19: TOXICOLOGIC PATHOLOGY IN WILDLIFE AND ZOO ANIMALS

Learning Objectives

1. Recognize lead toxicosis patterns in waterfowl, raptors, and California condors with attention to conservation implications.
2. Identify anticoagulant rodenticide toxicosis in predators with attention to second-generation compound residues.
3. Interpret environmental contaminant exposure including organochlorines, PFAS, and heavy metals in wildlife populations.
4. Recognize algal toxin, cyanotoxin, and marine biotoxin exposures with attention to associated wildlife mortality events.
5. Apply the Comparative Necropsy Pattern callout structure to toxicologic disease recognition.
6. Coordinate ancillary toxicologic diagnostics including tissue-appropriate sample selection and reference laboratory submission.

Toxicologic pathology in wildlife and zoo animals represents one of the most substantial areas of wildlife disease practice because environmental contamination, agricultural chemical exposure, and anthropogenic pollution produce documented wildlife disease at population-relevant scales. The pathologist working toxicologic cases requires familiarity with the major toxicant classes, their characteristic gross and histopathologic patterns, appropriate sample selection for toxicologic analysis, and the regulatory and public health implications of specific toxicant exposures. Wildlife toxicology has driven substantial regulatory intervention including bans of specific pesticides and environmental protection measures with catastrophic wildlife impact as the motivating evidence. The chapter addresses the major toxicologic categories encountered in wildlife pathology practice.

The chapter organizes toxicologic pathology into four operational domains. Lead toxicosis addresses the ongoing exposure of waterfowl, raptors, and condors with substantial conservation implications. Anticoagulant rodenticide toxicosis covers the recurring wildlife exposure documented in predator populations. Environmental contaminants including organochlorines, PFAS, and heavy metals addresses the broader spectrum of environmental exposure. Algal toxins and cyanotoxins completes the chapter with attention to marine and freshwater biotoxin exposures.

Lead Toxicosis: Waterfowl, Raptors, Condors

Waterfowl Lead Poisoning

Waterfowl lead poisoning historically produced substantial mortality across affected populations through ingestion of spent lead shot from hunting activities. Regulatory intervention with the 1991 nationwide ban on lead shot for waterfowl hunting substantially reduced the disease burden while lead shot ingestion continues to be documented in some populations from historical contamination and, in some cases, from continued use of non-compliant shot. Additional lead sources including lead fishing tackle and environmental contamination contribute to ongoing exposure. Necropsy recognition includes lead shot identification in the ventriculus, characteristic anemia with pallor of tissues, and, on histopathology, characteristic renal tubular changes with acid-fast intranuclear inclusion bodies in renal tubular epithelium.

Raptor and Vulture Lead Poisoning

Raptor and vulture lead poisoning reflects exposure through consumption of lead-shot game animals or gut piles from hunter-processed carcasses. Bald eagles, golden eagles, condors, and other scavenger and predator species demonstrate substantial documented exposure with characteristic clinical and pathologic patterns. California condor lead exposure has been a leading factor in the recovery challenges for the species with sustained coordinated response including hunter education, non-lead ammunition promotion, and, in some jurisdictions, regulatory restrictions on lead ammunition. The pathology in raptors and vultures includes characteristic clinical signs (neurologic dysfunction, weight loss), gross findings (poor body condition, sometimes visible lead fragments in gastrointestinal tract), and histopathologic recognition.

Applied Case: Lead Toxicosis in a California Condor

A California condor (Gymnogyps californianus) housed in a managed care program as part of the coordinated species recovery program was found deceased. Clinical monitoring in the days before death had documented reduced activity and behavioral abnormalities suggesting potential lead exposure; blood lead measurement had returned elevated concentrations consistent with acute lead toxicosis. Chelation therapy had been initiated with limited response before death. Necropsy focused on characterization of the lead exposure and identification of source material. External examination demonstrated the anticipated poor body condition. Coelomic necropsy demonstrated a small metallic fragment consistent with lead shot within the ventriculus supporting the source identification. Lead concentration in liver, kidney, and bone confirmed substantial lead body burden. The final morphologic diagnosis was lead toxicosis with associated systemic effects; the etiologic diagnosis was lead exposure through consumption of contaminated food source. Institutional response included the coordinated species recovery program reporting pathway, characterization of exposure source and location to inform continued monitoring, and contribution to the ongoing surveillance dataset for California condor lead exposure supporting continued species recovery efforts.

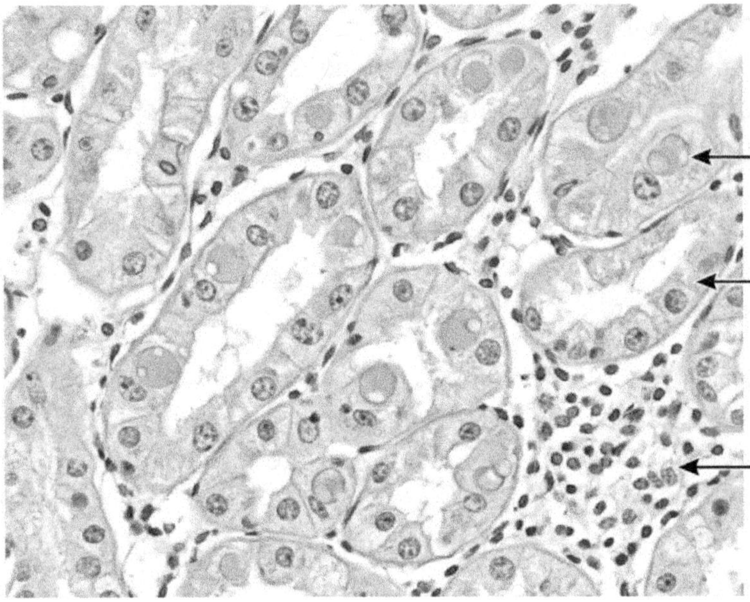

THE COMPARATIVE NECROPSY PATTERN SYSTEM — Lead Toxicosis Pattern in Waterfowl, Raptors, and Vultures

The Pattern: Poor body condition, characteristic clinical history of progressive weight loss and behavioral abnormalities, sometimes visible lead fragments in the gastrointestinal tract at necropsy, and, on histopathology, characteristic renal tubular changes with acid-fast intranuclear inclusion bodies indicating lead toxicosis.

Cross-Taxa Signature: Recognized across waterfowl (through lead shot ingestion), raptors including bald and golden eagles (through consumption of lead-shot game), vultures including California condors (with substantial recovery program implications), and other scavenging and predatory bird species with lead exposure. Also documented in some mammalian species with lead exposure including scavenging carnivores.

Diagnostic Anchor: Lead concentration in liver, kidney, or bone confirms lead body burden with species-appropriate reference concentrations. Blood lead concentration when antemortem samples are available provides additional characterization. Gross identification of lead fragments in gastrointestinal tract supports source identification when present.

Trap Logic: The look-alike is other causes of weight loss and neurologic disease including other toxicant exposure and various infectious and metabolic diseases distinguished by lead quantitation. Postmortem environmental lead contamination during necropsy handling requires exclusion by attention to sample collection technique.

Zoonotic/Reportable Flag: Not zoonotic. Lead exposure in federally protected species including bald eagles, golden eagles, and California condors requires coordinated reporting through US Fish and Wildlife Service and, in the case of California condors, the coordinated species recovery program. Environmental source characterization contributes to regulatory and management response.

Anticoagulant Rodenticide Toxicosis in Predators

Second-Generation Anticoagulant Exposure

Second-generation anticoagulant rodenticide toxicosis affects predator species through consumption of rodent prey containing rodenticide residues. Bald eagles, golden eagles, red-tailed hawks, great horned owls, mountain lions, bobcats, and other predator species have documented exposure with characteristic clinical and pathologic patterns. Second-generation compounds including brodifacoum, bromadiolone, difenacoum, and others produce more sustained hepatic residues than first-generation compounds and provide diagnostic utility for exposure characterization. The gross and histopathologic pattern includes multifocal internal hemorrhage with characteristic distribution and, in some individuals, chronic subclinical exposure detected through routine surveillance.

First-Generation Anticoagulant Exposure

First-generation anticoagulant rodenticide compounds including warfarin, chlorophacinone, and diphacinone produce similar clinical patterns to second-generation compounds but with shorter residue persistence complicating retrospective exposure characterization. Recognition of first-generation exposure requires appropriate ancillary workup with attention to compound-specific analysis. Wildlife exposure documentation has supported regulatory review of first-generation compound use in specific applications.

Regulatory Response to Wildlife Rodenticide Exposure

Regulatory response to wildlife anticoagulant rodenticide exposure has included substantial rulemaking at federal and state levels restricting specific compound use in some applications, coordinated wildlife surveillance datasets supporting characterization of exposure prevalence, and continued research supporting evidence-based regulatory decision-making. Wildlife pathology contributions to this response include case-by-case exposure documentation contributing to broader surveillance datasets.

Environmental Contaminants

Organochlorine Compounds

Organochlorine compound exposure remains relevant to wildlife pathology practice decades after regulatory restrictions on many compounds because of the environmental persistence of these compounds. DDT and its metabolites continue to be detected in some wildlife populations reflecting historical use. PCB compounds continue to be documented in marine mammals and other affected species. Recognition of organochlorine exposure at necropsy requires appropriate adipose tissue collection for compound-specific analysis.

PFAS and Emerging Contaminants

Per- and polyfluoroalkyl substances (PFAS) have emerged as substantial contaminants of wildlife health concern with documented exposure across a wide range of wildlife species and substantial ongoing research characterizing wildlife health implications. Wildlife PFAS exposure surveillance is a growing area of wildlife pathology contribution. Other emerging contaminants including neonicotinoid pesticides and various pharmaceutical residues in the environment continue to expand the toxicologic surveillance landscape.

Heavy Metals Other Than Lead

Heavy metals other than lead including mercury (substantial documented wildlife exposure with methylmercury as the specific toxic form), cadmium, and various other metals produce documented wildlife disease across affected populations. Recognition of heavy metal exposure at necropsy requires appropriate tissue selection and reference laboratory submission with species-appropriate reference concentrations.

Algal Toxins, Cyanotoxins, and Marine Biotoxins

Domoic Acid and Marine Biotoxins

Domoic acid toxicosis in California sea lions and other marine mammals is addressed in Chapter 9 as a leading example of algal biotoxin exposure. Marine biotoxin exposure across marine mammal and seabird species includes brevetoxin from red tide events, saxitoxin from paralytic shellfish poisoning-associated blooms, and other biotoxins with characteristic clinical and pathologic patterns.

Cyanotoxins and Freshwater Biotoxin Exposure

Cyanotoxin exposure from freshwater cyanobacterial harmful algal blooms produces documented wildlife disease across various species. Microcystin toxicosis produces characteristic hepatic disease with hepatic necrosis and hemorrhage. Anatoxin-a produces characteristic neurotoxic disease. Recognition of cyanotoxin exposure at necropsy requires appropriate ancillary workup and environmental context characterization.

THE COMPARATIVE NECROPSY PATTERN SYSTEM — Chapter 19 Toxicologic Pattern Foundations

Lead Toxicosis Pattern in Waterfowl, Raptors, and Vultures: Poor body condition and characteristic clinical history with renal tubular inclusion bodies confirming lead exposure. Anchor: lead quantitation in liver, kidney, or bone. Trap: other toxicant exposure and metabolic disease discriminated by quantitation. Flag: federally protected species require coordinated regulatory reporting.

Summary and Key Concepts

Lead toxicosis in waterfowl through spent lead shot ingestion, in raptors and vultures through consumption of lead-shot game, and in California condors with substantial recovery program implications represents one of the most substantial wildlife toxicologic issues.

Anticoagulant rodenticide toxicosis in predator species through consumption of rodent prey with rodenticide residues is documented across bald eagles, mountain lions, and other predator species with second-generation compounds providing diagnostic utility.

Environmental contaminants including organochlorines with historical persistence, PFAS as emerging contaminants, and heavy metals other than lead including methylmercury contribute to the wildlife toxicologic surveillance landscape.

Algal toxins including domoic acid in marine mammals, brevetoxin in marine wildlife, cyanotoxin exposure from freshwater harmful algal blooms with microcystin and anatoxin-a documented, and other biotoxin exposures require appropriate recognition and ancillary workup.

Wildlife toxicologic pathology has driven substantial regulatory intervention including lead shot restrictions, DDT and other organochlorine restrictions, and ongoing regulatory review of anticoagulant rodenticide use.

Wildlife pathology contributions to toxicologic surveillance support both individual case management and broader environmental protection response.

CHAPTER 20: NEOPLASIA IN NON-DOMESTIC SPECIES

Learning Objectives

1. Recognize species-specific tumor predispositions in captive and free-ranging non-domestic species.
2. Identify retroviral and viral oncogenesis patterns in wildlife populations.
3. Interpret comparative oncology findings across taxa with attention to translational implications.
4. Recognize population-level neoplasia surveillance patterns at Species Survival Plan facilities.
5. Apply the Comparative Necropsy Pattern callout structure to neoplastic disease recognition across taxa.
6. Coordinate ancillary neoplasia diagnostics including histopathologic characterization, immunohistochemistry, and molecular characterization.

Neoplasia in non-domestic species contributes substantially to the disease burden of aged captive populations and is recognized in a range of free-ranging wildlife contexts with varying epidemiologic significance. The pathologist working non-domestic neoplasia cases carries the interpretive burden of recognizing tumor patterns often against limited species-specific reference, applying comparative reasoning to species where the specific tumor entity has not been previously characterized, and integrating individual case findings with the growing population-level neoplasia surveillance datasets maintained at Species Survival Plan facilities. Comparative oncology has become a substantial research area with recognized translational implications for both animal and human oncology. The chapter addresses the range of neoplastic disease documented in non-domestic species with attention to species-specific patterns and to the interpretive frameworks that support recognition across unfamiliar taxa.

The chapter organizes non-domestic species neoplasia into four operational domains. Species-specific tumor predispositions address the recurring patterns documented in various captive species. Retroviral and viral oncogenesis covers the range of virally associated neoplasia. Comparative oncology findings address the cross-taxa comparisons that inform both wildlife pathology practice and comparative oncology research. Population-level neoplasia surveillance completes the chapter with attention to the Species Survival Plan surveillance datasets.

Species-Specific Tumor Predispositions

Neoplasia in Aged Captive Species

Neoplasia in aged captive species includes substantial documented tumor burden across captive nonhuman primates, captive great apes with well-characterized tumor patterns, captive large felids with recognized age-related tumor entities, captive avian species particularly aged psittacines with substantial documented neoplasia, and captive marine mammals with age-related tumor patterns. The specific tumor entities documented include gastric adenocarcinoma in aged lemurs and great apes (as noted in Chapter 8), thyroid neoplasia in aged captive felids, hepatocellular carcinoma in aged captive psittacines and other species, uterine leiomyoma in aged captive great apes, and numerous species-specific entities. Recognition and characterization of aged captive neoplasia contributes to institutional understanding of population age structure and to broader comparative oncology datasets.

Species-Specific Cancer Susceptibility Patterns

Species-specific cancer susceptibility patterns include the substantial documented lymphoma predisposition in captive ferrets, the multifocal cancer patterns documented in some captive rodent species, the lineage-clustered cancer patterns documented in captive great ape populations at some facilities, and the various species-specific patterns documented across captive collections. Some species demonstrate substantially elevated cancer prevalence relative to related species, and understanding of these predispositions supports both individual case interpretation and population-level management.

Ferret Lymphoma Case Series

Ferret lymphoma is documented at substantial prevalence in captive ferret populations with well-recognized clinical presentations, imaging findings, and histopathologic patterns. Multicentric lymphoma is the most common presentation. The disease has been extensively characterized in the veterinary literature with attention to clinical management, prognostic factors, and molecular characterization. Species-specific predisposition has been characterized with documented associations to age, husbandry factors, and, in some cases, viral etiologies. Case-by-case recognition contributes to ongoing characterization of ferret lymphoma epidemiology and management.

Retroviral and Viral Oncogenesis in Wildlife

Retroviral-Associated Neoplasia

Retroviral-associated neoplasia in captive and wild species includes feline leukemia virus-associated lymphoma and other neoplasia in captive felids, simian retroviral associations with lymphoproliferative disease in some captive nonhuman primates, avian retroviral neoplasia including reticuloendotheliosis virus-associated tumors and avian leukosis virus-associated disease, and other retroviral entities. Recognition of retroviral-associated neoplasia requires molecular or serologic characterization of the associated retrovirus complemented by histopathologic characterization of the specific neoplastic pattern.

Papillomavirus and Herpesvirus Associations

Papillomavirus and herpesvirus associations with wildlife neoplasia include documented associations of papillomavirus with characteristic proliferative lesions in various species, herpesvirus associations with fibropapillomatosis in free-ranging sea turtles (chelonid herpesvirus 5 in green turtle fibropapillomatosis), and various other viral-neoplasia associations. Fibropapillomatosis in green sea turtles has been characterized as a substantial wildlife disease entity with characterized viral etiology and documented conservation impact.

Emerging Viral-Neoplasia Associations

Emerging viral-neoplasia associations continue to be recognized through molecular characterization of clinical specimens. Various novel viral sequences have been identified in association with specific neoplastic entities across taxa. The interpretive challenge in emerging viral-neoplasia recognition parallels other emerging infectious disease recognition requiring integration of molecular findings with histopathologic characterization to distinguish causative association from incidental viral presence.

Comparative Oncology Findings Across Taxa

Cross-Species Cancer Pattern Recognition

Cross-species cancer pattern recognition supports both wildlife pathology practice and broader comparative oncology research. Similar tumor entities recur across mammalian taxa with variable species-specific patterns. The comparative reasoning framework that supports interpretation of tumor entities in unfamiliar species draws on the extensive human and domestic species oncology literature complemented by the growing wildlife oncology literature. Species-specific modifications to the standard interpretive framework support accurate recognition of tumor entities across captive collections.

Peto Paradox and Cancer Resistance in Wildlife

The Peto paradox observation that cancer prevalence does not scale with body size and lifespan across species has motivated substantial research into wildlife cancer resistance mechanisms. Large-bodied species including elephants demonstrate documented cancer resistance mechanisms including TP53 gene amplification supporting enhanced tumor suppressor function. Naked mole rats demonstrate extraordinary cancer resistance with characterized molecular mechanisms. Cetaceans demonstrate documented longevity with modest cancer prevalence relative to body size. Wildlife pathology contributions to characterizing cancer patterns across taxa support this research.

Translational Comparative Oncology

Translational comparative oncology draws on wildlife cancer characterization to inform both animal welfare and human oncology research. Wildlife tumor characterization has contributed to human cancer research through identification of novel tumor entities, characterization of tumor development mechanisms, and identification of potential therapeutic targets. The comparative oncology field represents a growing area of wildlife pathology contribution to broader biomedical research.

Population-Level Neoplasia Surveillance

Species Survival Plan Cancer Surveillance

Species Survival Plan cancer surveillance across captive collections supports characterization of tumor patterns in specific species with documented age structure, dietary and husbandry factors, and, in some cases, genetic contribution. Coordinated surveillance across multiple institutions provides population-level datasets that no single collection can generate. Individual necropsy findings contribute to these datasets supporting broader species management decisions including breeding recommendations, medical intervention protocols, and identification of environmental or dietary contributors to disease patterns.

Applied Case: Hepatocellular Carcinoma in an Aged Captive Amazon Parrot

An aged captive Amazon parrot in a Species Survival Plan managed collection had been under long-term care with routine health monitoring including periodic imaging assessment. Antemortem imaging had identified a discrete hepatic mass approximately three months before death; supportive care was elected given the age and species considerations. Necropsy focused on characterization of the hepatic mass and identification of any additional pathology. Systematic necropsy demonstrated a large solitary tan hepatic mass approximately 3 cm in maximum diameter with areas of central necrosis. Histopathology confirmed moderately differentiated hepatocellular carcinoma with characteristic trabecular growth pattern. Immunohistochemistry with hepatocyte-specific markers supported the diagnosis. The final morphologic diagnosis was primary hepatocellular carcinoma of the liver. Institutional response included coordinated reporting through the Species Survival Plan pathway contributing to the ongoing psittacine tumor surveillance dataset. The case reinforced the recognition of hepatocellular carcinoma as an age-related tumor entity in captive psittacines and contributed to the broader population-level tumor characterization for the species.

THE COMPARATIVE NECROPSY PATTERN SYSTEM — Species-Specific Tumor Pattern Recognition in Aged Captive Populations

The Pattern: Recognition of characteristic species-specific tumor entity in aged captive individual with appropriate correlation to species-specific tumor patterns documented at Species Survival Plan facilities.

Cross-Taxa Signature: Recognized across captive species with variable species-specific tumor predispositions. Gastric adenocarcinoma in aged lemurs. Thyroid neoplasia in aged captive felids. Hepatocellular carcinoma in aged psittacines. Multicentric lymphoma in captive ferrets. Uterine leiomyoma in aged captive great apes. Various other species-specific patterns.

Diagnostic Anchor: Histopathologic characterization with immunohistochemistry supporting specific tumor identification. Molecular characterization when needed. Correlation with species-specific tumor patterns from surveillance datasets.

Trap Logic: The look-alike is other primary or metastatic tumor entities distinguished by histopathologic characterization. Another look-alike is non-neoplastic mass lesions distinguished by histopathologic architecture and immunohistochemistry.

Zoonotic/Reportable Flag: Not zoonotic in most cases. Institutionally reportable at Species Survival Plan facilities for population-level tumor surveillance and management.

THE COMPARATIVE NECROPSY PATTERN SYSTEM — Chapter 20 Neoplasia Pattern Foundations

---

Species-Specific Tumor Pattern Recognition in Aged Captive Populations: Recognition of species-specific tumor entities across captive collections with characterized predispositions. Anchor: histopathologic characterization with immunohistochemistry. Trap: other tumor entities discriminated by architectural features. Flag: institutionally reportable for SSP surveillance.

Summary and Key Concepts

Species-specific tumor predispositions across captive nonhuman primates, captive great apes, captive large felids, captive avian species, captive ferrets, and captive marine mammals demonstrate characterized patterns supporting individual case interpretation.

Retroviral and viral oncogenesis includes feline leukemia virus, simian retroviral associations, avian retroviral neoplasia, papillomavirus associations including fibropapillomatosis in green turtles, and emerging viral-neoplasia associations.

Comparative oncology findings across taxa support both wildlife pathology practice and broader translational research including characterization of the Peto paradox and cancer resistance mechanisms in large-bodied and long-lived species.

Population-level neoplasia surveillance at Species Survival Plan facilities generates datasets no single collection can provide with individual necropsy findings contributing to broader species management decisions.

Wildlife tumor characterization has translational implications for both animal welfare and human oncology research supporting the growing comparative oncology field.

Individual necropsy characterization of neoplastic disease contributes to both individual case management and to broader population-level and comparative oncology datasets.

CHAPTER 21: TRAUMA, HUMAN-WILDLIFE CONFLICT, AND ANTHROPOGENIC INJURY

Learning Objectives

1. Recognize vehicle collision pathology in wildlife populations with attention to fracture patterns and mechanism reconstruction.
2. Identify firearm and projectile injury pathology with attention to chain of custody for potential legal cases.
3. Interpret entanglement, bycatch, and fisheries interaction injury in marine wildlife.
4. Recognize predator-prey and intraspecific trauma patterns across wildlife populations.
5. Apply the Comparative Necropsy Pattern callout structure to traumatic injury recognition.
6. Coordinate with federal law enforcement partners for cases with potential legal implications.

Trauma, human-wildlife conflict, and anthropogenic injury constitute a substantial proportion of wildlife pathology caseload with individual case pathology recognition supporting both individual case interpretation and broader documentation of human-wildlife interactions with potential regulatory and management implications. The pathologist working traumatic cases carries the interpretive burden of reconstructing injury mechanism from lesion pattern, distinguishing antemortem from postmortem tissue changes, and, in cases with potential legal implications, maintaining chain of custody documentation supporting downstream investigative use of the necropsy findings. The chapter addresses the major categories of traumatic and anthropogenic injury encountered in wildlife pathology practice.

The chapter organizes traumatic and anthropogenic injury into four operational domains. Vehicle collision pathology addresses the substantial wildlife mortality caused by road traffic. Firearm and projectile injury interpretation covers cases with legal implications requiring specific documentation approach. Entanglement, bycatch, and fisheries interaction addresses marine wildlife injury from fishing activities. Predator-prey and intraspecific trauma completes the chapter with attention to natural traumatic injury patterns.

Vehicle Collision Pathology

Fracture Pattern Recognition

Fracture pattern recognition in vehicle collision cases supports interpretation of the collision mechanism and, in some cases, characterization of the vehicle-wildlife interaction. Long bone fractures with characteristic distribution reflect the impact vector, associated soft tissue injury reflects the specific tissue disruption, and skin abrasion patterns reflect the direction of impact. Recognition of characteristic vehicle collision patterns distinguishes these cases from other traumatic mechanisms. Documentation of the specific patterns supports downstream use for management planning including identification of high-risk wildlife-vehicle interaction locations.

Species-Specific Vehicle Collision Patterns

Species-specific vehicle collision patterns reflect the biology of the specific wildlife species. Deer collision patterns include characteristic long bone fractures and associated soft tissue injury with specific distribution reflecting the collision mechanism. Small mammal collision patterns include characteristic crushing injury with specific distribution. Avian collision patterns include characteristic soft tissue and skeletal injury reflecting the specific interaction. Recognition of species-specific patterns supports interpretation of the specific collision mechanism.

Firearm and Projectile Injury Interpretation

Projectile Wound Recognition

Projectile wound recognition includes entrance wound characterization with specific features distinguishing entrance from exit wounds, projectile path characterization through anatomic structures with associated tissue disruption, and projectile identification when metallic material is recovered from the wound. Documentation includes photographic recording of external and internal wound features supporting downstream interpretive use. Radiographic examination of the carcass supports identification of retained projectile material even when external wound characteristics are limited.

Chain of Custody in Investigative Cases

Chain of custody in investigative wildlife cases including firearm-injury cases is addressed in Chapter 3 with detailed protocols. For federally protected species (bald eagles, golden eagles, migratory birds, marine mammals, endangered species) with traumatic mortality, chain of custody initiation at case receipt with subsequent documentation of all specimen transfers supports downstream investigative use. Coordination with US Fish and Wildlife Service law enforcement or NOAA Fisheries Office of Law Enforcement is initiated for cases with investigative potential.

Applied Case: Bald Eagle Gunshot Injury Investigation

A bald eagle carcass was submitted for necropsy from a state wildlife area with the initial finding notation of possible gunshot injury based on external examination by the recovery party. The submission was designated as investigative with chain of custody initiated at case receipt including notification of the US Fish and Wildlife Service law enforcement agent for the region. Necropsy was performed under investigative case protocol with photographic documentation preceding coelomic entry. External examination identified a small circular wound in the ventral thoracic region consistent with projectile injury with associated feather disruption pattern suggesting entrance wound. Radiographic examination of the carcass identified retained metallic material in the thoracic cavity. Coelomic necropsy demonstrated the projectile path through the thoracic wall, through pulmonary parenchyma, and terminating in the thoracic cavity with retained projectile material recovery. The projectile was recovered intact and archived per chain of custody protocols. The final morphologic diagnosis was penetrating projectile injury with resulting acute hemorrhage and death. Federal investigative case handling proceeded with the recovered projectile providing critical evidence for the subsequent federal wildlife law enforcement investigation.

THE COMPARATIVE NECROPSY PATTERN SYSTEM — Fatal Trauma Pattern Recognition in Wildlife With Legal Implications

---

The Pattern: Recognition of characteristic trauma pattern consistent with defined injury mechanism (vehicle collision, projectile injury, entanglement, predator interaction) with appropriate documentation supporting individual case interpretation and, in federally protected species, downstream investigative use.

Cross-Taxa Signature: Recognized across wildlife species with variable species-specific patterns reflecting the specific traumatic mechanism and species biology. Vehicle collision patterns in cervids, small mammals, and other affected species. Projectile injury patterns across affected species. Entanglement patterns in marine wildlife including turtles, marine mammals, and seabirds. Predator-prey patterns across various species.

Diagnostic Anchor: Documentation of vital reaction at wound sites distinguishing antemortem from postmortem tissue disruption. Documentation of directional injury pattern supporting mechanism interpretation. Radiographic examination when appropriate for retained material identification.

Trap Logic: The look-alike is postmortem scavenger predation superimposed on antemortem disease death producing gross tissue disruption without a fatal traumatic mechanism. Discrimination: postmortem scavenger damage lacks vital reaction; antemortem trauma demonstrates vital reaction with mechanism-consistent pattern.

Zoonotic/Reportable Flag: Federally protected species with traumatic mortality require coordinated reporting through appropriate federal law enforcement (US Fish and Wildlife Service Office of Law Enforcement, NOAA Fisheries Office of Law Enforcement) with chain of custody initiated at case receipt for investigative cases.

Entanglement, Bycatch, and Fisheries Interaction

Marine Mammal Entanglement

Marine mammal entanglement in fishing gear including gillnets, longlines, pot and trap gear, and derelict fishing gear produces documented mortality across pinniped, cetacean, and sirenian species. Entanglement produces characteristic dermatologic patterns including circumferential wounds at gear contact sites, distal extremity ischemic changes when gear compromises circulation, and, in prolonged entanglement, secondary chronic disease from impaired feeding or reduced mobility. Recognition of entanglement at necropsy contributes to the coordinated marine mammal stranding response and supports characterization of fisheries-wildlife interaction burden.

Sea Turtle Bycatch and Fisheries Interaction

Sea turtle bycatch in various fisheries produces documented mortality across affected species with characteristic pathology patterns including drowning injury with characteristic pulmonary changes, hook and line injury with specific gastrointestinal and cutaneous patterns, and gill net entanglement injury. Federal protection of sea turtle species under the Endangered Species Act supports coordinated response to bycatch cases with implications for both individual case management and broader fisheries management.

Seabird Fisheries Interaction

Seabird fisheries interaction includes longline hook injury, gillnet entanglement, and other patterns documented across affected species. Federal protection of migratory bird species under the Migratory Bird Treaty Act supports coordinated response to bycatch cases with implications for fisheries management.

Predator-Prey and Intraspecific Trauma

Predator-Prey Injury Recognition

Predator-prey injury recognition supports interpretation of the specific predator species responsible when characteristic bite marks, claw patterns, or feeding patterns are identified. Documentation of the specific injury pattern supports downstream interpretation and, in cases involving livestock or other management-relevant contexts, may contribute to management response. Distinguishing predation from scavenger consumption of a previously deceased animal requires attention to vital reaction at wound sites.

Intraspecific Trauma

Intraspecific trauma including breeding-related fighting injury, territorial disputes, and other intraspecific interactions produces documented wildlife injury and mortality across various species. Recognition of intraspecific injury patterns supports characterization of wildlife behavioral ecology and, in some captive contexts, may inform husbandry decisions about group composition and enclosure design.

THE COMPARATIVE NECROPSY PATTERN SYSTEM — Chapter 21 Traumatic Injury Pattern Foundations

---

Fatal Trauma Pattern Recognition in Wildlife With Legal Implications: Trauma patterns with mechanism reconstruction across vehicle collision, projectile injury, entanglement, and predator-prey categories with appropriate documentation supporting investigative use. Anchor: vital reaction distinguishing antemortem from postmortem. Trap: postmortem scavenger damage discriminated by absent vital reaction. Flag: federally protected species require coordinated federal law enforcement reporting.

Summary and Key Concepts

Vehicle collision pathology contributes substantial wildlife mortality with characteristic fracture patterns and species-specific presentations supporting mechanism interpretation and management planning.

Firearm and projectile injury interpretation requires specific documentation approach with chain of custody initiation for federally protected species supporting downstream investigative use.

Marine wildlife entanglement, bycatch, and fisheries interaction produces documented mortality across marine mammals, sea turtles, and seabirds with implications for both individual case management and broader fisheries management response.

Predator-prey and intraspecific trauma produces recognizable patterns supporting characterization of wildlife behavioral ecology and, in some contexts, management decisions.

Coordination with federal law enforcement partners including US Fish and Wildlife Service Office of Law Enforcement and NOAA Fisheries Office of Law Enforcement supports investigative cases with potential legal implications.

Wildlife pathology contributions to trauma characterization support both individual case interpretation and broader documentation of human-wildlife interactions relevant to regulatory and management response.

CHAPTER 22: MARINE MAMMAL PATHOLOGY

Learning Objectives

1. Recognize cetacean-specific pathology patterns including morbillivirus, Brucella ceti, and marine debris ingestion.
2. Identify pinniped-specific pathology patterns including phocine distemper virus and neonatal disease.
3. Interpret sirenian and marine fissiped pathology patterns.
4. Recognize stranding investigation patterns and unusual mortality event coordination.
5. Apply the Comparative Necropsy Pattern callout structure to marine mammal disease recognition.
6. Coordinate with NOAA Fisheries Marine Mammal Health and Stranding Response Program for cases and population health surveillance.

Marine mammal pathology represents one of the most specialized and coordinated areas of wildlife pathology practice with the substantial infrastructure of the NOAA Fisheries Marine Mammal Health and Stranding Response Program supporting nationwide case investigation and population health surveillance. The pathologist working marine mammal cases contributes to individual case interpretation, coordinated surveillance for unusual mortality events, and characterization of marine mammal population health across affected regions. The chapter addresses the major taxonomic groupings and their characteristic disease patterns with attention to the coordinated response framework that supports marine mammal pathology practice.

The chapter organizes marine mammal pathology into four operational domains. Cetacean-specific pathology addresses the disease patterns documented across dolphin, whale, and porpoise species. Pinniped-specific pathology covers the harbor seals, gray seals, elephant seals, sea lions, and walruses. Sirenian and marine fissiped pathology addresses the manatees, dugongs, sea otters, and polar bears. Stranding investigation and population health completes the chapter with attention to the coordinated response framework.

Cetacean-Specific Pathology

Cetacean Morbillivirus and Related Viral Disease

Cetacean morbillivirus has produced substantial documented unusual mortality events across bottlenose dolphin populations and other affected species with detailed coverage in Chapter 12. The pathology pattern includes interstitial pneumonia with syncytia, meningoencephalitis, and immunosuppression. Related viral diseases including cetacean gammaherpesvirus and other viral agents contribute to the cetacean disease burden.

Cetacean Brucellosis and Bacterial Disease

Cetacean brucellosis caused by Brucella ceti and related bacterial diseases contribute to the cetacean disease burden with detailed coverage in Chapter 14. Cetacean pneumonia caused by various bacterial pathogens produces documented mortality. Marine mammal-specific bacterial pathogens including Streptococcus phocae and various other agents contribute to the differential.

Marine Debris and Environmental Contaminant Exposure

Marine debris ingestion in cetaceans produces documented mortality across affected species with variable species-specific patterns. Environmental contaminant exposure including persistent organic pollutants and heavy metals contributes to cetacean disease burden with variable presentations. Recognition contributes to broader ocean health surveillance.

THE COMPARATIVE NECROPSY PATTERN SYSTEM — Cetacean Stranding Pattern Recognition and Coordinated Response

The Pattern: Cetacean stranding with systematic necropsy assessment across infectious disease, environmental contaminant, marine debris, and traumatic injury differentials with coordinated reporting through the NOAA Fisheries Marine Mammal Health and Stranding Response Program.

Cross-Taxa Signature: Recognized across cetacean species with variable species-specific presentations. Bottlenose dolphins, common dolphins, harbor porpoises, and various other species demonstrate documented stranding pathology across affected geographic regions.

Diagnostic Anchor: Systematic marine mammal necropsy assessment with standardized sampling protocols. Coordinated reporting through NOAA Fisheries regional coordinators supports individual case management and broader surveillance.

Trap Logic: The look-alike is stranding of individual origin without population-level significance versus stranding as part of unusual mortality event requiring different response scale. Recognition of stranding pattern in temporal and spatial context supports appropriate response.

Zoonotic/Reportable Flag: Marine mammal Brucella species are zoonotic. Marine mammal cases require reporting through NOAA Fisheries with unusual mortality event declarations following detection of outbreak patterns.

Pinniped-Specific Pathology

Phocine Distemper Virus

Phocine distemper virus has produced substantial documented pinniped mortality with detailed coverage in Chapter 12. The pattern includes characteristic morbillivirus pathology comparable to canine distemper virus and cetacean morbillivirus patterns.

Neonatal Pinniped Disease

Neonatal pinniped disease including maternal separation, malnutrition, and infectious disease produces documented mortality with substantial rehabilitation program response. Recognition at necropsy contributes to characterization of neonatal survival factors.

Pinniped Trauma and Fisheries Interaction

Pinniped trauma including boat strike, entanglement in fishing gear, and other anthropogenic injury produces documented mortality with coordinated response through the marine mammal stranding network. Recognition supports both individual case management and broader anthropogenic injury surveillance.

Sirenian and Marine Fissiped Pathology

Manatee Pathology

Manatee pathology includes cold stress syndrome in Florida manatee populations during winter cold events with characteristic clinical and pathologic patterns, boat strike injury with substantial documented mortality across affected populations, red tide biotoxin exposure with characteristic neurologic and other pathology, and various infectious and non-infectious disease patterns. The coordinated response framework for manatee cases includes state and federal partners supporting comprehensive case management and population surveillance.

Sea Otter Pathology

Sea otter pathology includes toxoplasmosis with documented association to freshwater outflow contamination, sarcocystosis with similar associations, various infectious disease patterns, and environmental contaminant exposure. Sea otter cases contribute to both individual case management and broader marine ecosystem health surveillance.

Stranding Investigation and Population Health

NOAA Fisheries Coordination

NOAA Fisheries Marine Mammal Health and Stranding Response Program coordination supports comprehensive marine mammal case investigation with regional coordinators managing case flow, standardized necropsy and sampling protocols, coordinated reporting for unusual mortality events, and integration with research and policy applications. Wildlife pathology contributions to this framework support both individual case management and broader marine mammal population health surveillance.

Unusual Mortality Event Framework

Unusual mortality event framework provides structured response to marine mammal mortality patterns exceeding baseline levels. Declaration of unusual mortality events triggers enhanced surveillance response including expanded necropsy and sample collection, coordinated interpretation across affected regions, and, when applicable, coordinated research response to characterize the specific etiology. Wildlife pathology contributions to unusual mortality event investigation support characterization of the specific disease dynamics.

Applied Case: Unusual Mortality Event Response for Bottlenose Dolphins

A coastal region experienced elevated bottlenose dolphin stranding rates during a summer period exceeding baseline levels sufficient to trigger unusual mortality event declaration. Coordinated response through the NOAA Fisheries regional coordinator included expanded necropsy and sampling from strandings, coordinated reporting across the network of participating laboratories, and coordinated interpretation supporting characterization of the specific etiology. Cases demonstrated the classical cetacean morbillivirus pathology with interstitial pneumonia, meningoencephalitis, and characteristic syncytia and viral inclusion bodies. Molecular characterization confirmed cetacean morbillivirus with subsequent characterization of the specific strain contributing to the coordinated surveillance dataset. The unusual mortality event response supported comprehensive characterization of the specific event and contributed to the broader understanding of cetacean morbillivirus epidemiology in North American cetacean populations.

THE COMPARATIVE NECROPSY PATTERN SYSTEM — Chapter 22 Marine Mammal Pattern Foundations

---

Cetacean Stranding Pattern Recognition and Coordinated Response: Cetacean stranding with systematic assessment and NOAA Fisheries coordinated reporting. Anchor: standardized marine mammal necropsy protocols with coordinated reporting. Trap: individual stranding versus UME requires temporal-spatial context assessment. Flag: Brucella zoonotic and UME reporting through NOAA Fisheries.

Summary and Key Concepts

Cetacean-specific pathology includes morbillivirus with documented unusual mortality events, Brucella ceti and bacterial disease, and marine debris and environmental contaminant exposure across affected species.

Pinniped-specific pathology includes phocine distemper virus, neonatal disease and rehabilitation program contribution, and anthropogenic injury including entanglement and boat strike.

Sirenian pathology including manatee cold stress, boat strike, and red tide biotoxin exposure and sea otter pathology including toxoplasmosis with freshwater outflow associations contribute to the marine mammal disease landscape.

NOAA Fisheries Marine Mammal Health and Stranding Response Program coordination supports comprehensive case investigation and population health surveillance with regional coordinators managing case flow and standardized protocols.

Unusual mortality event framework provides structured response to elevated mortality patterns with enhanced surveillance and coordinated interpretation.

Wildlife pathology contributions to marine mammal case investigation support both individual case management and broader marine ecosystem health surveillance.

CHAPTER 23: AVIAN PATHOLOGY IN ZOO AND FREE-RANGING POPULATIONS

Learning Objectives

1. Recognize order-specific pathology considerations across Psittaciformes, Passeriformes, Anseriformes, and Falconiformes.
2. Identify ratite-specific pathology patterns in captive and wild populations.
3. Interpret emerging avian disease surveillance patterns.
4. Apply the Comparative Necropsy Pattern callout structure to avian disease recognition across orders.
5. Coordinate ancillary avian diagnostics including species-appropriate pathogen panels.
6. Contribute to broader avian disease surveillance including HPAI and other reportable disease response.

Avian pathology in zoo and free-ranging populations represents one of the largest categories of wildlife pathology practice reflecting the substantial avian species diversity in captive and wild contexts and the range of disease processes affecting these populations. The pathologist working avian cases carries the interpretive burden of recognizing order-specific disease patterns, applying comparative reasoning across avian orders, and coordinating appropriate ancillary workup for the anticipated differential. Avian pathology contributes to individual case management, collection-level biosafety at zoological facilities, coordinated response to reportable disease including HPAI (Chapter 13), and broader avian conservation surveillance. The chapter addresses order-specific considerations and emerging disease patterns.

The chapter organizes avian pathology into three operational domains. Order-specific considerations address Psittaciformes, Passeriformes, Anseriformes, and Falconiformes. Ratite pathology covers the captive ostrich, emu, cassowary, and rhea populations. Emerging avian disease surveillance completes the chapter with attention to the ongoing recognition of new avian disease entities.

Order-Specific Considerations: Psittaciformes, Passeriformes, Anseriformes, Falconiformes

Psittaciformes

Psittaciformes pathology in captive collections includes substantial documented disease across species with recognized susceptibilities. Beak and feather disease virus infection (Chapter 12) produces substantial documented disease in cockatoos, African grey parrots, and other affected species. Psittacid herpesvirus 1 (Pacheco disease) produces peracute mortality in outbreak settings. Aspergillosis (Chapter 15) affects captive psittacines with substantial impact in African grey parrots and other affected species. Atherosclerosis and cardiovascular disease including vascular mineralization affect aged captive psittacines. Hepatic disease including hepatocellular carcinoma in aged individuals and various infectious hepatic disease patterns. Pulmonary disease including aspergillosis and pulmonary mineralization. Neurologic disease including proventricular dilation syndrome associated with avian bornaviruses. Recognition of these disease patterns supports individual and collection-level management of captive psittacine populations.

Passeriformes

Passeriformes pathology in captive and wild populations includes various infectious disease entities with species-specific patterns. West Nile virus disease (Chapter 9) affects passerine species with variable susceptibility. Mycoplasma gallisepticum has produced documented population-level disease in wild passerine species including house finches with substantial outbreak documented in eastern North America. Trichomoniasis affects columbid and other affected species. Various avian pox viruses and other infectious disease patterns are documented. Recognition of passerine disease supports both individual case management and broader wildlife health surveillance.

Anseriformes

Anseriformes (waterfowl) pathology in captive and wild populations includes substantial disease burden across affected species. Highly pathogenic avian influenza (Chapter 13) has produced substantial documented mortality across waterfowl populations during the current panzootic. Avian cholera (Pasteurella multocida) produces documented outbreak events with substantial mortality. Duck plague (Anatid herpesvirus 1) produces characteristic pathology in outbreak settings. Botulism (Clostridium botulinum) produces documented outbreak events particularly in warm weather conditions. Lead toxicosis (Chapter 19) affects waterfowl through ingestion of spent lead shot. Various other infectious and non-infectious disease patterns contribute to the waterfowl disease burden.

Falconiformes and Other Raptors

Falconiformes and other raptor pathology includes substantial documented disease across captive and wild raptors. Aspergillosis affects captive raptors with substantial impact particularly in rehabilitation facilities. West Nile virus disease affects various raptor species. Trichomoniasis affects raptors through pigeon or dove prey consumption. Lead toxicosis (Chapter 19) affects raptors through consumption of lead-shot game with substantial documented impact. Anticoagulant rodenticide toxicosis (Chapter 19) affects predator raptors through rodent prey consumption. Trauma including window strike, vehicle collision, and other anthropogenic injury produces documented mortality.

THE COMPARATIVE NECROPSY PATTERN SYSTEM — Multifocal Hepatic Necrosis Pattern in Captive Avian Species

The Pattern: Multifocal to coalescing hepatic necrosis in captive avian species with variable clinical and histopathologic patterns supporting recognition of specific viral, bacterial, or fungal etiology.

Cross-Taxa Signature: Recognized across captive avian orders with variable etiologic profiles. Psittacid herpesvirus 1 (Pacheco disease) in psittacines. Duck viral hepatitis in Anseriformes. Falconid herpesvirus in Falconiformes. Owl herpesvirus in Strigiformes. Yersinia pseudotuberculosis across captive avian species. Chlamydia psittaci in psittacines and other affected species. Aspergillosis with hepatic involvement.

Diagnostic Anchor: Histopathologic characterization for viral inclusion bodies (herpesvirus intranuclear, adenovirus intranuclear), bacterial organisms (gram-negative rods for Yersinia, characteristic organisms for other bacterial etiologies), or fungal hyphae (Aspergillus dichotomous branching). Molecular characterization confirms specific etiology.

Trap Logic: The look-alike is multifocal necrosis of toxic etiology distinguished by absence of infectious organisms and by history of potential toxicant exposure. Another look-alike is postmortem autolytic pallor discriminated by symmetric distribution and absent inflammatory response.

Zoonotic/Reportable Flag: Chlamydia psittaci is zoonotic. Some bacterial etiologies carry occupational health implications. Yersinia species carry variable zoonotic potential. Recognition triggers appropriate biosafety and reporting response.

Ratite Pathology

Ostrich, Emu, Cassowary, and Rhea Pathology

Ratite pathology in captive populations includes various infectious disease patterns, degenerative conditions, and species-specific entities documented across captive collections. Mycobacterial disease has been documented in captive ratites. Salmonella species produce enteric disease. Various parasitic infections including nematode disease produce documented pathology. Traumatic injury including limb fractures produces substantial documented mortality in captive ratites given the species biology and management challenges. Recognition of ratite disease patterns supports collection-level management of these captive species.

Emerging Avian Disease Surveillance

Ongoing HPAI Surveillance

Ongoing HPAI surveillance across captive and wild avian populations is addressed in Chapter 13 with detailed protocols. Continued vigilance for HPAI cases and coordinated reporting through USDA APHIS and state animal health authorities remains a critical component of avian pathology practice.

Emerging Pathogen Recognition

Emerging pathogen recognition in avian populations continues through ongoing molecular characterization and coordinated surveillance. Recent decades have seen recognition of numerous novel avian pathogens with variable clinical significance. Wildlife pathology contributions through case-by-case recognition and coordinated surveillance support the ongoing characterization of emerging avian disease.

Applied Case: House Finch Mycoplasma Gallisepticum Outbreak

The historical emergence of Mycoplasma gallisepticum in wild house finch populations in eastern North America during the mid-1990s represented a well-documented example of emerging wildlife disease recognition. Substantial population impact occurred with characteristic conjunctivitis and associated debilitation. Coordinated surveillance response through state and federal wildlife health authorities characterized the disease dynamics and contributed to broader understanding of wildlife infectious disease emergence. The case series continues to inform wildlife pathology practice and represents a template for coordinated response to emerging avian disease. Recognition of similar patterns in subsequent decades has continued to support wildlife health surveillance across affected populations.

THE COMPARATIVE NECROPSY PATTERN SYSTEM — Chapter 23 Avian Pattern Foundations

---

Multifocal Hepatic Necrosis Pattern in Captive Avian Species: Multifocal hepatic necrosis across captive avian orders with variable viral, bacterial, or fungal etiologies. Anchor: histopathologic characterization for inclusion bodies or organisms with molecular confirmation. Trap: toxic etiology and postmortem autolysis discriminated by absence of infectious organisms and inflammatory response. Flag: Chlamydia psittaci zoonotic and other bacterial etiologies carry occupational health implications.

Summary and Key Concepts

Psittaciformes pathology includes substantial documented disease across species with beak and feather disease virus, Pacheco disease, aspergillosis, atherosclerosis, and various other patterns.

Passeriformes pathology includes West Nile virus, Mycoplasma gallisepticum in wild house finches, trichomoniasis, and various infectious disease entities.

Anseriformes pathology includes HPAI with substantial current impact, avian cholera, duck plague, botulism, lead toxicosis, and various other patterns.

Falconiformes and other raptor pathology includes aspergillosis in rehabilitation facilities, West Nile virus, lead and anticoagulant toxicosis, and traumatic injury.

Ratite pathology in captive ostrich, emu, cassowary, and rhea populations includes various infectious disease and traumatic injury patterns.

Emerging avian disease surveillance including ongoing HPAI response supports both individual case management and broader avian conservation surveillance.

CHAPTER 24: REPTILE AND AMPHIBIAN PATHOLOGY

Learning Objectives

1. Recognize chelonian pathology patterns including chelonian herpesvirus, ranavirus, and mycobacterial disease.
2. Identify squamate pathology patterns including inclusion body disease, snake fungal disease, and various infectious entities.
3. Interpret anuran and caudate amphibian pathology including chytridiomycosis and ranavirus.
4. Recognize crocodilian pathology patterns in captive and wild populations.
5. Apply the Comparative Necropsy Pattern callout structure to reptile and amphibian disease recognition.
6. Coordinate with appropriate authorities for reportable reptile and amphibian disease.

Reptile and amphibian pathology represents a specialized area of wildlife pathology practice with substantial disease burden across captive and free-ranging populations and, in some cases, catastrophic conservation implications. Amphibian populations globally have experienced substantial declines with chytridiomycosis (Chapter 15) as a leading factor and ranavirus contributing to the disease burden. Reptile populations face substantial anthropogenic pressures including habitat loss, illegal trade, and emerging infectious diseases including snake fungal disease. The pathologist working reptile and amphibian cases contributes to individual case management, coordinated conservation surveillance for affected populations, and characterization of the ongoing disease dynamics. The chapter addresses the major taxonomic groups and their characteristic disease patterns.

The chapter organizes reptile and amphibian pathology into four operational domains addressing chelonians, squamates, anurans and caudates, and crocodilians. Each grouping demonstrates characteristic disease patterns supporting recognition across the taxonomic diversity encountered in wildlife pathology practice.

Chelonian Pathology

Chelonian Herpesvirus and Ranavirus

Chelonian herpesvirus 1 and 3 produce stomatitis-rhinitis-conjunctivitis syndrome and systemic disease across affected captive and free-ranging chelonian species. Ranavirus disease (Chapter 15) produces characteristic multifocal necrosis with intracytoplasmic viral inclusion bodies across chelonian species. Fibropapillomatosis in green sea turtles caused by chelonid herpesvirus 5 has substantial documented population impact with characteristic proliferative dermatologic lesions.

Chelonian Mycobacterial and Bacterial Disease

Chelonian mycobacterial disease (Chapter 3, Chapter 14) produces characteristic granulomatous disease with substantial biosafety implications. Various bacterial pathogens including Salmonella species contribute to chelonian disease burden with substantial zoonotic implications.

Marine Turtle Pathology

Marine turtle pathology includes marine debris ingestion (Chapter 8) with substantial documented mortality across species, fibropapillomatosis with viral etiology, and various infectious and non-infectious disease patterns. Federal protection of marine turtle species supports coordinated response through NOAA Fisheries.

Squamate Pathology

Inclusion Body Disease and Reptarenavirus

Inclusion body disease in captive Boidae caused by reptarenaviruses produces characteristic clinical and pathologic patterns including intracytoplasmic eosinophilic inclusion bodies in various tissues, neurologic clinical signs, and, in advanced cases, mortality. The disease has substantial impact on captive python and boa collections with ongoing coordinated response including antemortem screening and biosecurity protocols.

Snake Fungal Disease

Snake fungal disease caused by Ophidiomyces ophiodiicola (Chapter 10, Chapter 15) produces characteristic dermatologic disease in captive and free-ranging snakes with expanding geographic distribution. Recognition supports collection biosecurity and coordinated conservation response for affected wild populations.

Squamate Neoplasia and Infectious Disease

Squamate neoplasia includes various tumor entities documented in captive collections with age-related distribution. Infectious disease including bacterial, viral, and parasitic disease produces documented squamate mortality with variable species-specific patterns.

Anuran and Caudate Amphibian Pathology

Chytridiomycosis

Chytridiomycosis caused by Batrachochytrium dendrobatidis and B. salamandrivorans (Chapter 15) produces catastrophic amphibian population impact with substantial coordinated conservation response including active biosecurity to prevent further pathogen spread and captive assurance colony maintenance for particularly vulnerable species.

Amphibian Ranavirus

Amphibian ranavirus disease (Chapter 2, Chapter 15) produces characteristic multifocal necrosis and cutaneous ulceration across affected species with substantial documented mortality events.

Other Amphibian Disease

Other amphibian disease includes various bacterial infections including Aeromonas species-associated red leg syndrome, parasitic infections, environmental contaminant exposure, and various species-specific patterns. Amphibian population health is a substantial conservation concern requiring coordinated pathology contributions.

THE COMPARATIVE NECROPSY PATTERN SYSTEM — Ranavirus Pattern Across Ectothermic Vertebrates

---

The Pattern: Multifocal hepatic and splenic necrosis with intracytoplasmic viral inclusion bodies across chelonian and anuran species indicating ranavirus disease with substantial conservation implications.

Cross-Taxa Signature: Recognized across chelonian species (Frog virus 3-like ranavirus), anuran species (Frog virus 3), caudate species (Frog virus 3, Ambystoma tigrinum virus), and, in some cases, fish species (Santee-Cooper ranavirus, epizootic hematopoietic necrosis virus). The pattern crosses ectothermic vertebrate classes in a way few other agents do.

Diagnostic Anchor: Polymerase chain reaction targeting ranavirus major capsid protein gene confirms the agent. Histopathologic identification of intracytoplasmic basophilic viral inclusions with hepatic and splenic necrosis.

Trap Logic: Chelonian herpesvirus 3 discriminated by intranuclear inclusions. Chytridiomycosis in amphibians discriminated by fungal thalli in epidermis.

Zoonotic/Reportable Flag: Ranavirus is a WOAH-notifiable disease of amphibians. Not zoonotic. Detection triggers reporting through state wildlife health veterinarian and USDA APHIS with coordinated conservation response.

Crocodilian Pathology

Crocodilian Disease Patterns

Crocodilian disease patterns in captive and wild populations include various infectious disease entities, traumatic injury, and species-specific conditions. West Nile virus disease has been documented in captive crocodilians with substantial documented outbreak events. Various bacterial pathogens contribute to crocodilian disease burden. Traumatic injury including fighting-related trauma and captive-related injury produces documented mortality. Coordinated response for crocodilian cases follows appropriate authorities depending on the specific context.

Ranavirus Pattern Across Ectothermic Vertebrates: Multifocal hepatic and splenic necrosis with intracytoplasmic viral inclusions across chelonians, anurans, caudates, and some fish. Anchor: PCR for ranavirus major capsid protein gene. Trap: chelonian herpesvirus discriminated by intranuclear inclusions; chytridiomycosis discriminated by fungal thalli. Flag: WOAH-notifiable with coordinated conservation response.

Summary and Key Concepts

Chelonian pathology includes herpesvirus and ranavirus disease, mycobacterial and bacterial disease, and marine turtle-specific disease including marine debris ingestion and fibropapillomatosis.

Squamate pathology includes inclusion body disease in captive Boidae, snake fungal disease in captive and free-ranging snakes, and various infectious and neoplastic disease.

Anuran and caudate amphibian pathology is dominated by chytridiomycosis and ranavirus with catastrophic population implications and substantial coordinated conservation response.

Crocodilian pathology includes West Nile virus disease with documented captive outbreaks, various infectious disease, and traumatic injury.

Reptile and amphibian pathology contributions support both individual case management and coordinated conservation surveillance for affected populations.

Emerging disease recognition including snake fungal disease and continued ranavirus surveillance remains critical for reptile and amphibian conservation practice.

CHAPTER 25: FISH AND AQUATIC INVERTEBRATE PATHOLOGY

Learning Objectives

1. Recognize teleost pathology patterns in aquarium and free-ranging populations.
2. Identify elasmobranch pathology patterns in captive collections.
3. Interpret coral, cephalopod, and aquatic invertebrate pathology with attention to species-specific patterns.
4. Apply the Comparative Necropsy Pattern callout structure to fish and aquatic invertebrate disease recognition.
5. Coordinate ancillary fish and aquatic invertebrate diagnostics including species-appropriate pathogen panels.
6. Contribute to broader aquatic animal health surveillance.

Fish and aquatic invertebrate pathology represents a growing area of wildlife pathology practice reflecting the substantial captive aquarium collections at zoological institutions, expanding recognition of aquatic disease dynamics, and coordinated response to aquatic disease outbreaks affecting wild populations. The pathologist working aquatic cases requires specialized technique and knowledge of the diverse taxonomic groups encountered including teleosts, elasmobranchs, corals, cephalopods, and various other invertebrates. The chapter addresses the major groups and their characteristic disease patterns.

The chapter organizes fish and aquatic invertebrate pathology into three operational domains. Teleost pathology addresses the range of infectious and non-infectious disease documented in captive and wild teleost populations. Elasmobranch pathology covers the captive shark and ray populations. Coral, cephalopod, and aquatic invertebrate pathology completes the chapter with attention to the specialized taxonomic groups.

Teleost Pathology in Aquarium and Free-Ranging Populations

Teleost Infectious Disease

Teleost infectious disease includes various viral pathogens including infectious salmon anemia virus, viral hemorrhagic septicemia virus, and various other viral entities with characteristic patterns; bacterial pathogens including Mycobacterium species (Chapter 14), Aeromonas species, and various other bacterial entities; fungal pathogens; and parasitic entities including monogenean gill parasites, protozoal ectoparasites, and various endoparasites. Coordinated surveillance for World Organisation for Animal Health-notifiable fish diseases supports both individual case management and broader aquatic animal health protection.

Teleost Non-Infectious Disease

Teleost non-infectious disease includes environmental disease from water quality inadequacies, nutritional disease with species-specific requirements, neoplasia in aged captive individuals, and traumatic injury. Water quality-associated disease including ammonia toxicity, chlorine toxicity, and low dissolved oxygen produces characteristic patterns. Nutritional disease including specific vitamin and mineral requirements produces species-specific patterns.

Gill Pathology Recognition

Gill pathology recognition (Chapter 2) supports interpretation of teleost disease through characteristic patterns including lamellar hyperplasia, clubbing, and necrosis with distribution informing the specific etiology. Wet-mount microscopy of gill filaments before formalin fixation identifies specific parasitic agents. Histopathology confirms specific lesion patterns.

THE COMPARATIVE NECROPSY PATTERN SYSTEM — Mycobacterial Disease Pattern in Captive Teleosts

The Pattern: Chronic disease in captive teleost with characteristic granulomatous pathology across multiple organs and acid-fast bacilli identifiable on histopathology indicating mycobacterial disease (typically Mycobacterium marinum or related species).

Cross-Taxa Signature: Recognized across captive teleost species with recognized predispositions in various species. The disease is particularly prominent in some aquarium collections with documented outbreaks. Wild fish populations may harbor the pathogen with variable clinical significance.

Diagnostic Anchor: Histopathologic identification of granulomatous inflammation with acid-fast bacilli confirmed by Ziehl-Neelsen staining. Mycobacterial culture with species identification provides definitive characterization.

Trap Logic: Other granulomatous disease including fungal or foreign body granulomas discriminated by fungal stains and appropriate characterization.

Zoonotic/Reportable Flag: Mycobacterium marinum is zoonotic with occupational exposure risk in aquarium personnel including characteristic cutaneous fish tank granuloma disease. Recognition supports occupational health awareness for exposed personnel.

Elasmobranch Pathology

Elasmobranch Infectious and Non-Infectious Disease

Elasmobranch pathology in captive shark and ray collections includes various infectious disease entities, degenerative conditions, and species-specific patterns. Ancillary workup requires specialized approach reflecting the cartilaginous anatomy and unique physiology of the group. Necropsy technique for elasmobranchs (Chapter 2) requires specialized approach including spiral valve intestine examination and cartilaginous vertebrae assessment.

Elasmobranch Reproductive Disease

Elasmobranch reproductive disease includes various patterns documented in captive collections with implications for captive breeding programs. Egg case disease, dystocia in oviparous and viviparous species, and various other patterns require appropriate recognition.

Coral, Cephalopod, and Aquatic Invertebrate Pathology

Coral Disease

Coral disease affects captive coral collections and wild reef populations with substantial documented mortality events. Various coral disease entities have been characterized including bleaching-associated disease, black band disease, and various other patterns. Recognition requires specialized approach with whole-animal fixation and cross-sectional examination. Wildlife pathology contributions to coral disease surveillance support broader reef ecosystem health monitoring.

Cephalopod Pathology

Cephalopod pathology in captive octopus and cuttlefish collections includes various infectious and non-infectious disease patterns. Cephalopod necropsy technique (Chapter 2) requires specific approach including mantle cavity, gill, and heart complex examination. Various infectious disease entities have been documented with characterization ongoing.

Other Aquatic Invertebrate Disease

Other aquatic invertebrate disease including crustacean disease, echinoderm disease, and various other invertebrate patterns contributes to the broader aquatic disease landscape. Recognition supports individual case management and broader aquatic ecosystem surveillance.

THE COMPARATIVE NECROPSY PATTERN SYSTEM — Chapter 25 Fish and Aquatic Invertebrate Pattern Foundations

---

Mycobacterial Disease Pattern in Captive Teleosts: Chronic granulomatous disease across multiple organs in captive teleosts with acid-fast bacilli. Anchor: histopathology with Ziehl-Neelsen staining and mycobacterial culture. Trap: other granulomatous disease discriminated by appropriate stains. Flag: Mycobacterium marinum zoonotic with occupational exposure risk.

Summary and Key Concepts

Teleost pathology in aquarium and free-ranging populations includes various infectious, non-infectious, and neoplastic disease with specialized recognition patterns.

Elasmobranch pathology in captive shark and ray collections requires specialized approach reflecting cartilaginous anatomy and unique physiology.

Coral disease affects captive and wild reef populations with substantial documented mortality and coordinated surveillance response.

Cephalopod pathology in captive octopus and cuttlefish collections requires specialized necropsy technique and characterization.

Fish and aquatic invertebrate pathology contributions support both individual case management and broader aquatic ecosystem health surveillance.

Mycobacterial disease in captive teleosts represents a substantial concern with recognized zoonotic implications for aquarium personnel.

CHAPTER 26: EMERGING DISEASES AND ONE-HEALTH INTERFACE PATHOLOGY

Learning Objectives

1. Recognize emerging disease detection patterns and coordinated surveillance response.
2. Identify one-health cross-species transmission events with attention to zoonotic implications.
3. Interpret climate-driven disease range expansion patterns.
4. Recognize wildlife pathology and public health reporting responsibilities.
5. Apply the Comparative Necropsy Pattern callout structure to emerging disease recognition.
6. Coordinate with One Health surveillance frameworks integrating wildlife, domestic animal, and human health.

Emerging diseases and the one-health interface pathology represent an increasingly prominent area of wildlife pathology practice reflecting the recognition that wildlife health, domestic animal health, and human health are fundamentally interconnected. Recent decades have seen substantial emerging infectious disease recognition including HPAI H5N1 mammalian spillover (Chapter 13), SARS-CoV-2 in various wildlife species, monkeypox in captive nonhuman primates, and various other emerging pathogens with wildlife components. Wildlife pathology contributions to emerging disease recognition support both individual case management and broader public health surveillance. The chapter addresses the framework for emerging disease recognition and the coordinated response required for cases at the human-wildlife interface.

The chapter organizes emerging disease and one-health pathology into four operational domains. Emerging disease detection and surveillance addresses the framework for recognizing new disease entities. One-health cross-species transmission events covers the specific cross-species transmission recognition. Climate-driven disease range expansion addresses the growing recognition of climate change impacts on disease distribution. Wildlife pathology and public health reporting completes the chapter with attention to the coordinated reporting frameworks.

Emerging Disease Detection and Surveillance

Molecular Approaches to Emerging Disease Recognition

Molecular approaches to emerging disease recognition including metagenomic next-generation sequencing, consensus polymerase chain reaction for pathogen families, and coordinated surveillance datasets support ongoing recognition of novel pathogens in wildlife populations. The past two decades have seen substantial expansion in emerging pathogen identification with substantial implications for both wildlife and human health. Recognition of novel pathogens through molecular characterization complements traditional pathology approaches supporting comprehensive characterization of emerging disease.

Coordinated Surveillance Networks

Coordinated surveillance networks including the USGS National Wildlife Health Center, state wildlife health programs, coordinated marine mammal stranding networks, and various species-specific surveillance programs support ongoing emerging disease detection. Wildlife pathology case-by-case contributions to these networks support both individual case management and broader surveillance datasets. Integration with domestic animal and human health surveillance provides the One Health framework for comprehensive disease surveillance.

Applied Case: SARS-CoV-2 in White-Tailed Deer Surveillance

The recognition of SARS-CoV-2 infection in white-tailed deer populations across North America during 2020-2022 represented a substantial emerging disease event with implications for both wildlife health and pandemic response. Coordinated surveillance response through USDA APHIS Wildlife Services, state wildlife agencies, and academic partners characterized the distribution and dynamics of infection. Wildlife pathology contributions supported characterization of individual case implications and broader population-level dynamics. The case series continues to inform understanding of the SARS-CoV-2-wildlife interface and represents a template for coordinated response to emerging pathogen recognition in wildlife populations. Ongoing surveillance supports characterization of continued viral dynamics in wildlife populations.

One-Health Cross-Species Transmission Events

Zoonotic Disease Recognition

Zoonotic disease recognition across wildlife populations supports both individual case management and broader public health surveillance. Recognition of specific zoonotic pathogens including HPAI (Chapter 13), rabies, hantavirus, and various other zoonotic entities in wildlife supports appropriate biosafety and public health response. The One Health framework integrates wildlife, domestic animal, and human health surveillance supporting comprehensive characterization of zoonotic disease dynamics.

Wildlife-Livestock Interface Disease

Wildlife-livestock interface disease including bovine tuberculosis in wild cervids, brucellosis at the Yellowstone ecosystem interface, and various other interface diseases requires coordinated response between wildlife and agricultural authorities. Wildlife pathology contributions support both wildlife management and agricultural disease control. Recognition of specific interface disease patterns supports appropriate management response.

Wildlife-Human Interface Disease

Wildlife-human interface disease including specific occupational exposure risks (marine mammal Brucella, elephant tuberculosis, HPAI, various others) requires appropriate occupational health response for exposed personnel. Recognition supports appropriate personnel protection and public health follow-up when warranted.

THE COMPARATIVE NECROPSY PATTERN SYSTEM — Emerging Disease Recognition Pattern in Wildlife Pathology Practice

The Pattern: Recognition of unusual pathology pattern, unusual mortality event, or characterized novel pathogen infection in wildlife species triggering coordinated surveillance response and characterization.

Cross-Taxa Signature: Recognized across wildlife species with variable presentations. Recent decades have seen HPAI mammalian spillover, SARS-CoV-2 in various species, chronic wasting disease geographic expansion, chytridiomycosis, white-nose syndrome, and various other emerging disease recognition events.

Diagnostic Anchor: Systematic characterization including gross pathology, histopathology, and molecular characterization with metagenomic approaches for novel pathogen identification. Coordinated reporting through appropriate surveillance networks supports broader characterization.

Trap Logic: Distinguishing emerging pathogen recognition from incidental molecular findings requires integration of pathology with molecular characterization and appropriate case-control comparisons.

Zoonotic/Reportable Flag: Emerging disease recognition triggers appropriate coordinated response with state and federal wildlife health authorities, USDA APHIS for animal health implications, and public health authorities for human health implications. Biosafety escalation for suspect emerging pathogens precedes continued tissue handling.

Climate-Driven Disease Range Expansion

Vector-Borne Disease Range Expansion

Vector-borne disease range expansion associated with climate change has been documented across various pathogen-vector-host systems. Tick-borne disease including Lyme disease and various other tick-borne pathogens has demonstrated documented geographic range expansion. Mosquito-borne disease including West Nile virus and various arboviral diseases has demonstrated range expansion. Wildlife pathology contributions to characterizing these range expansions support both individual case interpretation and broader climate-disease surveillance.

Marine Disease Range Expansion

Marine disease range expansion including harmful algal bloom expansion and various marine pathogen range shifts has been documented with implications for marine wildlife populations. Wildlife pathology contributions support characterization of these dynamics.

Temperature-Sensitive Disease Recognition

Temperature-sensitive disease including chytridiomycosis dynamics associated with temperature ranges and various other temperature-sensitive disease patterns require ongoing recognition supporting characterization of climate-disease interactions.

Wildlife Pathology and Public Health Reporting

Coordinated Reporting Frameworks

Coordinated reporting frameworks including USDA APHIS reportable disease frameworks, state animal health authority reporting, NOAA Fisheries marine mammal reporting, US Fish and Wildlife Service coordination for federally protected species, and public health authority coordination for zoonotic disease support comprehensive wildlife disease reporting. Wildlife pathology contributions to these frameworks support both individual case management and broader surveillance.

Wildlife Pathology in the One Health Framework

Wildlife pathology in the One Health framework provides the wildlife health surveillance component of the integrated wildlife-domestic animal-human health surveillance approach. Coordinated response to emerging disease and cross-species transmission events requires integration of wildlife pathology contributions with domestic animal veterinary practice and human public health response. The pathologist's contribution to individual case recognition supports the broader coordinated response framework.

The Ongoing Contribution of Wildlife Pathology

The ongoing contribution of wildlife pathology to emerging disease recognition, one-health surveillance, and public health protection represents a substantial component of the discipline's professional role. Individual case-by-case recognition combined with coordinated surveillance response supports both individual animal welfare and broader public and animal health protection. The chapter closes the book with recognition of this substantial ongoing contribution and the ongoing need for coordinated wildlife pathology practice at the increasingly recognized interfaces of wildlife, domestic animal, and human health.

THE COMPARATIVE NECROPSY PATTERN SYSTEM — Chapter 26 Emerging Disease and One Health Pattern Foundations

---

Emerging Disease Recognition Pattern in Wildlife Pathology Practice: Systematic characterization of unusual pathology, mortality events, or novel pathogen infection with coordinated surveillance response. Anchor: comprehensive characterization with molecular approaches and coordinated reporting. Trap: incidental molecular findings distinguished from causative disease. Flag: coordinated response with wildlife, animal health, and public health authorities.

Summary and Key Concepts

Emerging disease detection through molecular approaches and coordinated surveillance networks supports ongoing recognition of novel pathogens in wildlife populations.

One-health cross-species transmission events including zoonotic disease, wildlife-livestock interface disease, and wildlife-human interface disease require coordinated response across affected sectors.

Climate-driven disease range expansion including vector-borne disease, marine disease, and temperature-sensitive disease represents a growing area of surveillance requirement.

Coordinated reporting frameworks integrate USDA APHIS, state animal health authorities, NOAA Fisheries, US Fish and Wildlife Service, and public health authorities in comprehensive wildlife disease surveillance.

Wildlife pathology in the One Health framework provides the wildlife health surveillance component of integrated wildlife-domestic animal-human health surveillance.

The ongoing contribution of wildlife pathology to emerging disease recognition and coordinated response represents a substantial component of the discipline's professional role at the increasingly recognized human-wildlife-domestic animal interface.

THE COMPARATIVE NECROPSY PATTERN MASTER ATLAS

The Comparative Necropsy Pattern Master Atlas consolidates every Comparative Necropsy Pattern introduced across the chapters into a structured indexed reference organized by lesion type and by taxonomic group. Each entry carries the Pattern name, Cross-Taxa Signature summary, Diagnostic Anchor, Trap Logic key, and Zoonotic/Reportable status. The Atlas is designed for use at the cutting board or before signout as a rapid reference for cross-taxa pattern recognition. Chapter cross-references support return to the parent chapter for detailed mechanism and evidence.

Master Index by Lesion Type

Hepatic Patterns

Cross-Taxa Hepatic Necrosis of Herpesviral Origin — Multifocal necrosis with Cowdry type A intranuclear inclusions across nonhuman primates (herpes B, callitrichid herpesvirus), elephants (elephant endotheliotropic herpesvirus), captive psittacines (psittacid herpesvirus 1), and other affected taxa. Diagnostic Anchor: intranuclear inclusion body morphology with immunohistochemistry or PCR. Trap: bacterial hepatic necrosis discriminated by neutrophil-rich exudate and gram-stainable organisms. Zoonotic/Reportable: herpes B in macaques is a hard-stop biosafety concern. Chapter 1, Chapter 6, Chapter 12.

Multifocal Random Hepatic Necrosis Signaling Systemic Infectious Disease — Discrete random hepatic necrotic foci indicating hematogenous infectious agent across mammalian, avian, and reptile taxa. Diagnostic Anchor: histopathologic characterization for inclusions with agent-specific molecular workup. Trap: bacterial hepatic necrosis discriminated by response pattern. Zoonotic/Reportable: variable by specific etiology. Chapter 6.

Multifocal Hepatic and Splenic Necrosis Signaling Yersinia Disease — Necrotic foci with gram-negative bacterial rods across captive birds, primates, and mammals. Diagnostic Anchor: culture with species identification. Trap: herpesvirus disease discriminated by inclusion bodies. Zoonotic/Reportable: Yersinia pestis is a select agent. Chapter 14.

Multifocal Hepatic and Splenic Necrosis Signaling HPAI Mammalian Spillover — Systemic hemorrhagic pattern with meningoencephalitis in HPAI-exposed mammals. Diagnostic Anchor: influenza A PCR with H5 subtyping. Trap: bacterial septicemia discriminated by absent encephalitis. Zoonotic/Reportable: federally reportable with public health implications. Chapter 1, Chapter 13.

Fixation-Artifact Pattern Masking Multifocal Necrosis — Central autolytic change mimicking multifocal necrosis. Diagnostic Anchor: recognition of pattern with fixation history review. Trap: true multifocal necrosis discriminated by variable focus size and inflammatory response. Zoonotic/Reportable: not itself infectious. Chapter 3.

Iron Storage and Metabolic Patterns

Hepatic Hemosiderosis Across Frugivorous Primates and Perissodactyls / Dietary Iron Storage Disease — Periportal-to-midlobular hepatocyte cytoplasmic hemosiderin across lemurs, marmosets, black rhinoceros, tapirs, frugivorous bats. Diagnostic Anchor: Prussian blue confirmation with quantitative iron measurement. Trap: hemolytic hemosiderosis discriminated by Kupffer cell dominance. Zoonotic/Reportable: institutionally reportable at SSP facilities. Chapter 1, Chapter 6.

Cachexia With Serous Fat Atrophy Across Free-Ranging Ungulates — Gelatinous adipose atrophy across cervids, bovids, suids, camelids. Diagnostic Anchor: pericardial adipose gelatinous transition. Trap: postmortem autolytic softening discriminated by symmetry. Zoonotic/Reportable: CWD and mycobacterial disease reportable. Chapter 1.

Nutritional Secondary Hyperparathyroidism — Rubber jaw and skeletal deformity in captive juvenile reptiles, birds, and mammals from dietary calcium-phosphorus imbalance. Diagnostic Anchor: histopathology demonstrating fibrous osteodystrophy. Trap: rickets discriminated by growth plate architecture. Zoonotic/Reportable: institutionally reportable for dietary review. Chapter 10, Chapter 18.

Cardiovascular Patterns

Ventricular Wall Thickness Recognition Across Endothermic and Ectothermic Taxa — Species-appropriate anatomic reference before pathologic interpretation. Diagnostic Anchor: comparative anatomic reference. Trap: normal species-specific variation misread as pathology. Zoonotic/Reportable: not applicable. Chapter 4.

Dilated Cardiomyopathy Pattern Across Nonhuman Primates and Captive Felids — Globoid, flabby heart with thinned walls across taxa. Diagnostic Anchor: myocardial fiber attenuation with preserved valvular architecture. Trap: volume overload from valvular disease. Zoonotic/Reportable: institutionally reportable at SSP facilities. Chapter 4.

Vascular Mineralization Pattern in Captive Psittacines and Aged Non-Domestic Mammals — Gritty mineralization within vessel walls with medial concentric distribution. Diagnostic Anchor: histopathology with von Kossa. Trap: postmortem mineralization artifact. Zoonotic/Reportable: institutionally reportable at SSP psittacine facilities. Chapter 4.

Fibrinous Pericardial Effusion Pattern Signaling Septic Pericarditis — Fibrinous exudate with pericardial thickening across mammals, birds, and reptiles. Diagnostic Anchor: cytology with culture. Trap: hemorrhagic effusion from trauma or hemangiosarcoma. Zoonotic/Reportable: chlamydial or mycobacterial etiology triggers biosafety response. Chapter 4.

Respiratory Patterns

Faveolar Lung Consolidation Pattern in Reptiles Versus Alveolar Consolidation in Mammals — Firm mucoid consolidation in reptile faveolar lungs versus mammalian hepatization. Diagnostic Anchor:

species-appropriate architectural reference. Trap: normal faveolar architecture misread as consolidation. Zoonotic/Reportable: reptile mycobacterial and Salmonella pneumonias carry biosafety implications. Chapter 5.

Cross-Taxa Bronchopneumonia Pattern Signaling Bacterial Pneumonia — Cranioventral airway-centered consolidation across taxa. Diagnostic Anchor: culture of fresh lung tissue. Trap: aspiration pneumonia discriminated by foreign body reaction. Zoonotic/Reportable: variable by specific etiology. Chapter 5.

Air Sacculitis Pattern in Avian Necropsy Across Orders — Air sac thickening on in-situ examination before organ displacement. Diagnostic Anchor: air sac sampling before coelomic disruption. Trap: postmortem air sac desiccation. Zoonotic/Reportable: HPAI and mycobacterial etiologies trigger biosafety escalation. Chapter 2.

Pulmonary Mineralization Pattern in Captive Psittacines — Multifocal firm mineralized foci with dietary imbalance. Diagnostic Anchor: histopathology with von Kossa. Trap: granulomatous mineralization discriminated by architecture. Zoonotic/Reportable: institutionally reportable for dietary intervention. Chapter 5.

Aspiration Pattern Recognition Across Taxa — Cranioventral consolidation with foreign material and giant cells. Diagnostic Anchor: identifiable foreign material or foreign body reaction. Trap: primary bacterial pneumonia discriminated by absent foreign material. Zoonotic/Reportable: oil-spill aspiration in federally protected species requires regulatory coordination. Chapter 5.

Aspergillosis Pattern in Captive Avian Species — Pulmonary and air sac nodules with dichotomously branching hyphae. Diagnostic Anchor: histopathology with GMS and culture. Trap: other fungal disease discriminated by morphology. Zoonotic/Reportable: institutionally reportable for husbandry review. Chapter 15.

Renal and Urinary Patterns

Reniculate Kidney Architecture Recognition in Marine Mammal Necropsy — Multi-lobar reniculate architecture in cetaceans and pinnipeds as normal anatomy. Diagnostic Anchor: anatomic reference. Trap: normal architecture misread as pathology. Zoonotic/Reportable: not applicable. Chapter 7.

Ethylene Glycol Toxicosis Pattern Across Wildlife Carnivores — Renal tubular calcium oxalate crystals. Diagnostic Anchor: birefringent crystals with ethylene glycol quantitation. Trap: dietary oxalate nephropathy. Zoonotic/Reportable: environmental antifreeze source warrants mitigation. Chapter 7.

Visceral Gout Pattern in Captive Birds and Reptiles — Chalky urate deposition on coelomic serosal surfaces. Diagnostic Anchor: gross recognition with histopathology and foreign body giant cell response. Trap: postmortem urate artifact discriminated by absent inflammatory response. Zoonotic/Reportable: institutionally reportable for husbandry review. Chapter 7.

Gastrointestinal Patterns

Compartmentalized Stomach Anatomy Recognition in Ruminants, Camelids, and Cetaceans — Species-specific compartment identification prerequisite to interpretation. Diagnostic Anchor: anatomic reference. Trap: compartment misidentification. Zoonotic/Reportable: not applicable. Chapter 8.

Systemic Salmonellosis Pattern in Wild Ruminants and Captive Reptiles — Enterocolitis with systemic granulomatous lesions with species-specific clinical significance. Diagnostic Anchor: culture with lesion confirmation. Trap: commensal reptile carriage. Zoonotic/Reportable: zoonotic across all taxa. Chapter 8.

Marine Debris Ingestion Pattern in Marine Turtles and Marine Birds — Retained anthropogenic material with mucosal injury. Diagnostic Anchor: material identification with antemortem injury correlation. Trap: incidental postmortem transit. Zoonotic/Reportable: federally protected species require regulatory coordination. Chapter 8.

Gastric Adenocarcinoma Pattern in Aged Captive Nonhuman Primates — Gastric mass with transmural involvement and metastasis in aged lemurs and great apes. Diagnostic Anchor: histopathologic characterization. Trap: non-neoplastic gastric ulceration. Zoonotic/Reportable: institutionally reportable at SSP facilities. Chapter 8.

Neurologic Patterns

Meningoencephalitis Pattern Recognition Across Mammalian and Avian Taxa — Meningeal and parenchymal inflammatory infiltrate across taxa. Diagnostic Anchor: histopathology with molecular pathogen panels. Trap: agonal meningeal congestion. Zoonotic/Reportable: rabies and arboviral encephalitides carry public health obligations. Chapter 9.

Chronic Wasting Disease Pattern in Free-Ranging and Captive Cervids — Cervid carcass with progressive neurologic decline requiring prion testing. Diagnostic Anchor: immunohistochemistry or ELISA on obex and retropharyngeal lymph node. Trap: other chronic weight loss diseases. Zoonotic/Reportable: federally reportable through USDA APHIS. Chapter 9, Chapter 17.

West Nile Virus Encephalitis Pattern in Corvids and Raptors — Nonsuppurative meningoencephalitis with brainstem involvement. Diagnostic Anchor: PCR with immunohistochemistry. Trap: EEE virus discriminated by molecular characterization. Zoonotic/Reportable: zoonotic contributing to public health surveillance. Chapter 9.

Meningoencephalitis Pattern Signaling HPAI Mammalian Spillover — Neurologic disease with organ necrosis in HPAI-exposed mammals. Diagnostic Anchor: influenza A PCR with H5 subtyping. Trap: rabies discriminated by PCR. Zoonotic/Reportable: reportable with public health implications. Chapter 13.

Musculoskeletal, Integumentary, and Ocular Patterns

Chytridiomycosis Pattern in Free-Ranging and Captive Amphibians — Amphibian epidermal thickening with fungal thalli from Batrachochytrium species. Diagnostic Anchor: histopathologic and molecular characterization. Trap: normal breeding-season changes. Zoonotic/Reportable: WOAH-notifiable amphibian disease. Chapter 10, Chapter 15.

Cataract Pattern Across Aged Captive Species — Lens opacification with variable etiologic profiles. Diagnostic Anchor: histopathologic characterization. Trap: postmortem lens changes. Zoonotic/Reportable: population-level clustering may indicate dietary or environmental factors. Chapter 10.

Endocrine, Reproductive, and Hematolymphatic Patterns

Diabetes Mellitus Pattern in Captive Nonhuman Primates and Captive Psittacines — Chronic hyperglycemia with metabolic consequences. Diagnostic Anchor: pancreatic islet histopathology with immunohistochemistry. Trap: stress hyperglycemia. Zoonotic/Reportable: institutionally documented for dietary review. Chapter 11.

Endometrial Hyperplasia and Pyometra Pattern in Captive Nonhuman Primates — Uterine cystic hyperplasia and purulent content with chronic cyclicity. Diagnostic Anchor: gross and histopathologic characterization. Trap: normal luteal phase changes. Zoonotic/Reportable: institutionally reportable for reproductive management. Chapter 11.

Granulomatous Lymphadenitis Pattern Signaling Mycobacterial Disease Across Taxa — Granulomatous lymph nodes with acid-fast bacilli. Diagnostic Anchor: acid-fast staining and mycobacterial culture. Trap: fungal granulomatous disease. Zoonotic/Reportable: TB and bovine TB federally reportable. Chapter 11, Chapter 14.

Infectious Disease Patterns

Beak and Feather Disease Pattern in Captive Psittacines — Feather dystrophy and beak abnormalities from psittacine circovirus. Diagnostic Anchor: PCR for beak and feather disease virus. Trap: polyomavirus infection. Zoonotic/Reportable: institutionally reportable. Chapter 12.

Cetacean Morbillivirus Pattern in Stranded Bottlenose Dolphins — Interstitial pneumonia with syncytia and meningoencephalitis during UME. Diagnostic Anchor: PCR with immunohistochemistry. Trap: Brucella infection. Zoonotic/Reportable: reportable to NOAA Fisheries. Chapter 5, Chapter 12, Chapter 22.

Multifocal Systemic Necrosis Pattern in HPAI-Affected Avian Species — Multifocal necrosis across affected avian species during current panzootic. Diagnostic Anchor: influenza A PCR with H5 subtyping. Trap: Newcastle disease and other viral disease. Zoonotic/Reportable: federally reportable. Chapter 13.

Ranavirus Pattern Across Ectothermic Vertebrates — Multifocal hepatic and splenic necrosis with intracytoplasmic viral inclusions across chelonians, anurans, caudates, and some fish. Diagnostic Anchor: PCR for major capsid protein gene. Trap: chelonian herpesvirus and chytridiomycosis. Zoonotic/Reportable: WOAH-notifiable. Chapter 2, Chapter 12, Chapter 15, Chapter 24.

Bacterial, Fungal, and Parasitic Disease Patterns

Granulomatous Visceral Pattern Signaling Mycobacterial Disease Across Taxa — Multifocal granulomatous lesions with acid-fast bacilli across mammalian, avian, reptile, and fish taxa. Diagnostic Anchor: histopathology with acid-fast staining and culture. Trap: fungal granulomatous disease. Zoonotic/Reportable: TB and bovine TB federally reportable. Chapter 14.

Multifocal Toxoplasma Necrosis Pattern in Captive Marsupials and New World Primates — Multifocal necrosis with tissue cysts and tachyzoites. Diagnostic Anchor: histopathology with immunohistochemistry and PCR. Trap: other systemic protozoal disease. Zoonotic/Reportable: zoonotic. Chapter 16.

Cerebrospinal Parelaphostrongylosis Pattern in Aberrant Cervid Hosts — CNS parasitic tract lesions in moose, elk, and captive artiodactyls. Diagnostic Anchor: histopathology and PCR. Trap: other tissue-migrant nematode disease. Zoonotic/Reportable: institutionally significant. Chapter 16.

Bile Duct Trematode Pattern in Wild Ruminants and Wild Carnivores — Bile duct dilation with recoverable adult flukes. Diagnostic Anchor: parasite recovery with identification. Trap: non-parasitic biliary hyperplasia. Zoonotic/Reportable: fascioliasis has zoonotic potential. Chapter 6.

Diagnostic Process and Recognition Patterns

Multifocal Organ Involvement Recognized During Systematic Necropsy — Concurrent lesions across three or more organs indicating hematogenous or systemic disease. Diagnostic Anchor: explicit noting of multifocal distribution in report. Trap: autolytic pseudo-multifocal pallor. Zoonotic/Reportable: multifocal patterns disproportionately reflect zoonotic agents. Chapter 2.

Fatal Trauma Pattern Recognition in Free-Ranging Mammals — Concurrent skeletal, soft tissue, and organ injury consistent with defined mechanism. Diagnostic Anchor: vital reaction at wound sites. Trap: postmortem scavenger predation. Zoonotic/Reportable: federally protected species require law enforcement notification. Chapter 2, Chapter 21.

Gill Pathology Pattern in Teleost Necropsy Interpretation — Lamellar hyperplasia, clubbing, or necrosis with distribution informing etiology. Diagnostic Anchor: wet-mount microscopy before formalin fixation. Trap: postmortem gill autolysis. Zoonotic/Reportable: several viral gill pathogens WOAH-notifiable. Chapter 2, Chapter 25.

Postmortem Interval Interpretation Across Necropsy Findings — Autolysis progression to date postmortem interval. Diagnostic Anchor: vital reaction at lesion margins. Trap: autolytic mucosal sloughing discriminated from antemortem enteritis. Zoonotic/Reportable: decomposed status does not exclude zoonotic pathogens. Chapter 2.

Systemic Inflammatory Response Pattern on Impression Smear Cytology — Degenerate inflammatory cells indicating systemic inflammation before histopathology. Diagnostic Anchor: same-day cytology directing workup. Trap: postmortem cytologic degeneration. Zoonotic/Reportable: cytologic bacterial rods trigger biosafety escalation. Chapter 3.

Zoonotic-Signature Pattern at Necropsy Case Receipt — Species-and-signal combinations requiring biosafety escalation before necropsy. Diagnostic Anchor: pattern-of-recognition with protocol activation. Trap: case without initial risk signals. Zoonotic/Reportable: hard-stop conditions require reporting to biosafety, animal health, and public health authorities. Chapter 3.

Chain-of-Custody Documentation Pattern for Investigative Wildlife Cases — Standardized documentation trail supporting investigative use. Diagnostic Anchor: documented control at every transfer point. Trap: retrospective chain-of-custody construction. Zoonotic/Reportable: federally protected species require federal law enforcement coordination. Chapter 3, Chapter 21.

Toxicologic and Other Recognition Patterns

Lead Toxicosis Pattern in Waterfowl, Raptors, and Vultures — Poor body condition with renal tubular inclusion bodies. Diagnostic Anchor: lead quantitation in liver, kidney, or bone. Trap: other toxicant exposure. Zoonotic/Reportable: federally protected species require coordinated regulatory reporting. Chapter 19.

Nutritional and Metabolic Disease Pattern Recognition in Captive Populations — Vitamin deficiency, mineral imbalance, storage disease, or lifestyle-related pathology. Diagnostic Anchor: pattern recognition with dietary history. Trap: primary infectious or neoplastic disease with secondary nutritional consequences. Zoonotic/Reportable: institutionally reportable for population-level review. Chapter 18.

Species-Specific Tumor Pattern Recognition in Aged Captive Populations — Recognition of species-specific tumor entities. Diagnostic Anchor: histopathologic characterization with immunohistochemistry. Trap: other tumor entities. Zoonotic/Reportable: institutionally reportable for SSP surveillance. Chapter 20.

Cetacean Stranding Pattern Recognition and Coordinated Response — Systematic assessment with NOAA Fisheries coordinated reporting. Diagnostic Anchor: standardized marine mammal necropsy protocols. Trap: individual stranding versus UME. Zoonotic/Reportable: Brucella zoonotic and UME reporting through NOAA Fisheries. Chapter 22.

Mycobacterial Disease Pattern in Captive Teleosts — Chronic granulomatous disease with acid-fast bacilli. Diagnostic Anchor: histopathology with Ziehl-Neelsen and mycobacterial culture. Trap: other granulomatous disease. Zoonotic/Reportable: Mycobacterium marinum zoonotic. Chapter 25.

Emerging Disease Recognition Pattern in Wildlife Pathology Practice — Recognition of unusual pathology or novel pathogen with coordinated surveillance response. Diagnostic Anchor: comprehensive characterization with molecular approaches. Trap: incidental molecular findings versus causative disease. Zoonotic/Reportable: coordinated response with wildlife, animal health, and public health authorities. Chapter 26.

Master Index by Taxonomic Group

Carnivores

Fatal Trauma Pattern in Free-Ranging Mammals (Ch 2, 21). Ethylene Glycol Toxicosis Pattern (Ch 7). Meningoencephalitis Pattern (Ch 9). Chronic Kidney Disease in Aged Captive Large Felids (Ch 7). Dilated Cardiomyopathy in Captive Felids (Ch 4). Hypertrophic Cardiomyopathy in Captive Felids (Ch 4). Aortic Dissection in Captive Cheetahs (Ch 4). Cheetah AA Amyloidosis (Ch 7). Rabies Pattern in Wild Carnivores (Ch 9). Canine Distemper in Captive Large Felids (Ch 12). HPAI Mammalian Spillover in Wild Carnivores (Ch 13). Meningioma in Aged Captive Grizzly Bear (Ch 9). Sarcoptic Mange Pattern in Wild Vulpine (Ch 10, 16). Lead Toxicosis in Scavenging Carnivores (Ch 19). Anticoagulant Rodenticide Toxicosis in Predators (Ch 3, 19).

Ungulates

Cachexia With Serous Fat Atrophy Across Free-Ranging Ungulates (Ch 1). Chronic Wasting Disease Pattern in Cervids (Ch 9, 17). Bovine Tuberculosis in Wild and Captive Artiodactyls (Ch 14). Brucellosis at Wildlife-Livestock Interface (Ch 14, 26). Bacterial Bronchopneumonia in Captive Giraffe (Ch 5). Elephant Endotheliotropic Herpesvirus in Elephant Calves (Ch 1, 6, 12). Elephant Tuberculosis (Ch 11, 14). Osteochondrosis in Captive Giraffe (Ch 10). Cerebrospinal Parelaphostrongylosis in Aberrant Cervid Hosts (Ch 9, 16). Iron Storage Disease in Captive Black Rhinoceros (Ch 6). Reticulopericarditis in Captive Ruminants (Ch 8).

Primates

Multifocal Hepatic Necrosis of Herpesviral Origin (Herpes B in Macaques, Ch 1, 12). Herpes B Zoonotic Signature Pattern (Ch 3). Gastric Adenocarcinoma in Aged Lemurs and Great Apes (Ch 8). Dilated Cardiomyopathy in Great Apes (Ch 4). Diabetes Mellitus in Captive Nonhuman Primates (Ch 11). Endometrial Hyperplasia and Pyometra in Nonhuman Primates (Ch 11). Uterine Leiomyoma in Aged Great Apes (Ch 11). Adrenal Cortical Adenoma in Aged Macaques (Ch 11). Toxoplasmosis in New World Primates (Ch 16). Mycobacterial Disease in Nonhuman Primates (Ch 14). Hepatic Hemosiderosis in Frugivorous Primates (Ch 1, 6).

Marine Mammals

Cetacean Morbillivirus Pattern in Bottlenose Dolphins (Ch 5, 12, 22). Reniculate Kidney Architecture Recognition (Ch 7). Domoic Acid Toxicosis in California Sea Lions (Ch 9, 19). Cetacean Aspiration in Stranded Dolphins (Ch 5). Brucella ceti in Harbor Porpoise (Ch 14). Phocine Distemper Virus in Pinnipeds

(Ch 12, 22). Marine Mammal Aspergillosis (Ch 15). Marine Mammal Erysipelothrix Disease (Ch 14). HPAI Marine Mammal Spillover in Pinnipeds (Ch 13). Marine Mammal Entanglement (Ch 21, 22). Manatee Cold Stress and Boat Strike (Ch 22). Sea Otter Toxoplasmosis (Ch 16, 22). Cetacean Stranding Coordinated Response (Ch 22).

Small Mammals, Rodents, and Marsupials

Multicentric Lymphoma in Captive Ferrets (Ch 11). Hyperadrenocorticism in Captive Ferrets (Ch 11). Toxoplasmosis in Captive Marsupials (Ch 16). Baylisascaris Zoonotic Recognition (Ch 16). Tyzzer Disease in Various Small Mammals (Ch 14).

Birds

Air Sacculitis Pattern in Avian Necropsy Across Orders (Ch 2). Multifocal Hepatic Necrosis in Captive Avian Species (Ch 12, 23). Pacheco Disease Outbreak in Psittacines (Ch 12). Beak and Feather Disease in Captive Psittacines (Ch 12). Aspergillosis in Captive African Grey Parrots (Ch 5, 15). Pulmonary Mineralization in Captive Psittacines (Ch 5). Vascular Mineralization in Captive Psittacines (Ch 4). Atherosclerosis in Captive Psittacines (Ch 4). Hepatocellular Carcinoma in Aged Amazon Parrots (Ch 6, 20). West Nile Virus in Corvids and Raptors (Ch 9). Avian Cholera in Waterfowl (Ch 14). HPAI Pattern in Affected Avian Species (Ch 13). Lead Toxicosis in Waterfowl and Raptors (Ch 19). Avian Pox in Passerines (Ch 12). Bald Eagle Rodenticide Toxicosis (Ch 3, 19). Bald Eagle Gunshot Investigation (Ch 21). Mycoplasma gallisepticum in House Finches (Ch 23, 26).

Reptiles

Faveolar Lung Consolidation in Reptiles (Ch 5). Ranavirus Pattern in Chelonians and Anurans (Ch 2, 24). Chelonian Necropsy Case (Aldabra Tortoise) with Mycobacterial Disease (Ch 1). Marine Turtle Debris Ingestion (Ch 8, 24). Visceral Gout in Captive Reptiles (Ch 7). Nutritional Secondary Hyperparathyroidism in Captive Juvenile Reptiles (Ch 10, 18). Inclusion Body Disease in Captive Boidae (Ch 24). Snake Fungal Disease Pattern (Ch 10, 15, 24). Salmonella Carriage in Reptiles Zoonotic Signature (Ch 8, 14). Reptile Adenovirus Disease (Ch 12). Fibropapillomatosis in Green Sea Turtles (Ch 20, 24).

Amphibians

Chytridiomycosis Pattern in Amphibians (Ch 10, 15, 24). Ranavirus Pattern in Anurans and Caudates (Ch 24). Aeromonas Red Leg Syndrome (Ch 24). Amphibian Population Health Surveillance (Ch 24).

Fish and Aquatic Invertebrates

Gill Pathology Pattern in Teleosts (Ch 2, 25). Mycobacterial Disease in Captive Teleosts (Ch 25). Elasmobranch Reproductive Disease (Ch 25). Coral Disease Patterns (Ch 25). Cephalopod Pathology (Ch 25).

Zoonotic and Reportable Pattern Quick-Reference

Hard-Stop Zoonotic Patterns (Immediate Biosafety Escalation Required)

Herpes B in macaques (Chapter 3). Rabies in wild carnivores and bats (Chapter 3, 9). Anthrax in ungulates (Chapter 3). HPAI in spillover-suspect mammals (Chapter 13). Yersinia pestis (Chapter 14). Francisella tularensis (Chapter 14). Highly pathogenic avian influenza in birds (Chapter 13).

Federally Reportable Wildlife Diseases

Highly pathogenic avian influenza (Chapter 13). Chronic wasting disease (Chapter 9, 17). Bovine tuberculosis in wildlife (Chapter 14). Foot-and-mouth disease in cloven-hoofed wildlife (Chapter 26). Newcastle disease (Chapter 12). Various OIE-notifiable fish diseases (Chapter 2, 25). Ranavirus (Chapter 2, 15, 24). Chytridiomycosis (Chapter 10, 15).

Federally Protected Species Requiring Law Enforcement Coordination

Bald eagles and golden eagles (Bald and Golden Eagle Protection Act, Chapter 3, 21). Migratory birds (Migratory Bird Treaty Act, Chapter 21). Marine mammals (Marine Mammal Protection Act, Chapter 21, 22). Marine turtles and other endangered species (Endangered Species Act, Chapter 21). Investigative case chain of custody protocols apply.

How to Use This Atlas

The Master Atlas is designed for use at the cutting board or before signout as a rapid reference for cross-taxa pattern recognition. Entries can be located either by lesion type (following the systematic organization above) or by taxonomic group. Each entry provides the Pattern name, brief Cross-Taxa Signature summary, Diagnostic Anchor, Trap Logic key, and Zoonotic/Reportable status. Chapter cross-references support return to the parent chapter for detailed mechanism, evidence, and applied case examples. The Atlas is not a substitute for chapter reading but supports the ongoing use of the Comparative Necropsy Pattern System as a scaffold for pattern recognition throughout wildlife pathology practice.

CONCLUSION

The pathologist who has worked through this book has walked a discipline that behaves differently from every other branch of veterinary diagnostic pathology. The taxonomic breadth is wider, the repetition-based pattern recognition is unavailable, the antemortem history is often absent, and the interpretive consequences of the necropsy findings extend beyond the individual case to population-level conservation management, coordinated regulatory response, and public health surveillance. What has been offered here is not a memorization framework but a cognitive one: cross-taxa reasoning applied through the Comparative Necropsy Pattern System as a scaffold on which recognition can be built even in unfamiliar species.

The Pattern callouts that recurred through the chapters were structured the same way for a reason. Hepatic necrosis of herpesviral origin across nonhuman primates, elephants, psittacines, and reptiles. Cachexia with serous fat atrophy across free-ranging ungulates. Iron storage disease across frugivorous mammals. Faveolar lung consolidation in reptiles versus alveolar hepatization in mammals. Avian air sacculitis across orders. Ranavirus across ectothermic vertebrates. Chytridiomycosis in amphibians. Granulomatous mycobacterial disease across taxa. Cetacean morbillivirus in stranded dolphins. HPAI mammalian spillover in exposed carnivores and pinnipeds. Chronic wasting disease in cervids. Each was written to the same five-part frame — Pattern, Cross-Taxa Signature, Diagnostic Anchor, Trap Logic, Zoonotic and Reportable Flag — so that the reader who has begun to recognize the shape of the Pattern block itself has begun to build the cognitive scaffold the book was written to deliver. That scaffold is now available for the next unfamiliar case, and the case after that.

Three interpretive habits stand out as the practical residue the discipline demands. Species-appropriate anatomic reference before pathologic interpretation is the first. The chelonian intraventricular muscular ridge is not a mass; the reniculate marine mammal kidney is not multifocal disease; the compartmentalized ruminant stomach is not four separate organs; the avian air sac system is not a distributed abnormality. Every one of these normal structures has been misread at some point by a pathologist reading a chelonian, a dolphin, a giraffe, or a parrot against a mammalian carnivore anatomic frame. The discipline requires the habit of asking what the species-appropriate normal is before asking what the observed lesion means.

Lesion-first reasoning when antemortem history is absent is the second habit. Morphologic characterization by distribution, by timing, and by pattern constrains the differential without species-specific memorization and is transportable across taxa. Multifocal random hepatic necrosis narrows the differential in a canine, a chelonian, a psittacine, and a marmoset in essentially the same way. What varies is the identity of the likely agents; what remains constant is the interpretive path. The pathologist who develops the habit of characterizing the lesion before naming the disease process will read across taxa faster than the pathologist who attempts to memorize species-specific patterns one taxon at a time.

Integration of individual case findings with coordinated surveillance frameworks is the third habit. Species Survival Plans, the NOAA Fisheries Marine Mammal Health and Stranding Response Program, USDA

APHIS reportable disease systems, the USGS National Wildlife Health Center, state wildlife health veterinarians, and, at the interface of animal and human health, public health authorities all depend on wildlife pathology's case-by-case contributions. The individual necropsy report is not the end of the case; it is the beginning of a downstream response that shapes breeding recommendations, dietary reformulation, biosecurity protocols, unusual mortality event declarations, regulatory rulemaking, and, in cases with zoonotic or select-agent implications, the coordinated public health response. Recognition of this integration is a component of contemporary wildlife pathology practice as much as recognition of the lesion pattern itself.

The coming decade in the discipline carries substantial ongoing recognition demands. Highly pathogenic avian influenza continues its unprecedented mammalian spillover trajectory with the possibility of further pandemic-relevant adaptation. Chytridiomycosis and white-nose syndrome continue their catastrophic amphibian and bat population impact. Chronic wasting disease continues its geographic expansion into new North American and European regions. Emerging pathogen recognition through metagenomic characterization continues to identify novel disease entities at a rate faster than the traditional pathology literature can absorb. Climate-driven disease range expansion continues to reshape the epidemiologic map for vector-borne and temperature-sensitive disease. Each of these places substantial demand on wildlife pathology practice, and the coordinated One Health surveillance framework in which the discipline participates continues to expand in importance for both animal and human health protection.

The Comparative Necropsy Pattern Master Atlas at the back of this book is the practical navigator for the reader returning to a specific case at the cutting board. Every Pattern introduced in the chapters is indexed twice: by lesion type when the reader knows what they are looking at but not what species is affected, and by taxonomic group when the reader knows the species but is reasoning through the differential. Zoonotic and reportable pattern flags support the biosafety and regulatory response that must precede continued dissection in specific cases. The Atlas was written to be scanned, not read; the parent chapters carry the mechanism and the evidence the Atlas summarizes.

A closing observation on the discipline's professional role. Wildlife pathology sits at an increasingly recognized interface where animal welfare, conservation biology, public health, and comparative medicine converge. Individual necropsy findings inform breeding management at Species Survival Plan facilities. They contribute to unusual mortality event characterization in marine mammal populations. They support regulatory intervention against environmental contaminants that have produced catastrophic population impact from DDT through lead shot through diclofenac through anticoagulant rodenticides. They provide the sentinel data that public health surveillance depends on for emerging zoonotic disease recognition. The pathologist working at this interface carries substantial professional responsibility, and the discipline's contribution to broader animal and human health protection continues to grow with each generation of practitioners.

For the resident preparing for ACVP Phase II, the reasoning framework developed here is the point. Wildlife and exotic content on the examination will not be predictable from the reader's specific rotation experience, but the cognitive scaffold that permits reasoning across an unfamiliar species is the same scaffold that supports diagnostic performance on the specific slide set the examination presents. For the diplomate practicing diagnostic pathology, the Master Atlas provides the rapid reference for cases that fall outside repetition-built familiarity. For the zoo veterinarian preparing samples or interpreting reports, the Pattern system supports translation across the veterinary-pathology interface. For the wildlife disease investigator, the coordinated surveillance framework contributions matter as much as the individual case interpretation. For the veterinary student on a pathology or wildlife rotation, the invitation is to build the cognitive scaffold now, because repetition-based recognition will follow later, but the framework for reasoning across taxonomic distance is available from the first case forward.

The book closes as it began: at the cutting board, with a specimen from a species the pathologist has not previously autopsied, and with the interpretive framework that makes that specimen tractable. The Comparative Necropsy Pattern System is not a shortcut around species-specific knowledge. It is the scaffold that supports the acquisition of species-specific knowledge one pattern at a time. The reader who has worked through this book has begun that acquisition. The rest is practice, and practice is what the discipline offers in abundance.